Respiratory Care Pocket Guide

10th Edition

Serving the Respiratory Profession since 1984

Dana F. Oakes
Scot N. Jones

RespiratoryBooks.com

a division of:
Health Educator Publications, Inc.
9220 Lake Carol Drive
Zebulon, North Carolina
United States of America
27597

Dana F. Oakes
BA, RRT, RRT-NPS
Educational Consultant

Formerly:
Director of Clinical Education
Respiratory Care Program
Columbia Union College
Tacoma Park, Maryland

Educational Coordinator/Instructor
Respiratory Care Department
Children's Hospital Nat. Medical Center
Washington, D.C.

Director of Respiratory Care
VA Medical Center
Washington, D.C.

Scot N. Jones
BA, RRT, RRT-ACCS
Educational Consultant

Formerly:
Clinical Coordinator
Respiratory Care Program
Broward College
Coconut Creek, Florida

Respiratory Care Supervisor
Respiratory Care Department
Vidant Medical Center
Greenville, NC

Copyright © 2021
10th edition
Health Educator Publications, Inc.
Copyright under the Uniform Copyright Convention. All rights reserved. No part of this book may be reproduced, stored in a retrieval system, or transmitted in any form or by any means, electronic, mechanical, photocopying, recording or otherwise, without written permission of the Publisher.
Printed in HONG KONG

ISBN 978-0-932887-64-1

RespiratoryBooks
A Division of Health Educator Publications, Inc.
9220 Lake Carol Drive
Zebulon, NC 27597

The Authors and Publisher have exerted every effort to ensure that the clinical principles, procedures, and practices described herein are based on current knowledge and state-of-the-art information available from acknowledged authorities, texts, and journals. Nevertheless, they cannot be considered absolute and universal recommendations. Each patient situation must be considered individually. The Authors and Publisher disclaim responsibility for any adverse effects resulting directly or indirectly from information presented in this book, undetected errors, or misunderstandings by the readers.

"I am sooooooo excited. I have been an RT for almost 40 years. I just finished the exam and I passed easily! No squeaking by. Wanted to personally thank you. I am really proud of myself...your program covers just what you need to know! I will be sure to recommend you to all my friends!"

-SANDY

Save 10% with code BlueBook1

Test Prep from the authors of Oakes' Pocket Guides

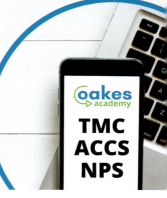

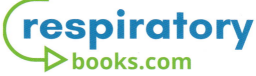

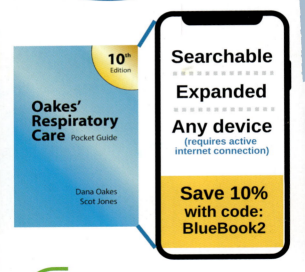

Assistant Editors

This is a team of incredible professionals whose impact on the journey of this edition can't be stated strongly enough. They tirelessly worked within a dynamic process with ever-changing timelines, in what has ended up being our most re-imagined edition ever. Thank you to each of you for your dedication to excellence.

Ameer Abdullah Alameer
Respiratory Care Practitioner
University of Imam Abdulrahman Bin Fasial (KSA)

Lori Badgley, MSRC, RRT
Lab Coordinator/Adjunct Faculty
Lincoln Land Community College
Springfield, Illinois, USA

Respiratory Therapist
Memorial Medical Center
Springfield, Illinois, USA

Greg Bishop, BSRT, RRT
Critical Care and Diagnostic Therapist
United Medical Group
Pikeville, Kentucky, USA

Respiratory Therapy Clinical Instructor
Southeast Kentucky Community and Technical College
Whitesburg, Kentucky, USA

Nicole L. Boylan
Respiratory Therapy Student
Pittsburgh Career Institute
Pittsburgh, Pennsylvania, USA

Student Intern
J.W. Ruby Memorial Hospital, WVU
Morgantown, West Virginia, USA

Misty Carlson, MS, RRT
Associate Professor
Director of Clinical Education Respiratory Care Program
School of Health Careers
College of Health and Public Services
Daytona State College
Daytona Beach, Florida, USA

Kelly L. Colwell, EdD, MRC, RRT, RRT-NPS, CPFT, AE-C
Assistant Professor of Health Professions
Program Director Respiratory Care, BSRC, BSRC Degree
Advancement and Polysomnography Programs
Graduate Program Director, Master of Respiratory Care, MRC
Youngstown State University
Youngstown, Ohio, USA

Wendy J. Dunlop, M.Ed., RRT
Associate Professor
former Director of Clinical Education
Reading Area Community College
Berks County, Pennsylvania, USA

Shaida Hashemi, BS
Respiratory Therapy Student (2019)
Grossmont College
El Cajon, California, USA

Deborah Ketchen, RRT
Respiratory Therapist
Pen Bay Medical Center
Rockport, Maine, USA

Kyle C. Mahan, MSM, RRT
Assistant Professor and Director of Clinical Education
Jefferson Community and Technical College

Adjunct Professor
University of Southern Indiana
UofL Health, Mary and Elizabeth Hospital
Louisville, Kentucky, USA

Elizabeth McGrane
Respiratory Therapy Student
Pittsburgh Career Institute
Pittsburgh, Pennsylvania, USA

Nia George, MAOM, RRT-RCP, COPD-E
Associate Dean of Curriculum
Independence University
Salt Lake City, Utah, USA

Nicole McKenzie, MHA, RRT
Program Director, Respiratory Care
The University of Toledo
Toledo, Ohio, USA

Angela S. Reid, MRC, RRT, RRT-ACCS
ACCS Respiratory Therapist
Mercy Health Hospital
Youngstown, Ohio, USA

Assistant Professor, Clinical Adjunct
Youngstown State University
Austintown, Ohio, USA

Stephen L. Richey, BA, RRT, RRT-NPS, FRAI
Respiratory Therapist
Evansville, Indiana, USA

Christopher Rowse, MS, RRT, RRT-ACCS, RPFT, RPSGT
Adjunct Faculty-Respiratory Care
Northern Essex Community College
Lawrence, Massachusetts, USA

Caleb L. Schrader, BSRT, RRT
CV/Transplant and NICU Respiratory Therapist
Kaiser Permanente Medical Center
Walnut Creek, California, USA

North Bay Medical Center
Fairfield, California, USA

Rochelle T. Stone, BS, RRT
Respiratory Care Practitioner
Wellspan Good Samaritan Hospital
Lebanon, Pennsylvania, USA

Stephen J. Valois, RRT, RRT-NPS, RRT-ACCS
Albany Medical Center
Albany, New York, USA

Charity SM. Zacarias, BS, RRT, RRT-NPS
Napa Valley Community College (2020)

Respiratory Therapist
UCSF Medical Center at Paranassus Heights
San Francisco, California, USA

Acknowledgement

Always first and foremost, we are thankful for our Lord, Jesus Christ, for allowing us to play a small part in our profession, for guiding our hands for so many years, and for the many who have used this pocket guide. To Him goes the glory.

Dedication

This 10th edition is dedicated to every healthcare provider hero that served in some capacity during the war on COVID-19, but in particular to the incredible Respiratory Therapist Heroes who served valiantly, who stepped into the unknown with fear but determination. We especially honor those who lost their lives during the journey. Never have we been prouder to be Respiratory Therapists.

Introduction

GOD was the first Respiratory Therapist – He gave us all the Breath of Life! We should be very proud of the Profession we have chosen, as we get to give the Breath of Life every day! 2020, the year of COVID-19, defined and proved RTs to be one of the most important, and in our eyes, one of the greatest professions of all time.

Oakes' Respiratory Care has been the #1 selling reference guide in Respiratory Therapy, since 1984. We are proud that Oakes' Books, over the last 37 years, have helped play a small role in developing the greatest Respiratory Therapists of all time.
Dana Oakes

This 10th edition is special. Not only does it mark nearly 40 years of being the top-rated pocket guide in an incredible profession, but what started as a normal (vigorous) edition update turned in to one of the most incredible re-imaginations ever. Every page has been researched, reformatted, and reconsidered with the input of an incredible team of assistant editors, including subject-matter experts, bedside clinicians, new graduates, and current students. This has been a powerful equation for a well-balanced, clinically relevant tool for all. Enjoy!
Scot Jones

CONTENTS

ASSESSMENT
- Clinical Assessment 1
- Acid-Base Assessment 2
- Chest Imaging 3
- Labs and Cultures 4
- Pulmonary Dynamics 5
- Pulmonary Function Testing 6
- Hemodynamics 7
- Cardiac Monitoring 8

INTERVENTIONS
- Respiratory Therapies 9
- Diseases and Disorders 10
- Pharmacology 11
- Resuscitation 12

Equations 13
Appendix .... A
Index I

TABLE OF CONTENTS

1 Clinical Assessment
- Health History/Interview 1-1
- Patient Approach 1-4
- Vital Signs 1-5
  - Respiratory Rate/Patterns 1-6
  - Heart Rate 1-9
  - Pulse Oximetry 1-10
  - Blood Pressure 1-11
  - Temperature 1-12
- Assessment 1-14
  - Head-to-Toe Assessment 1-15
  - Thoracic Diagrams 1-17
  - Auscultation 1-22
  - Dyspnea 1-26
  - Cardiovascular 1-28
  - Neurologic 1-30
  - Fluid and Electrolytes 1-32

2 Acid-Base
- Normal Values (Arterial/Venous) 2-2
- Sampling 2-3
- Venous Blood Gases 2-4
- Blood Gas Interpretation (Overview) 2-5
  - Steps of Interpretation 2-6
  - Disorders 2-9
    - Respiratory Acidosis 2-11
    - Respiratory Alkalosis 2-13
    - Metabolic Acidosis 2-15
    - Metabolic Alkalosis 2-17
  - ABG Accuracy Check 2-19

3 Chest Imaging
- Chest Radiograph (CXR)
  - Systematic Approach 3-2
  - Normal Radiographs 3-3
  - Abnormal Appearances/Causes 3-5
    - Segmental Infiltrates 3-9
    - Tube/Line Placement 3-10

Computerized Axial Topography Scan 3-11
Magnetic Resonance Imaging Scan 3-12
Thoracic Ultrasound 3-13

4 Labs and Cultures
Critical Lab Levels 4-2
Serum Electrolytes 4-3
Chemistry Panels 4-6
Complete Blood Count/Hematology 4-8
Coagulation 4-10
Other Lab Values 4-11
Microbiology 4-13
  Sputum Collection 4-14
  Sputum Characteristics 4-15
    By Disease 4-16

5 Pulmonary Dynamics
Ventilation
  Mechanics 5-2
  Pressures 5-3
  Compliance and Resistance 5-5
  Distribution of Ventilation 5-6
  Deadspace Ventilation 5-7
Perfusion
  Shunts 5-9
  Perfusion Zones 5-10
Ventilation/Perfusion 5-11

6 Pulmonary Function Testing
Average Pulmonary Function Values 6-2
Tests
  Volumes and Capacities 6-5
  Major Components 6-7
  Spirometry 6-8
  Flow-Volume Loop 6-11
  Other Volumes/Capacities 6-12
  Diffusion Across A-C Membrane 6-13
  Compliance and Resistance 6-14
  Respiratory Parameters 6-15

    Interpretation
        Basic PFT Interpretation Algorithm............................6-17
        Abnormal PFT Patterns 6-19
        Guidelines for Assignment of Severity.......................6-20

7 Hemodynamics
Hemodynamic Parameters 7-2
Oxygen Delivery...7-4
Blood Flow Through the Heart 7-5
Catheters/Lines Overview 7-6
Disease Entities (Pressure) 7-7
Right vs Left Heart Failure 7-8
Hemodynamic Presentation (Diseases)............................7-9

8 Cardiac Monitoring
Standard ECG Leads..8-2
    12-Lead 8-3
    15-Lead 8-3
ECG (Labeled) 8-4
Interpretation
    Basic Steps to Interpret...8-6
    ECG Paper 8-7
    Measuring Ventricular Rate 8-7
    By Rate...8-8
    By P Wave..8-8
    By PR Interval 8-8
    Summary of Basic Arrhythmias.......................................8-9
    Interpreting ECG Abnormalities 8-14
    Cardiac Ischemia..8-15

9 Respiratory Therapies
Aerosol Therapy
Types of..9-4
Bland Aerosol Administration 9-5
Aerosol Delivery Devices 9-6
Selection and Overview 9-8
Recommended Particle Sizes (MMADs)...........................9-9
Nebulizers 9-10
Metered-Dose Inhalers 9-12
Dry Powder Inhalers 9-13

Airway Management
- Bag-Valve-Mask (BVM) Ventilation 9-14
- Airway Adjuncts 9-15
- Endotracheal Tubes 9-16
- Mallampati Scoring 9-16
- Intubation 9-17
- Tracheostomy Tubes 9-20

Airway Clearance
- Overview 9-27
- Selecting 9-28
- Suctioning 9-29
- Directed or Therapeutic Coughing 9-33
- Active Cycle of Breathing 9-34
- Autogenic Drainage 9-35
- Diaphragmatic Exercises 9-36
- Diaphragmatic Strengthening 9-37
- Pursed-Lip Breathing 9-37
- Chest Physiotherapy 9-38
- AARC Guidelines 9-47
- Assistive Mechanical Devices 9-48
- Positive Expiratory Pressure (PEP) 9-49
- High-Frequency Oscillations 9-50
- Acapella 9-51
- Flutter Valve 9-51
- Intrapulmonary Percussive Ventilation 9-52
- Percussive Vests/Wraps 9-53
- Selection Algorithm 9-54
- ACCP Summary Recommendations 9-55

Humidity Therapy
- Overview 9-56
- Devices 9-57
- AARC Guidelines 9-58

Lung Expansion Therapy
- Overview and Selection 9-59
- Incentive Spirometry 9-60
- Intermittent Positive Pressure Breathing 9-63

Medical Gases
Cylinders
- Cylinder Color Standards 9-66
- Cylinder Duration Charts 9-67

Oxygen/Oxygenation
- Monitoring Oxygenation Status 9-68
  - Troubleshooting the Pulse Oximeter 9-69
  - Transcutaneous Monitoring 9-71
  - Lung Adequacy 9-72
  - Oxyhemoglobin Dissociation Curve 9-73
  - Oxygen and Carbon Dioxide Cascade 9-74
- Assessment of Oxygenation 9-75
  - Hypoxemia 9-76
  - Versus Hypoxia 9-76
  - Signs and Symptoms 9-77
  - Types and Causes 9-78
  - Diagnostic Algorithm 9-80
- Oxygen Therapy 9-81
- AARC Guidelines 9-82
- Oxygen Delivery Devices 9-83

Gases Measured/Used 9-89

10 Disease and Disorders
- Acute Coronary Syndrome (ACS) 10-4
- Acute Respiratory Distress Syndrome (ARDS) 10-5
- Alveolar Hypoventilation Syndromes 10-8
- Asthma 10-9
- Atelectasis 10-18
- Bronchiectasis 10-20
- Carbon Monoxide Poisoning 10-21
- Cardiac Tamponade 10-22
- Chronic Obstructive Pulmonary Disease (COPD) ... 10-23
- Cystic Fibrosis 10-32
- Diabetic Ketoacidosis 10-36
- Drowning 10-37
- Drug Overdose 10-38
- Fungal Disorders 10-39

Flail Chest	10-41
Heart Failure	10-42
Left-Sided (LHF, CHF)	10-43
Right-Sided (RHF, Cor Pulmonale)	10-44
Immunocompromised	10-45
Interstitial Lung Disease (ILD)	10-46
Lung Abscess	10-48
Neuromuscular Disorders	10-49
Oxygen Toxicity	10-52
Pleural Effusion	10-53
Pleuritis (Pleurisy)	10-54
Pneumonia	10-55
Pneumothorax (Air Leak Syndromes)	10-58
Pulmonary Edema	10-60
Pulmonary Embolism	10-61
Pulmonary Hypertension	10-62
Respiratory Failure	10-63
Restrictive Disease	10-64
Shock	10-65
Sleep-Disordered Breathing	10-66
Smoke Inhalation/Thermal Burns	10-67
Tracheoarterial Fistula	10-68
Tracheoesophageal Fistula	10-69
Trauma	10-70
Traumatic Brain Injury	10-71
Chest Trauma	10-72
Tuberculosis	10-73
Viral Infections	10-75

11 Pharmacology

Abbreviations Used in Drug Administration	11-4
JCAHO Do-Not-Use List	11-5
Drug Administration Procedures	11-6
Drug Calculations	
Solution and Dosage Problems	11-7
Conversion Within and Between Systems	11-8
Common Conversions	11-9
Receptors	
Alpha and Beta	11-10
Muscarinic	11-10
Drug Tables (by class and generic name)	
How to Use	11-11

Abbreviations Used 11-11
Anti-Asthma
    Mast Cell Stabilizers 11-12
    Antileukotrienes 11-13
Bronchodilators
    Short-Acting Beta Agonists (SABAs) 11-14
    Long-Acting Beta Agonists (LABAs) 11-17
    Ultra Long-Acting Beta Agonists (ULABAs) 11-19
    Short-Acting Muscarinic Antagonists (SAMAs) 11-20
    Long-Acting Muscarinic Anatgonists (LAMAs) 11-21
    Xanthines (Methylxanthines) 11-23
Alpha-1 Antitrypsin Deficiency Disorder 11-24
Anti-Infectives (Inhaled) 11-25
Mucoactives 11-31
Inhaled Analgesics 11-34
Inhaled Epinephrine 11-35
Phosphodiesterase Inhibitors 11-36
Pulmonary Vasodilators 11-37
Smoking Cessation 11-39
Steroids (Inhaled Corticosteroids) (ICS) 11-44
Combination Therapies 11-49
Drugs that Cause Respiratory Depression 11-56
Common Cardiac Drugs (by effect) 11-57

12 Resuscitation
Basic Life Support (in-Hospital) Algorithm 12-2
CPR Components (Summarized) 12-4
Automatic External Defibrillator (AED) 12-5
Opioid-Associated Life-Threatening Emergencies 12-6
Special Situations

13 Equations
Acid-Base 13-2
Oxygenation 13-4
Ventilation 13-12
Ventilator Calculations 13-15
Hemodynamics 13-20
Patient Calculations 13-26
Pulmonary Function 13-27
Miscellaneous 13-27

1 Clinical Assessment

Health History/Interview.....................................1-1
Patient Approach..1-4
Vital Signs..1-5
  Respiratory Rate/Patterns.................................1-6
  Heart Rate..1-9
  Pulse Oximetry...1-10
  Blood Pressure...1-11
  Temperature..1-12
Assessment...1-14
  Head-to-Toe Assessment................................1-15
  Thoracic Diagrams...1-17
  Auscultation...1-22
  Dyspnea...1-26
  Cardiovascular...1-28
  Neurological..1-30
  Fluid and Electrolytes.....................................1-32

Health History/Interview

Health History should be kept focused; be careful to maintain a neutral attitude (including body language) as you are interviewing the patient. Patients should know that your interest is medical in nature (not legal, etc.)

Demographics	Name, alias, age, occupation, weight/height, gender/identity
Chief Complaint	Primary reason for person needing care
History of Present Illness (HPI)	Basic chronological story (including symptoms) of what has led up to the chief complaint, including onset (how long), timing (frequency, duration of symptoms), and character (quality, quantity, severity)
Medical History	Including childhood diseases, all significant illness/injuries, hospitalizations, surgeries.

Health History (continued)

Family	Relevant history (about 4 generations back, both maternal and paternal)
Social	Hobbies, recreation, living arrangements, habits (alcohol, drugs, diet, exercise), recent travel, learning needs, significant others involved in care, cultural/religious needs
Emotional	Superficially: satisfaction with life, stressors, relationships, finances, mental health/illness (refer to nursing for anything serious)
Environmental/ Occupational	**Looking for triggers of respiratory symptoms:** <u>Occupational</u>: Farming, manufacturing, gases, smoke, chemicals, dust <u>Home</u>: Pets, smoking, mold, allergies <u>Regional</u>: Fungal exposures, outbreaks, etc. <u>Seasonal</u>: Pollen, wood stoves
Pulmonary	**While focused on Chief Complaint, explore all significant pulmonary history:** **Diseases/Disorders Known or Suspected:** Asthma, cancer, COPD (may call it bronchitis or emphysema), cystic fibrosis, pulmonary hypertension, sleep disorders (OSA, CSA) **Previous History of (esp. if required tx):** Pneumonia, pneumothorax, pleural effusions, respiratory viruses/bacterial infections/fungal infections, thoracic trauma **Smoking History:** Primarily tobacco/cigarettes Pack-Years = # yrs smoked x # packs per day quitting history, interventions used other smoking (vaping, marijuana, etc.)

Cardiovascular	Congenital heart disease, chronic chest pain (pleuritic vs , heart disease (CHF, MIs, etc.), hypertension, stroke, dysrhythmias, include any surgeries/procedures
Drugs/Medications	While a complete medication reconciliation isn't common, verifying relevant drugs (respiratory especially), dosages, compliance, and technique are important. This should include, without judgment, non-prescribed drugs and natural remedies (herbs, essential oils, etc.)
Sleep Health	Sleep problems known or reported by those who sleep near/with patient Daytime sleepiness Morning headaches Insomnia
Advance Directives	Ask about advance directives, including do-not-resuscitate and do-not-intubate status, as well as (medical) power of attorney. The team should ask clarifying questions early in treatment (know what the plan is).
Check Orders	Review physician orders and protocols

Patient Interactions

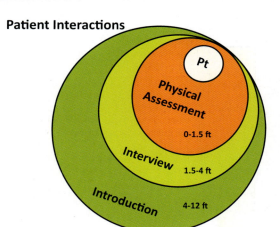

- **INTRODUCTION** *(establish a positive rapport, obtain patient's cooperation, determine overall patient condition, assess environment for safety)*
  - Confirm patient's identity
  - Use patient's "formal" name. Avoid overly friendly terms
  - Introduce yourself: give your role and purpose of visit
  - Be friendly, use eye contact

- **INTERVIEW** *(request information pertinent to chief complaint, gather medical history as needed, provide education)*
  - Avoid standing over patient/at foot of bed. Eye level is best
  - Maintain a relaxed style, communicate empathy
  - Be an active listener, don't interrupt, avoid judgment
  - Use an interpreter (or approved interp. technology) if needed
  - Be mindful of terminology being used (avoid jargon)

- **PHYSICAL ASSESSMENT** *(determine clinical status of patient, ensure ordered treatments are appropriate)*
  - Explain and request permission for touch (auscultation, etc)
  - Use minimal or no eye contact–keep touch to only that necessary for evaluation, minimize verbal "casual" talk, use only back of hand to touch breast tissue if needed
  - Use PPE to establish professional/infection barriers
  - Be aware of patient's response

Vital Signs: Normal and Abnormal Ranges

Age	Respiratory Rate (see pg 1-6)	Heart Rate (see pg 1-9)	Blood Pressure (see pg 1-11)
Adult	12-20	60-100	110-120/70-80
5-12 yrs	16-20	70-110	100/60
1-4 yrs	20-30	80-120	95/50
1st year	25-40	80-160	85/50
Newborn	30-60	90-180	75/40
Adult Abnormal ranges	< 12 = bradypnea > 20 = tachypnea	< 60 = bradycardia > 100 = tachycardia	< 90/60 = hypotension > 140/90 = hypertension

Respiratory Rate and Pattern

***Procedure**: best practice is to count respirations (or number of chest rises) while palpating the radial pulse for a full 60-seconds, especially if any irregularity in rhythm. Some clinicians count for 30-seconds, then multiply by 2.*

Observe and Record: Rate, Rhythm, Depth, Symmetry

Respirations Descriptive Terms

shallow	Slight rise and fall of chest *may indicate hypoventilation (assess further)*
normal	Baseline rise and fall - should be noticeable but not prominent - chest and abdomen rise and fall in synchrony
deep	Increased, almost exaggerated rise and fall *may indicate hyperventilation (assess further)*
paradoxical respirations	Opposite of normal: chest contracts during inhalation, expands during exhalation, out of sync with the abdomen (also called see-saw respirations, thoracoabdominal asynchrony) *may indicate diaphragm issue, including paralysis, severe distress, upper airway obstruction*

Respiratory Patterns

Eupnea is presented first as the normal baseline - all other patterns are presented alphabetically

Type	Pattern	Characteristics	Causes
Eupnea		Normal rate (12 - 20/min) Normal rhythm, Sighs 7/hr	Normal physiology
Agonal		Occasional reflex-driven gasps	Hypoxia/anoxia, cardiac arrest, cerebral ischemia
Apnea		Absence of breathing	Respiratory or cardiac arrest, ↑ICP
Apneustic		Long gasping inspirations with insufficient expiration	Lesions in the pneumotaxic center
Ataxic		Irregular, disorganized, varying depth	Stroke (CVA), trauma to the medulla
Biot's		Fast and deep breaths with periods of apnea, no set rhythm	Spinal meningitis, ↑ICP, CNS lesions or disease
Bradypnea		Slow rate (< 10/min), regular rhythm	Normal during sleep, brain tumors, diabetic coma, drugs (alcohol, narcotics), ↑ICP, metabolic alkalosis (limited), uremia

Assessment

Type	Pattern	Characteristics	Causes
Cheyne-Stokes		↑ Breaths (rate & depth) then decreasing breaths followed by periods of apnea (20-60 sec)	Normal in newborns/elderly, CHF, aortic valve lesion, dissecting aneurysm, ↑CO2 sensitivity meningitis, ↑ICP, cerebral anoxia, drug overdose (morphine), renal failure
Hypopnea		↓ Depth, normal rate, regular rhythm	Circulatory failure, meningitis, unconsciousness
Hyperpnea		↑ Depth, normal rate, regular rhythm	Exertion, fever, pain, respiratory disease
Kussmaul's		Fast and deep breaths like sighs with incomplete expiratory phase	DKA, severe hemorrhage, peritonitis, renal failure, uremia
Tachypnea		↑ Rate (> 25/min), regular rhythm	Anxiety (esp. asthmatics), atelectasis, brain lesions, drugs (aspirin), exercise, fear, fever, hypercapnia, hypoxemia, hypoxia, metabolic acidosis, obesity, pain

Assessment

Pulse (Heart Rate)
See Chapter 8 for ECG Rhythms

Procedure: *best practice is to palpate pulse (radial is usually first choice) for a full 60-seconds, especially if any irregularity in beat. Some clinicians count for 30-seconds, then multiply by 2.*

*An **apical pulse** can be auscultated by placing diaphragm of stethoscope over the heart (5th intercostal space, left of midclavicular line)*

Observe and Record: Rate, Rhythm, Strength

Pulse Strength (Intensity)

0	no palpable pulse (verify at carotid)
1+	faint but detectable
2+	slightly diminished versus normal
3+	normal (easily palpable)
4+	bounding pulse (anxiety, kidney disease, heart failure, fever, pregnancy)

(Common) Abnormal Pulse Rhythms

Pulsus alternans	Alteration of weak and strong pulses with regular beat *causes: often cardiac issue, though may be present with marked tachypnea*
Pulsus paradoxus	↓ Pulse strength during inspiration, ↑ pulse strength during expiration (a difference of more than 20 between inspiration and exhalation is significant) *causes: cardiac tamponade, COPD, acute asthma, hypovolemic shock*
Reverse Pulsus paradoxus	Opposite of pulsus paradoxus above: ↑ pulse strength during inspiration, ↓ pulse strength during expiration—often noted during positive pressure ventilation

Pulse Oximetry
the "5th Vital Sign" - SEE ALSO Pulse Oximetry, pg 9-68

An estimate of the proportion of hemoglobin that is saturated with oxygen. Usually within 3% of actual SaO$_2$ (arterial saturation) unless low (*SpO$_2$ estimate is very unreliable when SaO$_2$ is < 80)

	Physiol. Normal	Hypoxemia		
		Mild	Moderate	Severe
Adult	95-99%	91-94%	76-90%	< 75%*
Child	91-96%	88-90%	76-87%	< 75%*

Older adults may trend towards lower part of range—SpO$_2$ typically decreases with age

Alarms are often set at lower limit (93%, for example), and then high limit set at 99% (to trigger a reminder to wean supplemental oxygen)

Note that clinical ranges may vary some by age (neonates, etc.), disease (COPD, etc.), and clinical appropriateness (COVID-19, etc.)

Pulse Oximetry Quick Troubleshooting	
Check:	<ul><li>Good Perfusion?</li><li>Good Waveform?</li><li>Does HR of SpO$_2$ correlate with palpated pulse?</li><li>If monitored: does HR of SpO$_2$ and HR of ECG correlate?</li><li>Skin temperature at probe?</li></ul>
Try:	<ul><li>Switch position or type of probe</li><li>Replace probe</li><li>Warm body part with approved heat pack</li><li>Verify using ABG if necessary</li></ul>

Blood Pressure

120	Systolic	Pressure during left ventricular contraction
80	Diastolic	Pressure during ventricular relaxation
mm Hg		

Based mostly on compliance of aorta, ↓ CI with age

Adult Blood Pressure Categories

Category	Systolic	Diastolic
Hypotensive	< 90	< 60
Normal	< 120	< 80
Elevated	120-129	< 80
Hypertension Stage 1	130-139	80-89
Hypertension Stage 2	140+	90+
Hypertensive Crisis	> 180	> 120

- **Abnormal**
  - Inadequate (low) BP results in a lack of perfusion to vital organs (hypotensive)
  - Excessive (high) BP increases the risk of doing damage to blood vessels, including a risk of stroke (hypertensive)
  - Cuff too small (false ↑ BP); cuff too large (false ↓ BP)

- **Mean Arterial Pressure (MAP)**
  - MAP = [Systolic + 2(Diastolic)] / 3
  - Average pressure in systemic circulation
  - Normal is ~70 - 100 mm Hg
  - Measure of adequate perfusion-ability to deliver oxygen/blood to tissues throughout the body.
  - Maintain at 60 mm Hg or higher

- **Pulse Pressure**
  - Pulse Pressure = Systolic - Diastolic
  - Normal is around 40-50 mm Hg

Temperature

Normal Temperature Ranges

Place	Celsius Range	Fahrenheit Range
Core	36.5 – 37.5° C	97.7 – 99.5° F
Oral*	36.5 – 37.5° C	97.7 – 99.5° F
Axillary	35.9 – 36.9° C	96.7 – 98.5° F
Otic (tympanic)	37.1 – 38.1° C	98.7 – 100.5° F

*Cool or heated aerosol may affect temperature readings

Core Methods (most accurate):
- Rectal
- Pulmonary artery (PA) catheter
- Urinary bladder
- Esophageal

Peripheral Methods (may be influenced by other factors):
- Oral
- Tympanic membrane
- Temporal
- Axillary

Causes of Abnormal Temperatures

Hypothermia (decreases O_2 consumption)	Hyperthermia *(increases O_2 consumption)* rapid onset, difficult to control, doesn't respond to antipyretics
• Environmental exposure • Very young or very old • Brain/Spinal injuries • Shock • Anesthesia/Sedation • Therapeutic (MI) (targeted temperature management)	• Environmental exposure • Malignant (drug-related) • Brain/Spinal injuries
	Fever (usually responds to antipyretics)
	• Infection (w/ ↑ WBC)

Assessment

Inspection	Use of vision/smell/hearing to assess normal vs. abnormal. Assess for color, size, location, movement, texture, symmetry, odors
Palpation	Use of (generally) light touch to assess (for example, tracheal position). • Use gloves when in touch with membranes/fluids.
Percussion See pg 1-15	The technique of tapping your fingers (distal part of middle finger of dominant hand taps over distal part of middle finger of non-dominant hand) quickly/sharply against the chest wall to identify areas filled with air vs. fluid vs. solid. Listen to the sounds produced.
Auscultation See pg 1-22	The use of a stethoscope to listen to breath (upper airway/over trachea, and lower airway (anterior, lateral, and posterior chest wall) and heart sounds. • The area to be auscultated should be exposed, if possible • Warm the stethoscope diaphragm before touching skin • Ensure environment is as reasonably quiet as possible (mute television, etc.)
Other	• Reviewing the patient's medical record is a critical step in assessment. • Remember: numbers and imaging can mislead. Always use systematic assessment of the patient as a main guide in making clinical decisions.

Head-to-Toe Assessment

Assessment should be systematic, head-to-toe. This list is not exhaustive.

Arrival	
Check	- Is room safe? - Is patient in apparent distress? - Basic level of consciousness/anxiety - Response towards your arrival (cooperative vs. resistive, lack of communication)
General Impressions	- Vital signs - Age/weight/height - Physical/sensory needs - Diaphoresis (pain, respiratory distress, cardiac event, anaphylaxis, drug withdrawal) - Guarding/pain
Head	
Face	- Check the color (normal to ethnicity?) - Facial expression (alert, distress, fear, pain) - Flushed/red (rash, fever, anxiety/stress, WOB)
Eyes	Pupil response (fixed/dilated, pinpoint)
Nose/Nares	Nasal flaring (respiratory distress, esp children)
Lips/Gums	Color (blue = central cyanosis), pallor (hypotension, hypoxia, vasoconstriction)
Neck	
Sternocleidomastoid	Increased use may indicate increased WOB
Carotid pulse	Do not palpate unless CPR
Jugular Venous Distension (JVD)	Right-sided heart failure
Tracheal deviation	(either visualize or palpate): Shift towards: unilateral upper lobe collapse Shift away: lung tumor, pleural effusion, tension pneumothorax

Chest (see pg 1-28 for cardiovascular assessment/chest pain)	
Anterior-Posterior (AP)	Normal diameter is around 1/2 to 1/3 AP > 2/3 = barrel chest = sign of air-trapping
I:E Ratio	Normal 1:3 to 1:4 May be 1:4 or 1:5 with air-trapping
Resp Pattern	See pg 1-7 for patterns and definitions
Posture	Tripod (leaning on elbows) (COPD) Sitting upright
Rib angles	Normal = 45° (air-trapping = flattened)
Symmetry	left vs right (unilateral issue, right-mainstem intubation, pleural effusion, pneumothorax, flail chest, blocked chest drain), paradoxical (flail?)
Abnormalities	<u>Lesions</u>, <u>Contusions</u> (bruising) trauma? <u>Obesity</u>: can cause a restrictive disorder <u>Scars</u>: previous cardiac, thoracic surgeries, etc. <u>Spine</u>: Kyphosis, Lordosis, Scoliosis, Kyphoscoliosis <u>Sternum</u>: pectus carinatum (pigeon-chest, protrudes); pectus excavatum (funnel-chest)
Auscultate	See pg 1-22 for detailed information

Percussion See intro on pg 1-13	Note	Normal Areas	Abnormal Areas
	Flat	Thigh, muscle	Atelectasis, pleural effusion, pneumonectomy
	Dull	Heart, liver	Atelectasis, consolidation, cardiomegaly, fibrosis, pleural effusion, pulmonary edema
	Resonance	Normal Lung	
	Hyper-resonance	Abdomen	Acute asthma, emphysema, pneumothorax
	Tympany	Large gastric air bubble	Large pulmonary cavity, tension pneumothorax

Assessment 1-15

Tactile fremitus	Palpated: feeling vocal vibrations when patient says, "99" in a low-pitched voice.
	Decreased: Obstruction (COPD, secretions), restriction (shallow breathing) ET tube mal-positioned, barrier (pneumothorax, obesity, fibrosis, pleural effusion)
	Increased: Consolidation (atelectasis, fibrosis, pneumonia, tumor)
Accessory muscles	Increased muscle use: substernal/suprasternal, intercostal
	Respiratory *alternans*: chest wall breathing alternating with diaphragmatic breathing

Arms/Hands/Fingers

Turgor	Skin returns to shape after pinched gently: Slow to return may indicate dehydration
Digital clubbing	May be a sign of chronic hypoxia < 160° < 180° < 200°
Stains	Nicotine (yellowing)
Capillary refill	Pinch fingernail for 5 sec, if it takes more than 3 seconds for color to return, suspect decreased cardiac output/peripheral perfusion
Tremors	underlying neurological issue, alcohol/drug

Legs/Ankles/Feet

Pedal (Pitting) edema	Potential sign of heart failure			
	1+	rapid	3+	1-2 minutes
	2+	10-15 seconds	4+	> 2 minutes

Other

Observe	• Wounds, sores, bruising, rashes • Edema/ascites (abdomen, legs, etc.) • Cough/Sputum (see pg 4-15) • Subcutaneous emphysema (air trapped in tissue under skin, AKA crepitus) • Review pulmonary mechanics (see Ch 5)

Anterior view

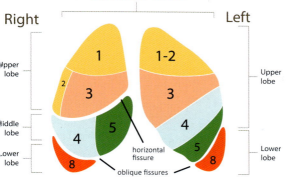

Upper Lobe	1	Apical
	2	Posterior
	3	Anterior
horizontal fissure		
Middle Lobe	4	Lateral
	5	Medial
oblique fissure		
Lower Lobe	8	Anterior Basal

Apical-Posterior	1-2	Upper Lobe
Anterior	3	
Superior	4	
Inferior	5	
oblique fissure		
Anterior Basal	8	Lower Lobe

anterior chest topography imaginary lines

Assessment 1-17

Posterior view

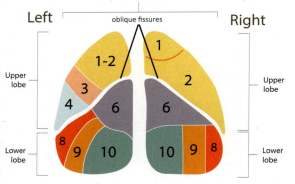

Upper Lobe	1-2	Apical-Posterior
	3	Anterior
	4	Superior Lingular
oblique fissure		
Lower Lobe	6	Superior
	8	Anterior Basal
	9	Lateral Basal
	10	Posterior Basal

	1	Upper Lobe
Apical		
Posterior	2	
oblique fissure		
Superior	6	Lower Lobe
Anterior Basal	8	
Lateral Basal	9	
Posterior Basal	10	

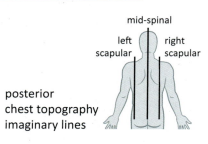

posterior chest topography imaginary lines

Assessment

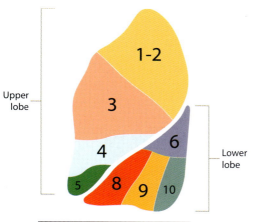

RIGHT Lateral Segments

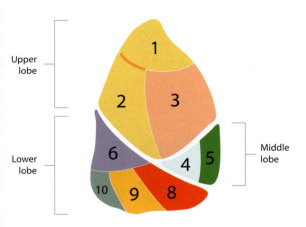

Upper Lobe	1	Apical
	2	Posterior
	3	Anterior
horizontal fissure		
Middle Lobe	4	Lateral
	5	Medial
oblique fissure		
Lower Lobe	6	Superior
	8	Anterior Basal
	9	Lateral Basal
	10	Posterior Basal

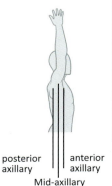

posterior axillary / anterior axillary / Mid-axillary

right lateral chest topography imaginary lines

Position of the Lungs and Heart

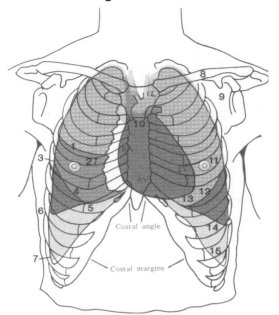

1. transverse fissure
2. 4th rib midclavicular
3. oblique fissure at 5th rib midaxillary
4. oblique fissure
5. lung border (expiration) 5th rib midclavicular
6. lung border (expiration) 8th rib midaxillary
7. pleural border 10th rib midaxillary
8. clavicles
9. scapula
10. aorta
11. nipple 4th intercostal space in male
12. oblique fissure
13. apex of heart PMI at 5th intercostal space
14. lung border (expiration) 8th rib midaxillary
15. pleural border 10th rib midaxillary

Assessment 1-21

Auscultation

Procedure: *systematically listen to breath sounds - best practice is to spend 5-10 seconds listening to each spot (use segment diagrams on 1-17 and following to guide you). Instruct patient to inhale deeply if able*

Observe and Record: Characteristics compared to normal

Normal Breath Sounds
These breath sounds are considered normal when they are auscultated in their expected location. When auscultated in an area NOT normally expected, they would then be considered abnormal (adventitious)

Thickness of lines below: indicate the strength/intensity of breath sounds
Steepness of lines below: indicate pitch (steeper = higher pitch)

Vesicular	expected over most lung areas; breezy-sounding; I:E should be 3:1
	inspiratory / expiratory *inspiratory is longer than expiratory / expiratory is low pitch, soft intensity*
Broncho-vesicular	expected over the carina on the anterior, between the upper scapulae on the posterior; breezy, tubular; I:E should be 1:1
	inspiratory / expiratory *insp/exp sounds are mostly equal / expiratory is medium pitch + intensity*
Bronchial	expected over the manubrium (upper portion of the sternum); hollow/tubular/loud; I:E should be 2:3
	inspiratory / expiratory *expiratory is longer than inspiratory / expiratory is high pitch, loud intensity*
Tracheal	expected breath sounds over the trachea; tubular/loud/harsh; I:E should be 5:6
	inspiratory / expiratory *insp/exp sounds are nearly equal / expiratory is high pitch, very loud*

Abnormal Breath Sounds

Descriptive Term	Common Causes
Decreased or Diminished *(absent if severe)*	↓**Airflow**: Obstruction: COPD, asthma, CF (air-trapping), secretions Restriction/Shallow Breathing: Drug OD, neuromuscular disorders, flail chest, significant sedation Artificial airway out of position: ET tube in right mainstem, above vocal cords, in esophagus; trach tube in false tract/tissue, not fully in stoma/airway **Barrier blocking sound**: Air: Air-trapping, COPD, pneumothorax Fat: Obesity Fibrosis: Pleural thickening Fluid: Pleural effusion, hemothorax Muscle: Hypertrophy
Crackles (sound like vibrations, mostly random/not continuous)	
Fine *(high-pitched "crackling" usually at end-inspiration)*	Atelectasis, fibrosis, pneumonia, pulmonary edema
Coarse *(loud, low-pitched "bubbling" or "gurgling" mostly during inspiration, but may also be expiratory if severe)*	Anything that causes secretions (COPD, cystic fibrosis, pneumonia, pulmonary edema)
Wheezes *(continuous sound, whistle-like, often during expiration though it may occur during inspiration, especially when severe)*	Bronchospasm (Asthma, COPD), airway obstructions (edema, tumor, foreign body, mucus plug, stenosis), cardiac wheeze

Assessment

Descriptive Term	Common Causes
Stridor *(continuous sound, loud, high-pitched, usually during inspiration, auscultated over trachea, sometimes heard without auscultating)*	If inspiratory, likely upper airway obstruction (edema such as with croup, epiglottitis, anaphylaxis, tumor, foreign body). If expiratory (less common), more likely the lower trachea, extubation edema, tracheal stenosis
Stertor *(noisy, low-pitched breathing during inhalation)*	Airway obstruction, usually above larynx, vibrations of the tissue of the nasopharynx/soft palate
Pleural or **Pericardial Rub** *(grating vibration, loud and harsh)*	<u>Pleural</u>: will correlate with inspiration and expiration: pleurisy, peripheral pneumonia, PE, tuberculosis <u>Pericardiac</u>: will correlate with heartbeat: pericarditis

Terms that are Debated*

There are a few terms that are used clinically sometimes, but are not officially endorsed by major organizations (ATS, ACCP) because the definition of the terms are considered to be overly subjective (studies have demonstrated a lot of variation in people using these terms)

Rhonchus (singular) Rhonchi (plural)	Continuous sound, snoring-like with low-pitch, a "low-pitched wheeze," may clear w/ cough
Fine Rales or Fine Rale Crepitation	Similar to fine crackles, a soft, higher-pitched discontinuous (sound is interrupted) "explosive" sound
Coarse Rales (sometimes Rhonchi)	Similar to coarse crackles, a loud, lower-pitched discontinuous (sound is interrupted) "explosive" sound

*Terms and descriptions in this section are based in part on *Murphy, Respiratory Care, 2008, Vol 53(3)*. ATS = American Thoracic Society; ACCP = American College of Chest Physicians

Voice Sounds (Vocal Resonance)

Voice Sound	Technique	Interpretation
Whispered pectoriloquy	Ask pt to whisper, "1-2-3" or "ninety-nine" while auscultating over trachea (to get a baseline sound). Then, listen over lung fields while having pt repeat whisper	<u>Negative</u>: Normal air-filled lungs filter out the words, should be indistinguishable <u>Positive</u>: Clearly identify the words while auscultating, indicates area of consolidation
Bronchophony	Ask patient to speak, "ninety-nine" while auscultating over trachea. Then, listen over lung fields as patient repeats	
Egophony	Ask patient to say a word with a long e sound, such as "bee" each time you put stethoscope on chest	<u>Negative</u>: All sounds are like "bee" - normal lung <u>Positive</u>: Sound like "ate" (long a sound) is heard over some area(s), indicates consolidation Note: may be falsely positive in areas of lung parenchyma

Assessment

Dyspnea

Dyspnea is difficulty breathing as perceived by the patient. While its causes are many, many center around pulmonary or cardiac issues.

- <u>Orthopnea:</u> difficulty breathing when lying down/recumbent (early symptom of heart failure, often improves if head of bed is increased)
- <u>Paroxysmal nocturnal dyspnea (PND):</u> sudden awakening from sleep with difficulty breathing (asthma, possibly heart failure, improves over time after sitting up)
- <u>Platypnea:</u> difficulty breathing when upright–sitting or standing. (multiple causes, including parenchymal diseases, hepato-pulmonary syndrome, cardiac shunts/defects, improves when lying down)
- <u>Positional dyspnea:</u> term used to describe trouble breathing at rest which improves with a position change

Assessing for Dyspnea

By nature, this is subjective (the perspective of the patient). You should look for objective clues as well (work of breathing/accessory muscle use, fever, diaphoresis, tachypnea, tachycardia, etc.)

- No matter what technique is used to evaluate dyspnea, be sure to ask patient to compare it to their baseline:
  - Mild, Moderate, Severe (compared to baseline)
  - Modified Borg Scale (see next page)
  - ATS Shortness of Breath Scale (see next page)

Causes of Dyspnea

Respiratory	Cardiac
Airway obstruction	Congestive heart failure
Asthma	Pericardial effusion
COPD	Cardiac shunt
Pneumonia	Valvular lesion
Pulmonary Embolus	
Pneumothorax	
Pleural Effusion	

Modified Borg Scale

Rating Value	Description of Dyspnea
0	Nothing
0.5	Very, very slight (barely noticeable)
1	Very slight
2	Slight
3	Moderate
4	Somewhat severe
5	Severe
6	
7	Very severe
8	
9	Very, very severe (hard to manage)
10	Maximal

ATS Shortness of Breath Scale

Grade	Degree	Description
0	None	Not troubled with SOB walking a slight hill
1	Mild	Troubled when walking on level ground or up a slight hill
2	Moderate	Walks more slowly than people of the same age on the level (because of SOB) or has to stop for breath when walking at own pace on level ground
3	Severe	Stops for breath after walking about 100 yds or a few minutes walking on level ground
4	Very Severe	Too breathless to leave the house; breathless when dressing

Cardiovascular Assessment

See also Chapter 7: Hemodynamics
See also Chapter 8: Cardiac Monitoring (ECGs)

Point of Maximal Impulse (PMI)

location where cardiac impulse can be most strongly palpated on the chest wall. Normal is 5th intercostal space, midclavicular line.

Abnormal:
- Decreased with air-trapping such as COPD
- Shifts toward a lobar collapse
- Shifts away from a pneumothorax
- Shifts left in cardiomegaly

Chest Pain

- Location: Front of chest (retrosternal) is common
- Radiating: May spread to neck, jaw, back, arm
- Characteristics:
  - Tight and crushing (often cardiac)
  - Pleuritic: chest pain exacerbated when inhaling/exhaling (rule out PE)
  - Angina: pressure/squeezing in chest, may radiate (symptom of coronary heart disease)
  - Palpitations (feelings of *bumping, skipping, throbbing*)
  - Other Causes: Pneumothorax, pleural effusion, cardiac tamponade, abdominal aortic aneurism, gastrointestinal (GERD, esophageal spasm, inflammation, etc.), psychiatric (panic attacks), musculoskeletal (pulled muscle, rib fracture, etc.)
- Request tests as clinically indicated (12-Lead ECG should be performed for most patients with chest pain)

Heart Sounds

1st Sound (S1)	• What you hear: the closure of atrioventricular valves (mitral/tricuspid) • loudest at the apex
	ventricular contraction (early systole)
2nd Sound (S2)	• What you hear: closure of aortic and pulmonic valves
	ventricular relaxation
3rd Sound (S3)	• Normal in children • Abnormal in adults: ventricular dilation such as with CHF • Referred to as a "ventricular gallop"
	rapid ventricular filling during diastole
4th Sound (S4)	• Audible in some healthy (esp older) adults • Abnormal in some: ventricular hypertrophy (hypertensive heart disease, aortic stenosis, hypertrophic cardiomyopathy) • Referred to as an "atrial gallop"
Murmurs	*sound of blood flow turbulence (may be due to a valve issue, but may be benign such as with exercise)* • Systolic: After S1 but before S2 • Diastolic: After S2 but before next S1 • Continuous

Grade	Sound	Precordial Thrill?*
I	faint	No
II	detectable, soft	No
III	moderately loud	No
IV	loud	Yes
V	very loud	Yes
VI	loudest (stethoscope off chest)	Yes

*Precordial thrill is palpated: a vibration feeling

Assessment

Neurologic Assessment

Motor Activity	Ability to cough/clear secretions
	Grip strength
	Motions: coordination, paralysis, tremors
	Ability to follow commands
	Posture: <u>Decorticate</u> – flexed arms, hands fisted
	              extended legs, plantar flexion
	        <u>Decerebrate</u>- extended arms,
	              extended legs, plantar flexion
	Pupil size and reaction

Mental Status	Emotional state, behavior, comfort, orientation LOC – See next page Alert and Oriented x3 (to person, time, place)

Modified Glasgow Coma Scale (GCS)
Scale from 3 (comatose) to 15 (fully alert)
Use as general guide with other assessment (under 8 maybe intubate)
Primarily designed for brain injury, but often used with others clinically.

Adult/Older Children	Score	Infant/Young Children
Eye Opening		
Spontaneous To speech To pain Not at all	4 3 2 1	Spontaneous To loud noise To pain Not at all
Verbal Response		
Oriented Confused Inappropriate Incomprehensible None	5 4 3 2 1	Smiles, coos, cries appropriately Irritable and cries Inappropriate crying Grunts and moans None
Motor Response		
Obeys commands Localizes pain Withdraws from pain Flexion to pain Extension to pain None	6 5 4 3 2 1	Spontaneous movement Withdraws to touch Withdraws from pain Flexion to pain Extension to pain None

Descriptive Terms for Levels of Consciousness (LOC)

Alert	Awake, oriented and responds appropriately
Confused	Inability to think clearly impaired judgment
Disoriented	Starting loss of consciousness disoriented to time/place
Lethargic	Sleepy, arouses easily, responds appropriately
Obtunded	Awakens only with difficulty, then responds appropriately
Stuporous	Does not completely awaken Responds only to deep pain Withdraws or pushes you away
Unresponsive	Responds only to deep pain, exhibits reflex
Comatose	No response, flaccid muscle tone

It is important to not only do a momentary check on LOC, but trend it against the baseline. An altered (worsening) level of consciousness can be an important clinical indicator:

Neurologic
- Overdose (intentional or unintentional)
- CVA (stroke)
- Intracerebral or subarachnoid hemorrhage
- Seizure
- Infection/fever (UTI, Sepsis, etc.)

Pulmonary
- Hypercarbia (CO_2 above baseline, usually significantly so, drowsy)
- Hypoxia (early: anxiety/confusion/restless, later: further decrease of LOC)

Assessment

Fluid and Electrolyte Assessment
Urine Output:

Average	1,200 mL/Day	~40 mL/hr or > 0.5 mL/kg/hr
Male	900-1,800 mL/Day	
Female	600-1,600 mL/Day	

Normal Electrolyte Values Affecting Muscles of Ventilation:

Potassium	K^+	3.5-5.0 mEq/L
Magnesium	Mg^{++}	1.3-2.5 mEq/L
Phosphate	PO^{4-}	1.4-2.7 mEq/L

Fluid Balance Assessment

Fluid Excess (Overload)	Fluid Deficit (Depletion)
↑ Body weight, ↑CO, ↑BP ↑ PAP, ↑ CVP , ↑ JVD Bounding pulse Pitting edema Edema (including pulmonary) Abdominal ascites Dyspnea/coarse crackles	↓ Body weight ↓ BP (positional) ↑ HR, ↓ PAP, ↓ CVP, ↓ JVD ↑ BUN, ↑Creatinine Poor peripheral pulse ↓ Skin turgor (not in elderly) Oliguria ↓ Capillary refill

Causes of Changes in Fluid Balance

↑Fluid (Hypervolemia)		↓Fluid (Hypovolemia)	
↑Intake	↓Output	↓Intake	↑Output

Iatrogenic (such as fluid resuscitation)	**↓Renal Perfusion:**
	  Heart failure
	  PPV (↓CO, ↑ADH)
	  Renal System
	  Malfunction
	  Blocked Foley
		Dehydration
		Starvation
		
		Fluid Shift:
		Burns
		Shock
			Burns
			Diarrhea
			Dialysis
			Hemorrhage
			Vomiting
			NG suction

2 Acid-Base

Normal Values (Arterial/Venous)	2-2
Sampling	2-3
Venous Blood Gases	2-4
Blood Gas Interpretation (Overview)	2-5
Steps of Interpretation	2-6
Disorders	2-9
Respiratory Acidosis	2-11
Respiratory Alkalosis	2-13
Metabolic Acidosis	2-15
Metabolic Alkalosis	2-17
ABG Accuracy Check	2-19

ABG Interpretation is an important element of patient assessment and clinical decision-making.

Basic classification is the process of deciding between Respiratory and Metabolic, Acidosis and Alkalosis, and then determining oxygenation status. At times, relying solely on basic classification might miss something in the bigger picture.

Interpretation is a more complete analysis of what is going on with the patient. It involves examining compensations and gaps to determine multiple disorders, a complete and thorough investigation.

This chapter is a reference for that, but a more complete pocket guide and instructional guide are available, *"Oakes' ABG Pocket Guide,"* and *"Oakes' ABG Instructional Guide"* (a two-book set).

Arterial and Venous Normal Values

A-V difference (right-most column) helps estimate the difference between an arterial sample and a venous sample.

Parameter	Arterial (ABG)		Venous* (peripheral VBG)		A-V Difference
	Norm	Range	Norm	Range	Average
pH *units*	pH_a 7.40	7.35-7.45	$pH_{\bar{v}}$ 7.36	7.31-7.41	0.04
PCO_2 *mm Hg*	$PaCO_2$ 40	35-45	$P\bar{v}CO_2$ 46	40-50	6
PO_2 (Room Air) *mm Hg*	PaO_2 100	80-100	$P\bar{v}O_2$ 40	30-50	55
O_2 Sat *%*	SaO_2 97	95-100	$S\bar{v}O_2$ 75	68-77	22
HCO_3^- *mEq/L*	24	22-26	24	23-27	1
TCO_2** *mEq/L*	25	23-27	25	23-27	none
BE *mEq/L*	0	+/- 2	0	+/- 2	none
O_2 content *mL/dL*	CaO_2 20	15-24	$C\bar{v}O_2$ 15	12-15	> 2

* See pg 2-4 (VBGs). Venous values depend on where the sample was drawn from. The above chart lists peripheral values. When analyzing a sample from a central line (CVP) or pulmonary artery (PA) catheter: (compared to ABG)

pH	▼ 0.03 - 0.05
PCO_2	▲ 3-8
HCO_3^-	▲ 2-3

Peripheral values may vary if peripheral circulation is compromised
All values may vary if hypotension, shock, or extreme acid-base imbalance

** TCO_2 is more a reflection of HCO_3^- than CO_2 [$TCO_2 = HCO_3^- + 0.03(PCO_2)$]

Acid-Base

Arterial Blood Gas Sampling

Indications	Need to evaluate: • **Oxygenation** (PaO_2, SaO_2, HbO_2, Hgb) • Ventilation ($PaCO_2$) • Acid-base (pH, $PaCO_2$, HCO_3^-) Note that ventilation and acid-base can be evaluated using a venous blood gas, but oxygenation requires an arterial gas
Contra-indications	• Hand puncture: negative Allen's test • Any limb site: infection, PVD, surgical shunt • Coagulopathy/anticoagulants (relative)
Hazards/ Complications	• Arterial occlusion • Arteriospasm • Contagion at site • Emboli (air/blood) • Hematoma • Hemorrhage • Pain • Trauma to vessel • Vasovagal response
Monitoring	*Patient*: RR, temperature, clinical appearance, position and/or activity level, puncture site (post sample) *O_2/vent therapy*: proper application of O_2 device, FIO_2 or flowrate, ventilator mode and settings *Procedure*: ease or difficulty, pulsatile blood return, air bubbles or clot
Clinical Quick Tips (not entire procedure)	• Palpate artery (radial is usually preferred, then brachial, then femoral if necessary) • Verify collateral circulation if radial (modified Allen Test - see pg 2-4) • Prepare syringe, insert gently but firmly, while palpating pulse, into artery. Bevel should be up during insertion. Flash of blood into syringe usually indicates arterial blood. • Apply pressure until bleeding has stopped • Prepare sample (carefully tap out air bubbles, roll gently to mix heparin)

Portions of this have been adapted from retired AARC Clinical Practice Guideline: Sampling for Arterial Blood Gas Analysis, ***Respiratory Care***, Volume 37, #8, 1992

Modified Allen Test
- Instruct patient to clench fist or close hand tightly for patient
- Occlude both ulnar and radial arteries
- Have patient relax hand (with arteries occluded), then remove pressure from ulnar artery only. Hand should flush to normal color within 15-seconds (positive). If not (negative test result), ulnar (collateral) circulation is considered inadequate for a radial ABG.

Venous Blood Gases (VBGs)
VBGs should only be considered when estimating pH, CO_2, and HCO_3^- to assess ventilation and acid-base. It does not provide an appropriate evaluation of oxygenation.

May be used as an alternative to ABGs in certain circumstances, particularly when unable to obtain an ABG:
- Diminished pulses
- Patient movement is excessive
- When a central line (but not arterial line) is present
- In cases of pain sensitivity, such as children (VBGs are generally regarded to be less painful than ABGs)

Sampling:
- Peripheral venous sample (venipuncture)
- Central venous sample (from a central line)
- Mixed venous sample (distal port of pulmonary artery catheter)

Interpretation
- See pg 2-2 for values and details on interpretation
- Assists in assessing ventilation and acid-base status (pH, PCO_2, HCO_3^-)
- The PO_2 (PvO_2) has minimal value (the oxygen has already been extracted by the tissues)
- The SO_2 (SvO_2) may be used as a guide to resuscitation during severe sepsis or shock
- VBGs are often used in combination with pulse oximetry (SpO_2) to complete the ventilation/oxygenation assessment.

ABG INTERPRETATION =

Classification

\+

Calculations

\+

Confirmation

A. Classification

Respiratory	
Acidosis	Alkalosis

Metabolic	
Acidosis	Alkalosis

B. Calculations

Calculate Compensation and Gaps:
Determine whether or not the body is compensating and whether or not other primary disorders exist.

Determine Oxygenation Status

C. Confirmation

Consistency with patient assessment, patient's baseline and check for accuracy: Determines validity of Classification and Calculations

KEYS to INTERPRETATION

1. Initial Technical Classification DOES NOT always equal a definitive ABG interpretation
2. Calculations are essential
3. Patient assessment is even more essential
4. Understanding a patient's baseline values are helpful
5. Always check for possible inaccuracies in the blood gas result
6. Trending ABGs over time is more helpful than a single ABG
7. ABG interpretation can lead to critical decisions–it is important to remember that errors are unacceptable.

Acid-Base

Steps of Acid-Base Interpretation

A) Classification (see chart next page)

Primary Problem
Step 1. Check pH: Acidosis or Alkalosis?

Primary Cause
Step 2. Check PaCO₂: is Respiratory the primary cause?
Step 3. Check HCO_3^- : is Metabolic the primary cause?

Compensation
Step 4. Is the body compensating?

Initial Classification
Step 5. *Technical Classification* and/or *Functional Classification*

B) Calculations

Step 6. Determine if compensation is appropriate or are there other *Primary Disorders*

	PaCO₂	pH	HCO_3^-
Respiratory Acidosis			
Acute	↑ 10	↓ 0.08	↑ 1
Chronic	↑ 10	↓ 0.03	↑ 4
Respiratory Alkalosis			
Acute	↓ 10	↑ 0.08	↓ 2
Chronic	↓ 10	↑ 0.03	↓ 5

	HCO_3^-	pH	PaCO₂
Metabolic Acidosis	↓ 1	↓ 0.015	↓ 1.2
Metabolic Alkalosis	↑ 1	↑ 0.015	↑ 0.7

Step 7. Determine Anion Gap and Bicarbonate Gap

  a. Anion Gap (AG): $AG = Na - (Cl + HCO_3^-)$
  b. Bicarbonate Gap (if an AG acidosis):

  $BG =$ Patient's $HCO_3^- + \Delta AG$
  BG Norm = 24 = AG Metabolic Acidosis
  < 20 = AG Met. Acidosis + Non AG Met. Acidosis
  > 28 = AG Met. Acidosis + Met. Alkalosis

Step 8. Determine Oxygenation (See pg 1-10)

C) Confirmation
Step 9. Systematically Assess Patient
Step 10. Check for Accuracy (errors)
Step 11. **Final Interpretations**

Primary Problem	Primary Cause			Compensation	Initial Classification
Step 1: Check pH	Step 2:		Step 3:	Step 4:	Step 5:
	Check PaCO₂ (35-45)	Respiratory primary problem?	Check HCO₃⁻ (22-26)	Metabolic primary problem?	Is the body compensating? (Yes/No)	Technical Classification (1)
Alkalosis > 7.45*	↑		↑	Yes	Yes (↑ $PaCO_2$)	PC Metabolic Alkalosis
	N		↑	Yes	-	Metabolic Alkalosis (UC)
	↓	Yes	↑	Yes	-	Mixed Respiratory Alkalosis & Metabolic Alkalosis
	↓	Yes	N,↓		(3)	Respiratory Alkalosis (UC)
	↓	Yes	↓		Yes (↓ HCO_3^-)	PC Respiratory Alkalosis
Normal 7.35-7.45	↑	Yes or compensating?	↑	Yes or compensating?	Yes (↑ $PaCO_2$)	FC Metabolic Alkalosis (7.41-7.45)
	↑	Yes or compensating?	↑	Yes or compensating?	Yes (↑ HCO_3^-)	FC Respiratory Acidosis (7.35-7.39)
	N		N		-	Normal or Mixed Disorder (2)
	↓	Yes or compensating?	↓	Yes or compensating?	Yes (↓ $PaCO_2$)	FC Metabolic Acidosis (7.35-7.39)
	↓	Yes or compensating?	↓	Yes or compensating?	Yes (↓ HCO_3^-)	FC Respiratory Alkalosis (7.41-7.45)

continued on next page

Primary Problem	Primary Cause				Compensation	Initial Classification
	↓	Yes	↑	↑	Yes (↑ HCO$_3^-$)	PC Respiratory Acidosis
	↑	Yes	↑	N, ↑	(3)	Respiratory Acidosis (UC)
Acidosis < 7.35 **	↑	Yes	↑	↓	-	Mixed Respiratory & Metabolic Acidosis
	N		Yes	↓	-	Metabolic Acidosis (UC)
	↓		Yes	↓	Yes (↓ PaCO$_2$)	PC Metabolic Acidosis

(1) Technical classification terminology:
  UC = Uncompensated (no compensation has occurred). Common usage leaves this designation off.
  PC = Partially Compensated (pH has returned part way back to normal range)
  FC = Fully Compensated (pH has returned back to normal range)

(2) Mixed Disorder (opposite disorders) = Respiratory Acidosis & Metabolic Alkalosis or Respiratory Alkalosis & Metabolic Acidosis
  (PaCO$_2$ and HCO$_3^-$ go in same direction and "apparent compensation" is greater than expected)

(3) The immediate change in HCO$_3^-$ from normal is due to the hydrolysis effect, rather than compensation.

* As pH moves towards 7.8 = ↑ CNS stimulation: irritability, arrhythmias, tetany, convulsions, respiratory arrest, death. Definitive therapy is indicated at pH > 7.6.

** As pH moves towards 7.0 = ↓ CNS stimulation: drowsiness, lethargy, coma, death. Definitive therapy is often considered at pH < 7.15.

ABG Disorders

Technical Class.	Functional Class.	Compensation Status
UC Respiratory Acidosis	Acute Respiratory Acidosis	**Kidneys**: Either not enough time to begin compensation or the kidneys are compromised
PC Respiratory Acidosis	Chronic Respiratory Acidosis	**Kidneys**: Either not enough time to fully compensate or compensation is maximal (chronic), but pH not back to normal range
FC Respiratory Acidosis	Chronic Respiratory Acidosis	**Kidneys**: Compensation is maximal (chronic) and full – pH is back to normal range (occurs only in very mild disorders)
UC Respiratory Alkalosis	Acute Respiratory Alkalosis	**Kidneys**: Either not enough time to begin compensation or kidneys are compromised
PC Respiratory Alkalosis	Chronic Respiratory Alkalosis	**Kidneys**: Either not enough time to fully compensate or compensation is maximal (chronic), but pH not back to normal range
FC Respiratory Alkalosis	Chronic Respiratory Alkalosis	**Kidneys**: Compensation is maximal (chronic) and full –pH is back to normal range (occurs in most disorders)
UC Metabolic Acidosis	Metabolic Acidosis*	**Respiratory**: system is compromised (rare that there is zero compensation) or such a mild change in HCO_3^- that any change in $PaCO_2$ is minimal.
PC Metabolic Acidosis	Metabolic Acidosis	**Respiratory**: Compensation is usually immediate and maximal, but pH is not back to normal range
FC Metabolic Acidosis	Metabolic Acidosis	**Respiratory**: This classification essentially *does not exist* because $PaCO_2$ generally does not return pH back to normal range. If pH is normal, there is usually a secondary respiratory disorder at work.
UC Metabolic Alkalosis	Metabolic Alkalosis	**Respiratory**: If there is no compensation, there is usually a secondary respiratory alkalosis
PC Metabolic Alkalosis	Metabolic Alkalosis	**Respiratory**: Compensation is usually immediate and maximal, but pH is not back to normal range
FC Metabolic Alkalosis	Metabolic Alkalosis	**Respiratory**: This class. really *does not exist* because $PaCO_2$ generally does not return pH back to normal range. If pH is normal, there is usually a secondary respiratory disorder at work.

NOTES

Functional Classification = common usage and function

Technical classification terminology:

UC = Uncompensated (no compensation has occurred). Common usage leaves this designation off.
PC = Partially Compensated (pH has returned part way back to normal range)
FC = Fully Compensated (pH has returned back to normal range)

A *corrected* blood gas disorder is one in which the pH is returned to normal range by altering the component primarily affected.
A *compensated* blood gas disorder is one in which the pH is returned towards normal range by altering the component not primarily affected.

Because of the limitations of the lungs or kidneys to "fully" compensate for most alterations of each other (i.e., completely return pH to normal), *"full"* or *"complete"* compensation is more appropriately referred to as *"maximal"* compensation.

Maximal Compensation = the body has completely compensated all it is designed to compensate – usually pH returns only 50% of the way back.
If the disorder is *mild*, maximal compensation may return the pH to within normal range, resulting in a *"full"* compensation (FC).
If the disorder is *moderate to severe*, maximal compensation will only return the pH part way back to normal range, resulting in a *"partial"* compensation (PC).

* The terms *"acute"* and *"chronic"* for metabolic disorders are often omitted because, *functionally*, there is usually no time distinction between acute and chronic metabolic disorders – the respiratory system compensation is usually immediate.
Also, because all metabolic disorders are essentially Partially Compensated, all metabolic disorders are simply termed Metabolic Acidosis or Metabolic Alkalosis, without any further descriptive terminology.

Respiratory Acidosis

Definition	$PaCO_2$ > 45 mm Hg (Hypercarbia or Hypercapnia)
Cause	Hypoventilation -or- Ventilatory Failure
Compensation	Slow ↑ in HCO_3^- (Renal ↑ in Base)
Treatment (Goal)	Improve ventilation, return pH to normal (Treat underlying cause, if able)

Overview of Parameter Changes

	pH	$PaCO_2$	HCO_3^-	K^+	Cl^-
Uncompensated (acute)	↓	↑	↑*	N	N
Partially Compensated (PC) (chronic)	↓	↑	↑	N	N
Fully Compensated (FC) (chronic)**	N	↑	↑↑	N ↑	↓

* The acute change from normal is due to the hydrolysis effect, rather than compensation.
** Rare. Maximal renal compensation commonly results in only partial correction of pH. pH only returns less than halfway back towards normal — unless a very mild respiratory acidosis.

Determining Compensation

Expected change in pH and HCO_3^- for Every 10 mmHg ↑ in $PaCO_2$

	Expected ↓ in pH	Expected ↑ in HCO_3^-
Acute	0.08 *	1
Partially Compensated	0.03-0.08	1-4
Maximally Compensated	0.03	4

*Other references may cite anywhere between 0.05 and 0.1

Signs and Symptoms of Respiratory Acidosis
(relative order of appearance, and varies with severity of acidosis)

General Stage	Common Symptoms (not exhaustive)
Early (Acute)	Hypoxemia (alveolar air equation) Tachypnea Dyspnea Anxiety, Agitation Tachycardia
Later (Acute) *(patient tires out)*	Headache Lethargy Worsening mental status Bradypnea Cardiac arrest Seizures/Coma/Death
Chronic	(HCO_3^- will begin to compensate) Arrhythmias Pulmonary hypertension Headache (esp in AM) Disturbed sleep
Acute on Chronic	Similar to acute symptoms listed above pH is more important to trend than $PaCO_2$ (if pt has an abnormal baseline)

Primary Causes of Respiratory Acidosis
(examples are in parentheses - Oakes ABG Pocket Guide has a detailed list)

- **Airway Obstruction** (Aspiration, Secretions, Bronchoconstriction)
- **Impaired Lung Tissue Function** (ARDS, Pneumonia)
- **Restrictive Disorders** (Obesity, Trauma, Deformities)
- **Central Nervous System Depression** (Drugs, Head Injury, Stroke)
- **Excessive CO_2 Production** (Burns, Fever, Sepsis)
- **Neuromuscular** (Injury, Electrolytes, Guillain Barré, Myasthenia Gravis)
- **Cardiovascular** (Cardiac Arrest, Cardiogenic Pulmonary Edema, Shock)
- **Other** (Air-trapping, Malnutrition, Mechanical Ventilation Settings)

Respiratory Alkalosis

Definition	$PaCO_2$ < 35 mm Hg (Hypocarbia or Hypocapnia)
Cause	Hyperventilation
Compensation	Slow ↓ in HCO_3^- (Renal ↓ in Base)
Treatment (Goal)	Reduce ventilation, return pH to normal (treat underlying cause, if able)

Overview of Parameter Changes

	pH	$PaCO_2$	HCO_3^-	K^+	Cl^-
Uncompensated (acute)	↑	↓	↓*	N	N
Partially Compensated (PC) (chronic)	↑	↓	↓	N	N
Fully Compensated (FC) (chronic)	N	↓	↓↓	N ↓	↑

* The acute change from normal is due to the hydrolysis effect, rather than compensation.
K^+ = Potassium Cl^- = Chloride

Determining Compensation

Expected change in pH and HCO_3^- for Every 10 mmHg ↓ in $PaCO_2$

	Expected ↑ in pH	Expected ↓ in HCO_3^-
Acute	0.08 *	2
Partially Compensated	0.03-0.08	2-5
Maximally Compensated	0.03	5

*Other references use 0.1

Acid-Base

Signs and Symptoms of Respiratory Alkalosis
(relative order of appearance, and varies with severity of alkalosis)

General Stage	Common Symptoms (not exhaustive)
Early (Acute)	Hyperventilation/Dyspnea Dizziness Parasthesia Anxiety Tachycardia Hyperkalemia
Later (Acute) *(patient tires out)*	Confusion Feeling of euphoria Hallucinations Seizures/Stupor Hypokalemia
Chronic	Arrhythmias Hypo/hyperchloremia Hypokalemia

Primary Causes of Respiratory Alkalosis

(examples are in parentheses - Oakes ABG Pocket Guide has a detailed list)

- **Hypoxemia** (most common cause)
- **Central Nervous System Disorders** (Drugs, Infection, Anxiety)
- **Metabolic** (Hypothermia, Sepsis, Fever)
- **Decreased Diaphragmatic Function** (Obesity, Pregnancy, Ascites)
- **Cardiovascular** (Shock, MI, PE, CHF)
- **Other** (High Altitude, Ventilator Settings)

Metabolic Acidosis	
Definition	$HCO_3^- < 22$ mEq/L
Cause	Increased Acid or Decrease in Base
Compensation	Hyperventilation (Lungs)
Treatment (Goal)	Address Metabolic Issue, when possible Consider Mechanical Ventilation if severely low pH

Overview of Parameter Changes

	pH	PaCO$_2$	HCO$_3^-$	K$^+$	Cl$^-$
Uncompensated (acute)	↓	↓	↓	↑	↑
Partially Compensated (PC) (chronic)*	↓	↓	↓	↑	↑
Fully Compensated (FC) (chronic)	N	↓	↓↓	N	N

* Rare. There is usually some degree of immediate (10 – 30 min) respiratory compensation (hyperventilation), unless there is respiratory impairment. Hence, there is usually no distinction between acute and chronic.
If there is no compensation, then the respiratory system is compromised.
In rapid changes of HCO$_3^-$, respiratory compensation may take 12-24 hours.

** This classification essentially does not exist because PaCO$_2$ generally does not return pH back to normal range (usually only ½ way back). If pH is normal, there is usually a secondary respiratory disorder at work.

Determining Compensation

Expected change in pH and PaCO$_2$ for Every 1 mEq/L ↓ in HCO$_3^-$

	Expected ↓ in pH	Expected ↓ in PaCO$_2$
Acute or Chronic	0.015	1.2 - 1.5 (max)**

* For ease of calculation, for every 1 mEq/L ↓ in HCO$_3^-$, the last digit of pH ↓ 1.5.
** Maximal compensation: PaCO$_2$ = last two digits of pH

Signs and Symptoms of Metabolic Acidosis

General Stage	Common Symptoms (not exhaustive)
Acute	Hyperventilation (compensation) Air hunger Dyspnea/Hyperpnea/Tachypnea Kussmaul's respiration (if DKA) Dry skin/mucous membranes Lethargy/Seizures/Coma/Death
Chronic	Arrythmias Dyspnea Muscle fatigue Hyperkalemia

Causes of Metabolic Acidosis

(examples are in parentheses - Oakes ABG Pocket Guide has a detailed list)

Anion Gap Metabolic Acidosis ($\uparrow$ acid): $\uparrow$ acid leads to $\uparrow$ Anion Gap
- **Increased Acid Production** (Lactic Acidosis [see below], Ketoacidosis)
- **Increased Acid Addition** (Toxins, Drugs)
- **Decreased Acid Excretion** (Dehydration, Renal Failure, Trauma)

Causes of Lactic Acidosis
- **Hypoxemia**
- **Under-delivery of O_2 to Tissue Cells** (Cardiac Arrest, Anemia, Carbon Monoxide Poisoning)
- **Over-consumption of O_2 by Tissue Cells** (Seizures, Sepsis, Shivering)
- **Non-Hypoxic Causes** (Diabetes, Severe Infection, Pancreatitis, Renal Failure)

Non-Anion Gap Metabolic Acidosis ($\downarrow$ base): $\downarrow HCO_3^- \rightarrow \uparrow Cl^-$
(Also called Hyperchloremic Metabolic Acidosis)
- **Increased Kidney Excretion** (Renal Tubular Acidosis)
- **Intestinal Loss** (Diarrhea, Enteric Drainage Tubes)
- **Infusion or Ingestion** (TPN, Carbonic Anhydrase Inhibitors)
- **Other** (Eucapnic Ventilation: normalized $PaCO_2$ after a prolonged period of hyperventilation)

Metabolic Alkalosis

Definition	HCO_3^- > 26 mEq/L
Cause	Decreased Acid or Increase in Base
Compensation	Hypoventilation (Lungs)
Treatment (Goal)	Address metabolic issue, when possible

Overview of Parameter Changes

	pH	$PaCO_2$	HCO_3^-	K^+	Cl^-
Uncompensated* (acute)	↑	↑	↑	↓	↓
Partially Compensated (PC) (chronic)	↑	↑	↑	↓	↓
Fully Compensated (FC)** (chronic)	N	↑	↑↑	N	N

* Rare. If there is no compensation there is usually a secondary respiratory alkalosis. There is usually no distinction between acute and chronic.

** This classification essentially does not exist because $PaCO_2$ generally does not return pH back to normal range (usually only ½ way back). If pH is normal, there is usually a secondary respiratory disorder at work.

Determining Compensation

Expected change in pH and $PaCO_2$ for Every 1 mEq/L ↑ in HCO_3^-

	Expected ↑ in pH*	Expected ↑ in $PaCO_2$**
Acute or Chronic	0.015	0.7 - 1.5 (max)**

* For ease of calculation, for every 1 mEq/L ↑ in HCO_3^-, the last digit of pH ↑ 1.5.

** Compensation (expected $PaCO_2$) is highly variable – anywhere between 0.25 – 1.0 with 0.7 the average (see below). Maximal compensation is rare and limited (see below). When maximal compensation does occur, $PaCO_2$ = last two digits of pH

Acid-Base

Signs and Symptoms of Metabolic Alkalosis

General Stage	Common Symptoms (not exhaustive)
Acute	Hypoventilation (compensation) Lightheadedness Headache Tingling/Numbness Tachycardia Palpitations Lethargy Seizures/Coma/Death
Chronic	Arrythmias Hypo/Hyperchloremia Hypokalemia Anxiety

Causes of Metabolic Alkalosis
(examples are in parentheses - Oakes ABG Pocket Guide has a detailed list)

Increased Base
- **Intestinal Intake** (Antacids, $NaHCO_3^-$)
- **Decreased Chloride** (Diarrhea, Cushing's Syndrome, severe hypokalemia)

Decreased Acid
- **Increased Kidney Excretion** (Chronic renal failure, diuretics, hypokalemia, hypochloremia, hypovolemia)
- **Intestinal Loss** (Nasogastric suctioning, vomiting)
- **Drugs** (Diuretics, systemic steroids)
- **Other** (Eucapnic ventilation - normalizing $PaCO_2$ of chronic retainer)

ABG Accuracy Check

Check Patient	Does ABG line up with patient's clinical condition? • Good ABG but pt in distress? • Poor ABG but pt in no distress? • Rising or normal $PaCO_2$ in severe distress (such as asthma)?
Check Lab Values	• HCO_3^- should be within 1-2 mEq/L of Total CO_2 (lab value) • A difference of more than 4 is a technical error • Actual HCO_3^- should = $24 \times PaCO_2/(80\text{-Last 2 digits of pH})$ - only works if pH 7.30-7.50
Check for Errors *Sampling Errors*	1. **Venous blood contamination** *Strong Suspicion if PaO_2 is 40 or less* 	Value	Venous	Effect of venous blood in sample
---	---	---
pH	7.31-7.41	Decreases pH
PCO_2	41-51	Increases PCO_2
PO_2	30-40	Decreases PO_2 | 2. **Air in Sample** (may vary with how much sample shaken, time to analysis, temperature of sample, volume of air) PaO_2 may be higher than expected $PaCO_2$ may be lower than expected | Value	Air	Effect of Air in Blood
---	---	---
PaO_2	159 mm Hg	Moves towards 159 (usually ↑)
$PaCO_2$	0 mm Hg	↓ $PaCO_2$ ↑ pH	 3. **Anticoagulant** (heparin): too much (same effect as air) 4. **Patient not on reported FIO_2** 5. **Patient not in a steady-state** (ABG sampled quickly after a change in status)

Acid-Base

Check for Errors (continued) **Measuring Errors**	**Measuring Errors** - Improper calibration, quality control - Documentation errors - Patient temperature entered incorrectly (such as with therapeutic hypothermia) - Wrong patient - Time delay in measuring (> 30 min) - Increased WBC or platelets (decreases PaO_2)
Check the PaO_2 FiO_2 Relationship	**Patient is on Room Air:** PaO_2 should be less than 130 mm Hg **Patient is on Supplemental Oxygen:** PaO_2 should be approximately 5 x FiO_2 **Always Question:** Was the O_2 mask actually on the patient? Was the cannula in nose? Was 100% O_2 being delivered temporarily on ventilator?
Check the PaO_2 SaO_2/SpO_2 Relationship	Relationship should correlate. Discrepancies indicate a problem with the ABG sample (sampling time delay, venous blood, air in sample) or a problem with pulse oximeter reading.
Check the PaO_2 $PaCO_2$ Relationship	On Room Air and at normal atmospheric pressure, PaO_2 + $PaCO_2$ should always be less than 150 mm Hg

3 Chest Imaging

Chest Radiograph (CXR) Interpretation
   Systematic Approach 3-2
   Normal Radiographs 3-3
   Abnormal Appearances/Causes 3-5
      Segmental Infiltrates 3-9
      Tube/Line Placement 3-10
Computerized Axial Topography Scan
   (CT Scan) 3-11
Magnetic Resonance Imaging Scan
   (MRI Scan) 3-12
Thoracic Ultrasound 3-13

IMAGING

Keys to Good Interpretation

1. Be Systematic
Regardless of the systematic approach you adopt, review every image in the same order, every time. One approach is on pg 3-2.

2. Be Aware
Images must be interpreted in context of the patient's status. They are clinical snapshots and can be misleading if viewed independently of the patient's condition.

3. Be Wary
Use caution in making decisions (such as pulling back an endotracheal tube) based solely upon a chest image. Body habitus, poor quality, and other factors can make locating tubes difficult at times.

Imaging   3-1

Systematic Approach to Interpreting a
Chest Radiograph see also: Abnormal Appearances on pg 3-5

1. **Confirm patient and medical record number**
2. **Confirm date and time**
3. **Identify type:** AP (from front) vs PA (from back) vs Lateral (side)
4. **Check quality:** about 4 vertebrae visible, inspiratory film?
   Exp film may show abnorm ↑ heart size, ↓ volume, ↑ interstitium
5. **Check rotation:** clavicles centered around vertebrae
6. **Systematically explore from Outside-to-Inside:**

Soft Tissue	Amount of tissue (obesity, breasts) Subcutaneous emphysema (crepitus)
Bones	Examine for fractures, especially clavicles, ribs. Obvious spinal deformity (kyphosis, etc.)?
Heart	Size: > 60% of thoracic width = abnormal[1] Identify: Major structures (ventricles, etc.)

Lungs	Expansion (7-9 ribs, mid-clavic. at diaphragm)
	 Find trachea, carina (midline?)
	 Find fissures, if visible
	 Find hila (L is above R)
	 Costophrenic and Cardiophrenic Angles (blunted ~fluid?)
	 Diaphragm: Right is slightly ↑ than Left (liver)
	 Elevated? Flattened (air trap)?
	 Parenchyma:
	   Haziness (~atelectasis)
	   Consolidation (air bronchograms at periphery)
	   Infiltrates (consolidation, localized or diffuse)
	   Pneumothorax (lack of vasc. markings)
	   General abnormalities (foreign objects, nodules, honeycombing, etc.)

Tubes Lines	ET tube (3-5 cm above carina) Trach tube (present or not) Gastric tube Chest tube(s) ECG leads Central catheter or PA catheter Identify others: pacemaker, vent circuit, etc.

[1] AP films (typical of critical care) over-estimate heart size.

Normal Chest Radiograph - Posterior-Anterior (PA)

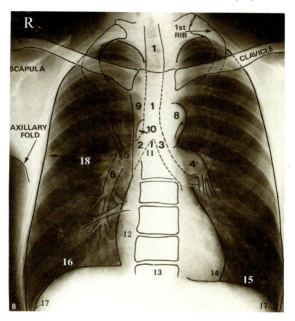

1. trachea
2. right mainstem
3. left mainstem
4. left pulmonary artery
5. right upper lobe pulmonary vein
6. right interlobar artery
7. right upper and lower lobe vein
8. aortic knob
9. superior vena cava
10. ascending aorta
11. carina
12. right atrium
13. right ventricle
14. left ventricle
15. left hemidiaphragm
16. right hemidiaphragm
17. costophrenic angle
18. minor fissure

Reprinted with permission from Fraser, R.H. and Pare, J.A.: *Organ Physiology: Structure and Function of the Lung*. Copyright 1977 by W.B Saunders, Co., Philadelphia

Normal Chest Radiograph - Lateral

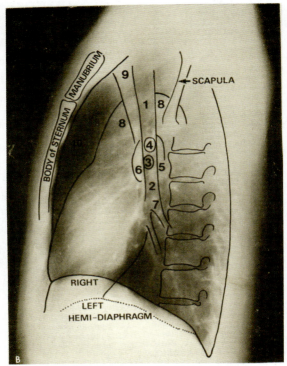

1. trachea
2. right intermediate bronchus
3. left upper lobe bronchus
4. right upper lobe bronchus
5. left interlobar artery
6. right interlobar artery
7. pulmonary veins
8. aortic arch
9. brachiocephalic vessels
10. substernal space

Reprinted with permission from Fraser, R.H. and Pare, J.A.: *Organ Physiology: Structure and Function of the Lung*. Copyright 1977 by W.B Saunders, Co., Philadelphia

Abnormal Appearances and Possible Causes

Appearances	Possible Causes
Air Bronchogram Can visualize airways out towards the periphery	Consolidated alveoli (pneumonia, etc.)
AP vs. PA Projection AP usually shows ↓ lung volumes, ↑ hemi-diaphragms, ↑ lung markings in bases, **heart enlarged**, scapula overlies upper fields, often rotated	Portable X-ray, AP usually taken for critical care patients. Be aware when looking at heart size in particular.
Butterfly Pattern	
Puffy cloudy appearance in central lung fields	Pulmonary edema
"Honeycomb" like cloudy appearance throughout lung fields	Interstitial edema
Costophrenic Blunting Normal costophrenic angles are easily identified, sharp angles. Blunting occurs when the angles become more blurred/blunted	Pleural effusion
Increased Heart Size*	
Right Ventricle Pulmonary artery is pushed towards left cardiac border, apex of heart is shifted upward	Cor pulmonale, pulmonary hypertension, ASD, VSD
Right Atrium May be difficult to view due to normal variations, look for enlargement of the right atrial shadow	Cor pulmonale, pulmonary hypertension

* Heart may appear falsely enlarged with AP projection - always use a PA view to confirm cardiac enlargement.

Imaging

Appearances	Possible Causes
Left Ventricle Rounding of left cardiac border, boot-shaped extension	Congestive Heart Failure
Left Atrium A projection (laterally) of the right cardiac border	Congestive Heart Failure
Kerley B Lines Perpendicular lines to pleura in the peripheral bases	Interstitial edema
Miliary Pattern Small, round <u>regular</u> densities	Tuberculosis Other disorders where alveoli fill with fluid/material
Nodular Pattern Small, soft tissue density masses (round or oval) - tend to be <u>irregular</u>	Neoplasm (tumors, etc.) Fungal infection Parasitic infection Rheumatoid arthritis
Peripheral Markings Decreased Decreased or absent markings in periphery	Pneumothorax (most common) Pulmonary hypertension Pulmonary embolism
Pulmonary Arteries Dilated May be antler-shaped, cloudiness at base	Pulmonary hypertension
"Loss of" **Silhouette Sign*** Loss of the normal silhouette of the heart, aorta, or diaphragm (*See diagram pg 3-8*)	May indicate airspace opacity, atelectasis, mass, or fluid in contact with heart/aorta. May help identify location of lesions.

Appearances	Possible Causes
Reticular (Interstitial) Pattern Linear "shadows" (fine or coarse)	Fine: Interstitial disorder (pulm. edema, pneumonitis) Sarcoidosis, fibrosis, inhalation injuries Coarse: Honeycombing (end-stage pulmonary fibrosis)
Reticulogranular Pattern Ground glass appearance, often with air bronchograms	ARDS, RDS The other reticular patterns (see above) may also appear in this pattern
Volume Decreased Decreased size of thoracic cage, elevated diaphragm, ↑ interstitial markings	Atelectasis, ↓ surfactant, ↓ compliance, abdominal issue pushing up diaphragm (ascites, etc.)
Volume Increased Increased size of thoracic cage (hyper-aeration), flattened diaphragm, ↓ interstitial markings	*Trapped air:* asthma, COPD, excessive set tidal volumes, ↑ (applied) PEEP or auto-PEEP, tension pneumothorax

* This is sometimes referred to as a *silhouette sign* even though it is technically the loss of the silhouette

Silhouette Sign

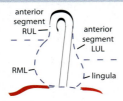

ANTERIOR STRUCTURES
(ascending aorta)
(heart)

Are Obliterated by Infiltrates in:
Anterior segment of RUL
Anterior segment of LUL, RML
+/or lingular

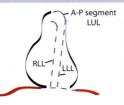

POSTERIOR STRUCTURES
(aortic knob)
(descending aorta)

Are Obliterated by Infiltrates in:
A-P segment of LUL, RLL, LLL

– – – Presence of silhouette sign

Segmental Infiltrates on the Chest X-Ray (CXR)

This diagram shows the relative location of infiltrates as they appear on a chest radiograph. Use this information for patient positioning, postural drainage, etc.

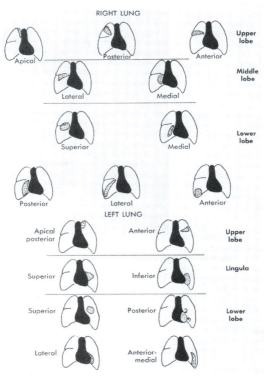

Reprinted with permission from Sheldon, R.L..In Scanlan, C.L., Spearman, C.B. and Sheldon, R.L., editors: *Egan's Fundamentals of Respiratory Therapy*, 6th ed. Copyright 1995 by the Mosby Yearbook, Inc., St. Louis

Common Chest Radiograph Findings by Disease/Disorder
See individual disease/disorder in Disease Chapter

Approximate Tube/Line Placement on Chest Radiograph

Line/Tube	Placement
Endotracheal Tube	Locate carina. ET tube tip should be approximately 3-5 cm above carina (adults) when neck is in a neutral position (~ 3 cm if flexed; ~7 cm if extended). If carina is not visible, use T2-T4 for positioning when neck is in a neutral position. Pediatrics: The trachea is shorter, ET tube tip may be as close as 1.5 cm from carina.
Tracheostomy Tube	Tip should be midline, about midpoint between carina and the upper end of the tracheostomy tube. Check for any presence of subcutaneous emphysema (suggesting tube tip is in the tissue)
CVP Line	Tip should be in superior vena cava, just before right atrium
PA Catheter	Tip should be in right or left pulmonary artery (about 5 cm distal to main pulmonary artery bifurcation)
NG or OG Tube	Tip and side hole should be beyond gastroesophageal junction
Chest Tube	Tip of radiopaque line should be within the pleural space and medial to the inner margin of the ribs. Positioning depends on whether collecting air or fluid

CT Scan of the Chest

Provides more details than a normal chest radiograph (x-ray), and allows for the display of anatomy in different planes (making the structures easier to view without being clouded by other structures), but at the cost of a greater exposure to radiation than a normal chest radiograph. Note that a highly detailed frontal image is usually available, as well as thin cross-sections, slice-by-slice.

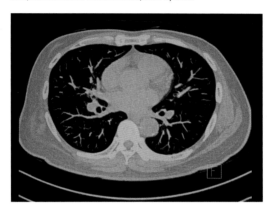

Indications
- Examine abnormalities found on a chest radiograph (CXR) that are difficult to differentiate. Example: atelectasis vs pneumonia (volumes can be much more apparent on CT scan).
- More closely examine and quantify the presence of a pleural effusion or pneumothorax (especially smaller ones)
- Suspicion of pulmonary embolus (CT Angiogram [CTA] with contrast)
- Screening for patients at high-risk of cancer

Instructions
Patients should be instructed, if possible, to take 3-4 deep breaths, then hold inspiration for 10-30 seconds (single breath-hold technique). If unable, multiple scans of 5-15 seconds can be taken.
Note: expiratory scans can be used when air-trapping or malacia is suspected.

MRI Scan of the Chest

Similar to a CT Scan, an MRI can provide detailed information not available in a normal chest radiograph (x-ray). Uses a strong magnet that results in a mathematical display.

Indications
- Examination of complex diaphragmatic and pleural disorders/diseases
- Examination of concerns related to the hilum and mediastinum
- Suspicion of pulmonary embolus
- Patients who should avoid contrast administration (renal dysfunction) as MRI doesn't absolutely require contrast

Considerations
An MRI contains a very strong magnetic field:
- Ensure (metal) O_2 tanks and other metal-based equipment do not enter the MRI room
- Only MRI-compatible ventilators should be in MRI room. Be sure to know limitations of such equipment (how close it can be to the magnet, for example).
- Be aware of the limitations of any specialized airways/tubes (while rare, some airways may have metal components)
- Ensure pockets are emptied of potential projectiles: scissors, stethoscope, etc.
- Check with MRI team regarding any personal piercings, implants, etc. prior to entering the MRI room
- If patient has an implanted cardiac device (ICD), check with MRI team
- Monitoring patients during an MRI can be challenging. Ensure ventilator screen is clearly visible from observation area
- Patients generally must be stable enough to handle being supine for a period of time.

Thoracic Ultrasound (USS)

Sound waves are transmitted and then the waves that reflect back are measured. More dense structures (like the ribs) are absorbed and appear darker, while less dense elements (like air in the lungs) reflect back and display as less dark. Ultrasonography can be used to identify abnormalities and to guide procedures (thoracostomy tube placement, central venous catheter placement)

Terminology

Anechoic (black on screen)	bone (hyperechoic rim), blood vessels, adipose (mostly anechoic)
Hypoechoic (gray on screen)	cartilage, muscles (striated pattern)
Hyperechoic (white on screen)	pleura (slide rhythmically with breathing), including pleural line
Lung sliding	a shimmering/moving of the pleural line synchronous with respirations (this is normal)
Lung pulse	a moving of the pleural line synchronous with cardiac pulsations

Considerations

- Ultrasound waves cannot pass through air so it is important that the transducer is tight against skin with adequate conducting gel
- The general procedure involves locating relevant anatomic landmarks (diaphragm, chest wall, lung, pleural line), then identifying and characterizing abnormalities
- Be aware of patient characteristics that can interfere with accurate findings (edema, musculature, obesity, intercostal muscle use, etc.)
- Colorized ultrasound can show fluid flow as well. Blue is flow away from probe, red is flow towards the probe (BART = Blue Away, Red Towards)

Imaging

Primary Indications/Findings (Pulmonary)*

Evaluation of pleural fluid (pleural effusions)	Aids in evaluating presence, volume, and characteristics. This includes identifying transudative vs. exudative, including empyemas.	
Preferred position is seated upright (fluid moves to dependent positions); if not capable use either supine or semi-supine position	**Anechoic**	favors a transudative process.
	Echogenicity (hypo- or hyperechoic)	favors an exudative process
	Septations* or areas of echogenicity	favors an exudative process
	*Septations are pockets of fluid - the septations (septum) are often visible during an ultrasound but not always with other imaging techniques.	
Evaluation of pleural surfaces *Preferred position matches that of pleural fluid, above*	May help identify pleural thickening present on the visceral and/or parietal surface. Note: can be misinterpreted as a pleural effusion; color doppler may help differentiate (fluid color sign = fluid movement/effusion)	
Evaluation for pneumothorax *Preferred position is in supine or semi-supine position (air is in least dependent position)*	• The presence of lung sliding/lung pulse excludes a pneumothorax diagnosis. The absence of each suggests a pneumothorax is possible but not definite. • Identification of B-lines or lung rockets (indication that lungs are fully expanded in that area) excludes pnuemothorax diagnosis	
Evaluation of lung consolidation	Usually only visible when consolidation extends to pleural surface Appears gray, with poor boundaries	
Diaphragm Strength	Thickness of diaphragm and length of excursion - this use of USS is being explored	

* Heart function and volume status can also be assessed using ultrasonography

4 Labs and Cultures

Critical Lab Levels 4-2
Serum Electrolytes 4-3
Chemistry Panels 4-6
Complete Blood Count/Hematology 4-8
Coagulation 4-10
Other Lab Values 4-11
Microbiology 4-13
  Sputum Collection 4-14
  Sputum Characteristics 4-15
    By Disease 4-16

Understanding Lab Values

1. **Normal ranges often vary.**
   There can be frustration in understanding and referencing "normal" lab values when they vary from resource to resource. Different lab equipment, reagents, and methods used for collection/analysis are primarily why. There can be such variation that some resources don't even provide normal ranges. This chapter references common (wide) ranges, but exact values should be referenced at the healthcare facility being used.

2. **Patients are more important than numbers.**
   As with most clinical numbers (ABGs, Labs, etc.), it is always important to interpret within the context of systematic patient assessment (do the numbers potentially reflect how the patient appears?).

Critical Lab Values

Lab values that are critical, when combined with systematic patient assessment, suggest the need for immediate action. This list is partial, chosen as they are directly relevant to respiratory therapy.

Lab	Lower Than	Greater Than
Bicarbonate mEq/L	< 10	> 40
Bilirubin mg/dL		> 15
Glucose mg/dL	< 40-50	> 400
Hematocrit %	< 22	> 64
Hemoglobin mg/dL	< 8	> 21
$PaCO_2$ mm Hg	< 20	> 60
pH	< 7.20	> 7.60
PaO_2 mm Hg	< 40	> 100*
Potassium mEq/L	< 2.5	> 6.1
Sodium mEq/L	< 120	> 160
White Blood Cell uL	< 2,000	> 40,000

* Neonate (due to concerns related to oxygen toxicity)

Serum Electrolytes

Essential for life-function, serum electrolytes help maintain balance (neutrality) both within cells (intracellular) and outside of cells (extracellular). An electrolyte imbalance will interrupt normal function and may become life-threatening. This section primarily addresses acute imbalance, not chronic.

Test	Range	Clinical Significance	Clinical Increases	Clinical Decreases
Na+ Sodium	**135-147 mEq/L** SI 135-147 mmol/L	Important extracellular cation, responsible for maintaining extracellular fluid volume and regulating cell membrane potential.	**(hypernatremia)** *Thirst, lethargy, weakness, irritability Later (> 158); seizures/ coma, death (> 180)* **Water loss** Dehydration, diabetes, skin (sweat), GI (vomiting, NG/OG drainage, diarrhea), urine **Sodium increase** Excessive intake (including sodium bicarbonate administration, hypertonic saline), Cushings syndrome, salt poisoning	**(hyponatremia)** *Early < 125-130: nausea, malaise Later < 115-120: headache, lethargy, obtunded, seizures/coma, respiratory arrest* **Water gain** Decreased kidney output, CHF, cirrhosis, renal insufficiency **Sodium decrease** Dehydration, trauma, diuretics/diuresis, adrenal insufficiency

Labs

Test	Range	Clinical Significance	Clinical Increases	Clinical Decreases
K+ Potassium	**3.5 - 5.0 mEq/L** SI 3.5 - 5.0 mmol/L	Important intracellular cation, maintains osmolality, affects muscle contraction, plays roles in nerve impulses, enzyme action, cell membrane function.	**(hyperkalemia)** *ECG changes (see chart left/below), ascending muscle weakness-to-paralysis (symptomatic > 6.5-7.0)* **Potassium Increase** Massive blood transfusion, TPN, drugs **Intracellular Shift (out)** Rhabdomyolysis, metabolic acidosis, drugs (incl. succinylcholine) **Impaired Excretion** Kidney disease (GFR < 30 mL/min), volume depletion (dehydration, bleeding, CHF)	**(hypokalemia)** *ECG Changes (flattened T-wave, ST-depression, U-wave appearance), (ascending) muscle weakness-to-paralysis, (symptomatic < 3.0)* **Potassium Loss** Severe/chronic diarrhea, NG suctioning, vomiting **Intracellular Shift (in)** Alkalosis, insulin, beta-adrenergic stimulation* (albuterol, terbutaline, dobutamine, etc.), MI, head injury, hypothermia **Increased Urinary Loss** Diuretics/diuresis (esp. with hypertension), polyuria, high-dose penicillin

K+ Level	ECG Change
5.5 - 6.5	tall, peaked t-waves
6.5 - 7.5	loss of p-waves
7.0 - 8.0	widened QRS complex
8.0 - 10.0	arrhythmias, asystole

The rate of rise in potassium is often a greater factor than the level itself

* This tendency of beta-adrenergics to decrease potassium is sometimes used clinically by administering albuterol in larger doses to lower potassium.

Test	Range	Clinical Significance	Clinical Increases	Clinical Decreases
Cl⁻ Chloride	**95 - 105** mEq/L SI 95-105 mmol/L	Principle extracellular anion, important in acid-base balance	(hyperchloremia) Cardiac decompensation, renal insufficiency	(hypochloremia) COPD, dehydration, DKA, diuretics, fever, metabolic acidosis
PO₄⁴⁻ Phosphate	**1.4 - 2.7** mEq/L SI 0.9-1.5 mmol/L	Major intracellular anion, important for bone health, nerve function, and muscle contraction	(hyperphosphatemia) Acute or chronic kidney disease, vitamin D toxicity	(hypophosphatemia) Alcoholism, severe sepsis, trauma, DKA, acute respiratory alkalosis, chronic diarrhea
Ca⁺⁺ Calcium	**4.5 - 5.8** mEq/L SI 1.2-2.6 mmol/L	Essential anion for bones, teeth, mucoproteins Role in cell membrane, muscle contraction and coagulation	(hypercalcemia) Acidosis, adrenal insufficiency, diuretics (thiazide), immobilization, sarcoidosis, tumors.	(hypocalcemia) Alkalosis, diarrhea, hypoproteinemia, osteomalacia, renal insufficiency, steroid therapy, vitamin D deficiency.
Mg⁺⁺ Magnesium	**1.5 - 2.4** mEq/L SI 0.8-1.2 mmol/L	Intracellular cation, important in ATP function, acetylcholine release at neuromuscular junction	(hypermagnesemia) Antacid ingestion, parathyroidectomy, renal insufficiency	(hypomagnesemia) Chronic alcoholism, diabetic acidosis, diarrhea, nasogastric suctioning, severe renal disease

Chemistry Panels

A Basic Chemistry Panel includes major electrolytes (sodium, potassium, and chloride), total CO_2, glucose, lactose, creatinine, and BUN. A Comprehensive Metabolic Panel also includes magnesium, phosphorus, and calcium. For organizational purposes we have presented all Serum Electrolytes in a separate section.

Test	Normal Range	Clinical Significance	Clinical Increases	Clinical Decreases
Bicarbonate (Total Carbon Dioxide, TCO_2, CO_2 Content)	23 - 30 mEq/L	Total CO_2 is serum bicarbonate + available CO_2 (95% of this is bicarb, so it is used to estimate serum bicarb, not CO_2 levels)	Metabolic Alkalosis or compensation to Respiratory Acidosis	Metabolic Acidosis or compensation to Respiratory Alkalosis
Blood Urea Nitrogen (BUN)	8 - 25 mg/dL SI 2.9-8.9 mmol/L (Indicator of kidney function)	End product of protein metabolism.	Adrenal or renal insufficiency, CHF, dehydration, ↓renal flow, N_2 metabolism, GI bleed, shock, urine obstruction.	Hepatic failure, low protein diet, nephrosis, pregnancy
Lactate	< 2 mmol/L (sample must be processed immediately, increases 0.4 every 30 minutes at room temp)	Indicates either anaerobic metabolism (increased production) or inability to clear (liver impaired)	Shock (esp hemorrhagic, septic), hypoxia (regional or systemic), liver impairment, dehydration, trauma	

Test	Normal Range	Clinical Significance	Clinical Increases	Clinical Decreases
Creatinine	**0.6 - 1.5** mg/dL SI .05–0.13 mmol/L	By-product of muscle metabolism	Nephritis, renal insufficiency, urinary tract obstruction (Indicator of kidney function)	Debilitation
Glucose	**80 - 120** mg/dL (fast) **< 180** (random) SI 3.5-5.5 mmol/L	Provides energy for cellular function **Noncritically Ill:** < 140 (fasting), or < 180 (random) **Critical Illness:** 140 - 180 mg/dL (insulin infusion) **Acute MI:** < 180 mg/dL	Eating/feeding, diabetes, infections, stress, steroids, trauma, uremia, pancreatic dysfunction, endocrine dysfunction	Symptoms usually when glucose < 55 mg/dL Insulin, excessive alcohol, critical illness (liver, kidney, etc.), adrenal gland dysfunction

Complete Blood Count (CBC)

Measures of the circulating red blood cells (erythrocytes), white blood cells (leukocytes), and platelets (thrombocytes).

Test	Normal Range	Clinical Significance	Clinical Increases	Clinical Decreases
Erythrocytes (Red Blood Cells) (RBCs)	**Male 4.6 - 6.2** million/mcL SI 4.6 - 6.2 x 10^{12}/L **Female 4.2 - 5.4** million/mcL SI 4.2 - 5.4 x 10^{12}/L	Oxygen- (and carbon dioxide-) carrying capacity	Primary polycythemia, secondary polycythemia (chronic hypoxia, severe diarrhea, dehydration)	Anemias, leukemia, bleeding, chemotherapy/radiation
Hemoglobin (Hgb)	**Male 13.5 - 16.9** g/dL SI 8.1-11.2 mmol/L **Female 12.5 - 16.0** g/dL SI 7.4-9.9 mmol/L	Grams of hemoglobin in 100 mL of whole blood	**Chronic hypoxias** COPD, CHF, living at a higher elevation, congenital heart disease, obesity hypoventilation, etc. **Hematologic diseases** polycythemia vera Dehydration Concentration of plasma	**Abnormal hemoglobins** methemoglobinemia, sickle cell disease **Decreased production** bone marrow production suppression, iron deficiency Bleeding
Hematocrit (Hct)	**Male 39 - 55%** SI 0.39 - 0.55 **Female 36 - 48%** SI 0.36-0.48	Percentage of blood volume occupied by RBCs		

Labs

4-8

Test	Normal Range	Clinical Significance	Clinical Increases	Clinical Decreases
Reticulocytes	Male 0.5-2.7% of RBCs Female 0.5-4.1% of RBCs	Immature red blood cell–provides information on bone marrow activity	↑ bone marrow activity, blood loss, infection, polycythemia (Rubra vera)	↓ bone marrow activity, leukemia, severe anemia, aplastic anemia
Leukocytes (WBCs)	Total: **5,000 - 10,000** / µL SI 5-10 x 10⁹/L	Blood cells which fight infection	**(leukocytosis)** Infection, surgery, trauma.	**(leukopenia)**
Neutrophils (DIFFERENTIAL)	40-75% (segs = mature) 0 - 6% (bands = immature)		Trauma, bacterial infections (bands may indicate an ongoing infection)	Bone marrow diseases
Lymphocytes	20 - 45%		Viral infections	
Monocytes	2 - 10%		Foreign material reaction	Immunodeficiencies
Eosinophils	0 - 6%		Allergic reactions (incl. asthma)	
Basophils	0-1%		Allergic reactions	
Platelet Count	**150,000 - 400,000** /µL SI 150-400 x 10⁹/L	Blood cells that play a vital role in clot formation	**(thrombocytosis)** Reactive causes (infection, blood loss, anemia, inflammation), autonomous causes (polycythemia vera)	**(thrombocytopenia)** < 50,000 = surgical concern < 20,000 = spont. bleeding Leukemia, viral infections (Hep C, rubella, varicella), HIV, sepsis

Coagulation Studies

Measures of clotting function: likelihood to either bleed (increased value) or clot (decreased value). See also Platelets, which play a vital role in clotting.

Test	Normal Range	Clinical Significance	Clinical Increases	Clinical Decreases
Bleeding Time	1-7 min SI 60-420 sec	Measure of platelet function	Aspirin, DIC, thrombocytopenia, uremia	
Prothrombin Time (PT)	10 - 14 sec	Time to clot (extrinsic coagulation)	Clotting factor defect, liver disease, lupus erythematosus	
Partial Thromboplastin Time (PTT, aPTT)	25 - 35 sec	Time to clot (intrinsic coagulation)	(Prolonged clotting) Liver disease, vitamin K deficiency, heparin (goal is to prolong), warfarin	Disseminated intravascular coagulation (DIC), advanced cancer, tissue inflammation
International Normalized Ratio (INR)	0.8 - 1.2	Calculation based on PT (above) that standardizes values between labs - (used for warfarin)	INR ~5 = likely to bleed Causes are often related to either drugs (warfarin, heparin), or underlying disease	INR < 0.6 = likely to clot
D-Dimer	< 400 ng/mL	fibrin fragments > 400 = PE possible < 400 = PE unlikely	PE, DVT, DIC, recent surgery, trauma, infection, liver disease, pregnancy, eclampsia, heart disease, cancer	anticoagulant therapy (false negative). If negative, likely not a PE

4-10 Labs

Other Clinical Lab Values

Test	Normal Range	Clinical Significance	Clinical Increases	Clinical Decreases
Alpha 1-anttitrypsin	< 200 mg/dL	One indicator of a genetic form of lung disease/COPD	Abscesses, arthritis, early inflammation, pneumonia.	Alpha-1 antitrypsin deficiency**
(Serum) Anion Gap	4 - 12 mEq/L	AG (Anion Gap) = $Na^+ - (Cl^- + HCO_3^-)$*** narrows causes of metabolic acidosis	Lactic acidosis (incl. hypoxia), ketoacidosis, drug ingestion (methanol, ethylene glycol, aspirin, etc.), chronic kidney disease	Monitor a "lack of increase," not a decrease: diarrhea, tube drainage, carbonic anhydrase inhibitors
B-type Natriuretic Peptide (BNP)	< 100 pg/mL	Secreted by heart in response to stretching by cardiac muscles, helpful for determining if dyspnea is heart failure or some other cause.	< 100: negative for heart failure 100-400: inconclusive (check for PE, LV hypertrophy, cor pulmonale) > 400: stronger indication of heart failure	

**May exhibit similar symptoms to COPD, often at an earlier age (30 yrs +) as well as liver impairment.

*** Anion Gap in some places includes K⁺ in the calculation (Na⁺ + K⁺), which raises normal range by 4 mEq/L

Labs

Test	Normal Range	Clinical Significance	Clinical Increases	Clinical Decreases
Troponin	Facilities use 2 different test possibilities: I = < 0.03 ng/mL T = < 0.1 ng/mL Use lab reference values, reported as "elevated" if > 99% of upper reference limit	Both specific and sensitive biomarker indicating myocardial injury.	Troponins are a snapshot and should be repeated to properly evaluate results: • > 1000 ng/L may indicate severe myocardial injury • Acute rise/fall in serial troponins: presence of acute myocardial injury (possibly coronary ischemia) • No notable rise/fall: perform 3rd troponin, consider other causes (renal failure, sepsis, resp. failure, stroke)	

Microbiology

Due to the respiratory nature of this pocket guide, this section directly addresses sputum culturing, but the general concept can be applied to urinalysis, blood analysis, wound cultures, etc.

Test	Sampling	Clinical Significance	Results
Gram Stain (sputum)	Single sputum sample obtained and placed in a sterile container.	Basic test to classify bacteria based upon gram negative vs. gram positive results (until culture and sensitivity)	**Gram + Including:** *Streptococcus, Staphylococcus* **Gram - Including:** *Klebsiella, Pseudomonas aeruginosa, Haemophilus influenzae*
Culture and Sensitivity (sputum)	Single sputum sample obtained and placed in a sterile container.	Identifies specific bacteria (usually with some terminology of how much was found), as well as antibiotic(s) that are effective in treating. If no growth in 24-48 hrs, consider virus, parasite, fungus, TB, Legionella, or *M. pneumoniae*	Identifies bacteria Identifies sensitivity to antibiotics (likelihood of bacteria to be treated by specific antibiotics)
Acid-Fast Smear and Culture	A series of 3 sputum samples (collected 8-24 hrs apart, at least one being early AM)	Determines the presence of acid-fast bacilli (most notably: *Mycobacterium tuberculosis*)	+ or - for presence of acid-fast bacilli. Note: false-positives are common, a + AFB is not absolute.

Sputum Collection	
Indications	To obtain sputum specimen for various laboratory testing
Contra-indications	Dependent on technique, may include: mental status, age (directed cough), excessive oral secretions (will contaminate)
Procedure	**Preparation** • Encourage extra fluids the day before • Schedule for early AM if possible **Collection** • Explain procedure to the patient • Help patient sit upright • Instruct patient to blow nose/rinse out mouth • Instruct to give strong cough and spit specimen into collection cup • Do not touch edge/inside of cup • If clear/watery, probably saliva • If thick/colorful, likely good sample • Typical quantity: routine (2-3 cc), TB and fungus (10-15 cc) • Should go to lab within 1 hour • Ideal specimen is obtained by bypassing oral cavity, directly into specimen container • Intubated: use sputum "trap" in-line with closed system

Sputum Induction	
Indications	If unable to obtain sample in traditional methods, you may need to induce
Contra-indications	(Relative) patients with history of bronchospasm, asthma, etc.
Procedure	• Brief application of 3-7% hypertonic saline (consider ultrasonic or high-output heated jet) • After nebulizing, following the procedure above for collection
Hazards	• May cause bronchospasm (administer SABA prior to hypertonic to help prevent)

Sputum Characteristics

Document amount, consistency, color, odor and anything else noteworthy (presence of mucous plugs, etc.). Also note any changes (better or worse) over time.

Normal Sputum Production

Amount	10-100 cc/day (most goes into esophagus)
Consistency	Thin
Color	Clear
Odor	None

Amount

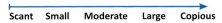

Scant   Small   Moderate   Large   Copious

Consistency
In addition to basic terms thin/thick:

viscous	thick/sticky
frothy	pink/frothy = pulmonary edema, CHF commonly

Color/Characteristic

blood (red/pink)	current bleeding (trauma, malignancy, PE, cancer)
brown/dark red	older blood
fetid	foul-smelling (may indicate anaerobic infection)
mucoid	clear/white, thick (often asthma)
purulent	yellow or green, thick, viscid, may have bad odor (pus cells = infection)
mucopurulent	*mucoid + purulent*
white/gray	asthma - see mucoid above, COPD, cancer, allergies, viral infection

Sputum Characteristics for Select Diseases

Disease	Mucoid (clear, thin, frothy)	Purulent (yellow or green, thick, viscid, strong odor, pus)	Mucopurulent (both mucoid and purulent)	Hemoptysis (bright red, frothy blood)	Currant Jelly (blood clots)	Rusty (mucopurulent with red tinge)	Prune Juice (dark brown, mucopurulent, strong odor)	Blood-Streaked	Pink, frothy (usually thin, bubbly appearance)
Viral Infections	×								
Tuberculosis	×	×	×	×					
Pulmonary embolus				×					
Pulmonary edema	×								×
Pneumonia – Staphylococcal		×							
Pneumonia – Pseudomonas		×	×					×	
Pneumonia – Pneumococcal		×				×	×	×	
Pneumonia – Mycoplasma	×								
Pneumonia – Klebsiella					×		×		
Neoplasm				×	×	×			
Lung cancer	×		×	×					
Lung abscess		×	×						
Emphysema	×		×						
Cystic Fibrosis			×						
Chronic Bronchitis	×		×						
Bronchiectasis		×		×		×			
Asthma	×		×						

5 Pulmonary Dynamics

Ventilation
    Mechanics 5-2
    Pressures 5-3
    Compliance and Resistance 5-5
    Distribution of Ventilation 5-6
    Dead Space Ventilation 5-7

Perfusion
    Shunts 5-9
    Perfusion Zones 5-10

Ventilation/Perfusion 5-11

Mechanics of Ventilation
Inspiration/Exhalation

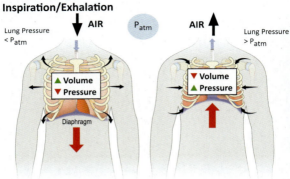

Inspiration	Exhalation
Active	**Passive (muscles relax)**
Boyle's Law: as volume increases, pressure decreases (with temp constant). This pressure decrease relative to the mouth/ambient air results in flow of air to the lungs	**Boyle's Law:** as volume decreases, pressure increases (with temp constant). This pressure increase relative to the mouth/ambient air results in flow of air out of the lungs
1. **Diaphragm/chest muscles contract** Diaphragm flattens down Ribs swing up 2. ▲ Intrathoracic volume 3. ▼ Intrathoracic (pleural) pressure + pleural cohesion 4. ▲ Intrapulmonary (lung) volume 5. ▼ Intrapulmonary (alveolar) pressure 6. Air moves ▼ gradient (in)	1. **Muscles relax + elastic recoil of the lungs** Diaphragm rebounds Ribs swing down 2. ▼ Intrapulmonary volume 3. ▲ Intrapulmonary pressure 4. Air moves ▼ gradient (out)

Volume and Pressure Changes During Spontaneous Breathing

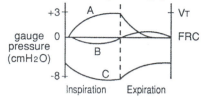

A: Lung Volume B: Alveolar Pressure C: Intrathoracic Pressure

Pressures and Pressure Gradients

For abbreviations and explanations see table on next page

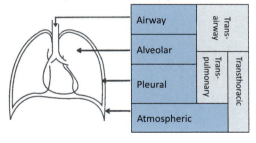

Abbreviation	Definition	Also Known As	Comments
Pressures			
P_{aw}	Airway Pressure	Mouth pressure (P_m)	Normally atmospheric (zero), unless positive airway pressure is applied
P_{alv}	Alveolar Pressure	Intrapulmonary pressure, alveoli pressure (P_A)	Varies during breathing cycle
P_{pl}	Pleural Space Pressure	Intrapleural pressure (P_{IP}) or intrathoracic pressure (P_{IT})	Varies during breathing cycle. Negative during quiet spontaneous breathing
P_{atm} or P_{bs}	Atmospheric Pressure	Atmospheric (barometric) pressure (P_B)	Normally zero unless negative pressure is applied
Pressure Gradients			
P_{ta}	Transairway pressure gradient: Pta = Paw - Palv	Pressure difference down the airway.	Responsible for gas flow into and out of the lungs.
P_{tp}	Transpulmonary pressure gradient: Ptp = Palv - Ppl	Pressure difference across the lung.	Responsible for degree of and maintenance of alveolar inflation or volume change.
P_{tt}	Transthoracic pressure gradient: Ptt = Patm - Palv	Pressure difference across the lung and chest wall.	Total pressure necessary to expand or contract the lungs and chest wall together.

Compliance and Resistance (Overview)

Static Compliance (Cstat)	Total compliance of lung and thorax $C_{LT} = \Delta V / \Delta P$
Dynamic Compliance (Cdyn)	Total impedance Cdyn = Cstat + Raw ($\Delta V/\Delta P$ when **actively** inhaling)
Airway Resistance (Raw)	Impedance to Airflow Raw = ΔP/flow = 0.6 - 2.4 cmH_2O/L/sec @ 0.5 L/sec (norm)
Time Constant (TC)	Filling or Emptying Time of the Lung (Cstat x Raw) - See pg 13-20
Time Constant Examples — Normal Lung Unit	TC = 0.1 L/cmH_2O x 2.0 cmH_2O/L/Sec = (0.1) x (4.0) = 0.4 sec
Time Constant Examples — Asthma	TC = 0.1 L/cmH_2O x 4.0 cmH_2O/L/Sec = (0.1) x (2.0) = 0.2 sec
Time Constant Examples — Fibrosis	TC = 0.05 L/cmH_2O x 2.0 H_2O/L/Sec = (0.05) x (2.0) = 0.1 sec

Compliance

(See page 13-18 for clinical equations)

Change in lung volume per unit change in pressure in the presence of flow (dynamic) or in the absence of flow (static)

- Ease of distention: how easily the lungs open
- Compliance is the inverse (opposite) of elastance
- ▲ Elastance = ▼ Compliance
- ▼ Elastance = ▲ Compliance

SEE FIGURE NEXT PAGE

Resistance/Compliance Diagram

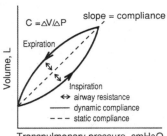

Distribution of Ventilation

Minute Ventilation ($\dot{V}_E$)	**Total air** moved in or out of the lungs in one minute $V_T \times f$ $\dot{V}_A + \dot{V}_D$
Alveolar Ventilation ($\dot{V}_A$)	Ventilation which **participates** in gas exchange $V_A \times f$ $\dot{V}_E - \dot{V}_D$
Dead Space Ventilation ($\dot{V}_D$)	Ventilation which **does not participate** in gas exchange $V_D \times f$ $\dot{V}_E - \dot{V}_A$

Dead Space Ventilation (Types of)

Physiological dead space =	Anatomical dead space +	Alveolar dead space +	Mechanical dead space
$V_{D_{phys}}$	$V_{D_{anat}}$	$V_{D_{alv}}$	$V_{D_{mech}}$
normal = $V_{D_{anat}}$ disease = > $V_{D_{anat}}$	~ 150 mL	abnormal	abnormal
This is the total dead space	Conducting passages Estimated at 1/3 the tidal volume or 1 mL/lb IBW (decrease by 50% if trach)	Alveoli without perfusion	Air in tubing that is rebreathed (rebreathes CO_2)
	Conducting Passages/ Airways	↑ V/Q mismatch (within units, between units) Venous admixture (pulmonary or cardiac cause)	Ventilator Circuit Flex tubing added to tubing/airway While seldom used today, mechanical dead space can be used to manipulate CO_2 levels to balance an ABG 12 in = ▲ CO_2 5 mm Hg

Dead Space Ventilation with Abnormal Perfusion

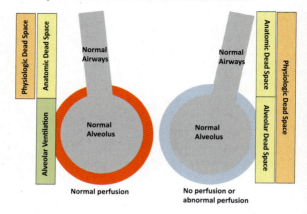

Distribution of Ventilation through Lung Regions

- Air moving into the lungs will go to gravity-dependent areas (Functional Residual Capacity)
- A deeper breath to near TLC will distribute more evenly
- Positive pressure breaths (ventilator) will take a path of least-resistance, usually uppermost areas.
  - With diseases/disorders lung units do not necessarily act as one similar unit with the same compliance/resistance, but are more heterogenous with varying compliance/resistance. Much of a tidal volume will go to the most compliant lung units (often the healthiest ones), risking damage with higher tidal volumes.

Perfusion

Total Perfusion ($\dot{Q}_T$)	Total perfusion of the lung	
	~ CO	$\dot{Q}c + \dot{Q}s$
Capillary Perfusion ($\dot{Q}c$)	Blood which **participates** in gas exchange	
Shunt ($\dot{Q}s$)	Blood which **does not participate** in gas exchange	

Shunts (Types of)

Physiological = Shunt	Anatomical + Shunt	Capillary Shunt
$\dot{Q}s_{phys}$	$\dot{Q}s_{anat}$	$\dot{Q}s_{cap}$
	2-5% Cardiac Output	
Total Shunt	Pleural, Thebesian (cardiac), and bronchial veins; congenital heart defects, atrial valve malformations, vascular lung tumors	Alveolar collapse/atelectasis, pneumothorax, airway obstruction, surfactant deficiency, lesions, secretions, edema, consolidation, diffusion defect

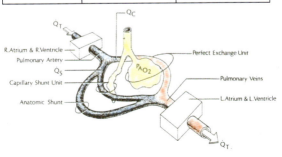

Perfusion Zones

Blood flow in and around the lungs is not equal but is driven by several factors:
- Cardiac output
- Alveolar pressure (volumes, esp. PEEP)
- Gravity

We can conceptualize this into "Zones" (conceptualized by John West, MD) which can then be manipulated therapeutically.

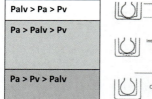
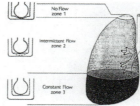

Pavl: alveolar pressure
Pa: arterial pressure
Pv: venous pressure

Body position has a significant effect on the distribution of pulmonary blood flow. The dark shaded areas represent greatest blood flow:

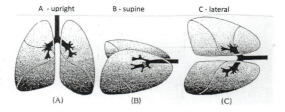

Above figures reprinted with permission from Shapiro, B, et.al.: Clinical Application of Arterial Blood Gases, 3rd Ed., Yearbook Publishers, 1982.

See Strategies, next page

Ventilation/Perfusion ($\dot{V}/\dot{Q}$)

This is a ratio of ventilation to perfusion. Perfectly equal would be 1.0 (for every unit of blood flow, it will receive a unit of gas flow) It is important to remember this is an average: actual $\dot{V}/\dot{Q}$ varies throughout the lungs.

Ventilation	Perfusion
(minute ventilation) = 4 L/min O_2	(perfusion) = 5 L/min blood
Normal = 4/5 or 0.8	

$\dot{V}/\dot{Q}$ Mismatch
There is normally a slight mismatch (explaining why 0.8 is normal, not 1.0), but this can worsen with diseases/disorders

Ventilation exceeds perfusion	Perfusion exceeds ventilation
Ventilation with reduced or no perfusion = dead space	Perfusion with reduced or no ventilation = shunt
V/Q > 0.8	V/Q < 0.8
• Heart failure • Pulmonary embolus • Emphysema • Pulmonary capillary damage	• Aspiration • Foreign body airway obstruction • Severe asthma • Pulmonary edema

Strategies for aligning $\dot{V}/\dot{Q}$

1. **Strategically position the patient**
   Place Bad Lung Up, Good Lung Down (BLU GLD, or Blue Gold) (unless infectious secretions in bad lung, then reverse this)
   Trial prone position to optimize $\dot{V}/\dot{Q}$
2. **Optimize alveolar recruitment** (the ventilation side of $\dot{V}/\dot{Q}$)
   Lung expansion, CPAP, PEEP, etc.
3. **Ensure adequate perfusion**
   Pulmonary vasodilators, minimize O_2 (which causes vasoconstriction), etc.

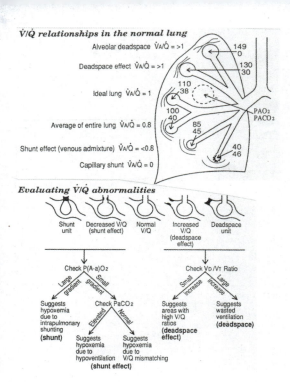

6 Pulmonary Function

Average Pulmonary Function Values 6-2

Tests
- Volumes and Capacities 6-5
- Major Components 6-7
- Spirometry 6-8
- Flow-Volume Loop 6-11
- Other Volumes/Capacities 6-12
- Diffusion Across A-C Membrane 6-13
- Compliance and Resistance 6-14
- Respiratory Parameters 6-15

Interpretation
- Basic PFT Interpretation Algorithm 6-17
- Abnormal PFT Patterns 6-19
- Guidelines for Assignment of Severity 6-20

Pulmonary Function Values

1. **Normal ranges often vary.**
   Most PFT parameters don't have a single normal value. An average (or normal) value can vary based on body surface area, age, height, sex, race, etc. Many organizations recommend the use of "Lower Limits of Normal," abbreviated LLN, instead of absolute numbers (such as < 80%)

Average Pulmonary Function Values

Spirometry outcomes are reported at BTPS (body temperature, ambient barometric pressures, saturated with water vapor)

Lung Volumes and Capacities see diagram on pg 6-5 for Vol/Cap relationships		Average Values
IC	Inspiratory Capacity	3.60 L
IRV	Inspiratory Reserve Volume	3.10 L
ERV	Expiratory Reserve Volume	1.20 L
VC	Vital Capacity	4.80 L
RV	Residual Volume	1.20 L
FRC	Functional Residual Capacity	2.40 L
TLC	Total Lung Capacity	6.00 L
RV/VC	Residual Volume/VC	33 %
RV/TLC	Residual Volume/TLC	20 %
Ventilation		**Average Values**
V_T	Tidal Volume ●	0.50 L
RR	Respiratory Rate ●	12 /min
$\dot{V}_E$	Minute Volume ●	6.00 L/min
V_D	Dead Space Volume	150 mL
$\dot{V}_A$	Alveolar Ventilation	4.20 L/min
V_D/V_T	Dead Space/Tidal Volume Ratio	0.30
Mechanics of Breathing		**Average Values**
FVC	Forced Vital Capacity ●	4.80 L
SVC	Slow Vital Capacity ●	4.80 L
FIVC	Forced Inspiratory Vital Capacity	4.80 L

● Indicates Values that can be Measured with Bedside Spirometry

FEV_T	Forced Exp Volume over Time (FEV_1, etc.) ●	(varies)
FEV 1%	Forced Exp Volume Ratio (1 sec)	83 %
FEV 3%	Forced Exp Volume Ratio (3 secs)	97 %
FEF 200-1200	Forced Expiratory Flow (at volume, often 200-1200) ●	400 L/min
PEF	Peak Expiratory Flow ●	600 L/min
FEF 25%-75%	Forced Midexpiratory Flow ●	4.70 L/sec
FIF 25%-75%	Forced Midinspiratory Flow	5.00 L/sec
$\dot{V}max\ 50$	Forced Expiratory Flow at 50% of FVC	5.00 L/sec
MVV	Maximal Voluntary Ventilation ●	170 L/min
C_L	Static Compliance of Lungs	0.2 L/cm H_2O
C_{LT}	Static Compliance of Lungs and Thoracic Cage	0.1 L/cm H_2O
Raw	Airway Resistance	1.50 cmH_2O/L/sec
MIP or NIF	Maximal Inspiratory Pressure (Negative Inspiratory Force) ●	- 80 mm Hg
MEP	Maximal Expiratory Pressure	120 mm Hg
Gas Distribution		**Average Values**
$\dot{V}_A$	Alveolar Ventilation	4.20 L/min
V_D/V_T	Physiological Dead Space Ratio	< 30
SBN_2	Single-Breath N_2 Test ΔN_2 from 750-1250 mL expired	< 1.5 % N_2
FRC (N_2)	Alveolar N_2 after 7 min of O_2	< 2.5 % N_2

Pulmonary Blood Flow		Average Values
CO	Cardiac Output	5.40 L/min
$\dot{Q}_T$	Total Perfusion of the Lung	5.20 L/min
$\dot{Q}S_{phys}$	Physiological Shunt	< 7%
$\dot{Q}S_{anat}$	Anatomic Shunt	< 3%
QC_{pul}	Pulmonary Cap. Blood Volume	75-100 mL
Alveolar Ventilation		**Average Values**
$\dot{V}_A$	Alveolar Ventilation	4.20 L/min
Gas Exchange		**Average Values**
$\dot{V}CO_2$	Carbon Dioxide Production	200 mL/min
$\dot{V}O_2$	Oxygen Consumption	250 mL/min
RQ	Respiratory Quotient	0.8 (tissue level)
RER	Respiratory Exchange Ratio (CO_2 output/O_2 uptake)	0.8 (end-tidal level)
Alveolar Gas		**Average Values**
PAO_2	Partial Pressure of Alveolar O_2	109 mm Hg
$PACO_2$	Partial Pressure of Alveolar CO_2	40 mm Hg
$P(A-a)O_2$	A-a Oxygen Gradient	33 mm Hg (on F_iO_2 1.0)
Arterial Blood		
CaO_2	Content of Arterial Oxygen	20 Vol %
$C\bar{V}O_2$	Content of Mixed Venous Oxygen	15 Vol %
$C(a-\bar{V})O_2$	Arterial-Venous difference of Oxygen Content	5 Vol %
DLCO	Diffusing Capacity (Single Breath)	25 mL/min/mm Hg

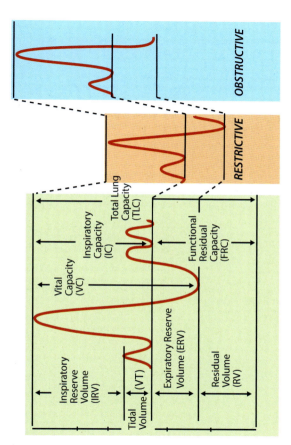

Volumes and Capacities (Overview)
(see 6-2 to 6-4 for values)
(see 6-8 for descriptions of maneuvers)

PFT 6-5

Volumes and Capacities Descriptions

These are generally measured during spirometry, although residual volume, by definition, can not be measured (spirometry is measured by exhalation, RV can not be exhaled). Other techniques are required (see pg. 6-7).

See diagram on pg 6-5 to help visualize these

Test	Description
Tidal Volume	Volume of gas moved in or out of the lungs in a normal resting breath
Inspiratory Reserve Volume	Maximum volume of gas inspired from end-tidal inspiration
Inspiratory Capacity	Maximum volume of gas inspired from resting expiratory level (V$_T$ + IRV)
Expiratory Reserve Volume	Maximum volume of gas expired from resting expiratory level
Vital Capacity	Maximum volume of gas expired after a maximum inspiration (IC + ERV)
Residual Volume (not measured)	Volume of gas in the lungs at the end of a maximum expiration
Total Lung Capacity (not measured)	Volume of gas in lungs at the end of a maximum inspiration
RV/TLC	Residual volume expressed as a percent of total lung capacity
Functional Residual Capacity	Volume in lungs at resting expiratory level (ERV + RV)
Thoracic Gas Volume	Volume of gas in entire thoracic cavity at resting expiratory level whether or not it communicates with the airways

Normal Values
- Normal values may vary within 20% of predicted.
- Values will change with position, age, sex, height, altitude, race/ethnicity.

Major Components of Pulmonary Function Testing

Spirometry *Provides both FVC and FEV, which are critical to PFT interpretation* *See pg 6-8 and beyond*	Measures (Expiratory) Flows and most Volumes (not RV) • Technique-dependent • Critical in assessing air-flow and volumes of lungs (including FVC, FEV_1)
Body Plethysmography Helium Dilution Nitrogen Washout *See pg 6-12*	Measures Residual Volume and derivatives • Particularly important for diseases that result in air-trapping (COPD, etc.)
Diffusing Capacity for Carbon Monoxide *See pg 6-13*	Measures DLCO (diffusion) • Provides further diagnosis of abnormal spirometry • Obstruction: asthma vs COPD • Restriction: ILD vs chest wall
Bronchodilator Responsiveness Testing	Determines the degree of responsiveness of bronchospasm after administration of a SABA (usually albuterol) Increase in the FEV_1 or FVC of > 12% + > 0.2 L indicates responsiveness
Bronchoprovocation Challenge *Used when suspected asthma with normal spirometry*	In some patients with reactive airways, PFTs can appear normal or near-normal unless provoked. Bronchial provocation (often using methacholine) may create bronchospasm which can then be measured.
Oximetry with Exercise or Sleep	Assesses dyspnea on exertion, adequacy of supplemental O_2, screens for sleep disorders (sleep test should be scheduled for further evaluation)

Spirometry

Can be obtained by lab-based spirometer or point-of-care spirometry. FVC and FEV_1 are perhaps the most important values to interpret and report. Note that volumes and capacities can be measured, except those that involve residual volume, including TLC (by definition it can't be exhaled) - see *Other Volumes/Capacities* for those.

PFT Measure	Description	Interpretation
Forced Vital Capacity (FVC)	**Most common spirometry test** Maximum volume of gas exhaled forcefully after a maximum inspiration (this is the total exhaled volume)	See algorithm on 6-17 for interpretation
Forced Expiratory Volume, timed (FEV_t) FEV_1	A volume of gas measured at a specific time interval during an FVC maneuver. The volume exhaled in the first second (FEV_1) is a critical value in interpretation.	*(see table below)*
Forced Expiratory Volume, percent FEV_1/FVC	The percent of gas forced out in 1 second (compared to total FVC) The FEV_1/FVC ratio (or simply, FEV 1%) is a critical value in interpretation	

Time	%	Normal	Obstructive	Restrictive
0.5	60			
1.0	83	>70%	<70%	>70% *usually*
2.0	94			
3.0	97	>95%	<95%	>95%

6-8 PFT

PFT Measure	Description	Interpretation
Forced Expiratory Flow 25-75% (FEF 25-75)	Average forced expiratory flow during the middle half of an FVC (mid-maximal expiratory flow)	Measures average flow through **smaller airways**. Normal = 4.7 L/sec (282 L/min). ↓ in early stages of obstr. disease. Normal in restr. disease.
Forced Expiratory Flow 200-1200 (FEF 200-1200, MEF)	Average FEF of one liter of gas after the first 200 mL is exhaled during an FVC (maximal expiratory flow)	Measures average flow in **larger airways**. Normal = 6-7 L/sec (400 L/min). ↓ = mech. problem or severe obstruction. Effort dependent.
Peak Expiratory Flow (PEF, FEFmax)	Maximum instantaneous flow attained during an FVC maneuver	Indication of ability to cough. Normal = 10 L/sec (600 L/min).
Peak Inspiratory Flow (PIF)	Maximum instantaneous flow attained during a forceful inspiration.	Helpful in distinguishing between obstruction vs. lack of effort (effort dependent). Normal = 5 L/sec (300 L/min). PIF > PEF in obstruction, PIF = PEF in restriction.
Maximum Voluntary Ventilation (MVV, MBC)	Total volume of gas a subject can breathe in and out with maximum effort in one minute (maximum breathing capacity).	Indicates efficiency of total pulmonary system: muscles, compliance, resistance, neurological coordination. Effort dependent. ↓ with moderate obstruction (exaggerates air-trapping) and severe restriction.

PFT Measure	Description	Interpretation
Slow Vital Capacity (SVC)	May be indicated when the FVC is abnormal and airway obstruction is apparent.	In normal lungs FVC = SVC Restrictive = ↓ FVC and SVC Obstructive = SVC is higher, potentially normal
Flow Volume Loop (Curve) (MEF + MIF)	Performed with spirometry, provides a waveform with volume on the horizontal (X) axis and flow on the vertical (Y) axis. 1. Maximal breath in 2. Forced expiration as hard and fast as possible 3. Maximal breath in as fast as possible	The shape of the loop can give valuable information about underlying lung processes See next page for Normal Loop and abnormal variations.

Flow-Volume Loop

(spontaneously-breathing patient - inspiration and exhalation are reversed with mechanical ventilation)

Note that a tidal volume loop (usually several) should show on the diagram. It has been left out to keep the labeled image easy to read.

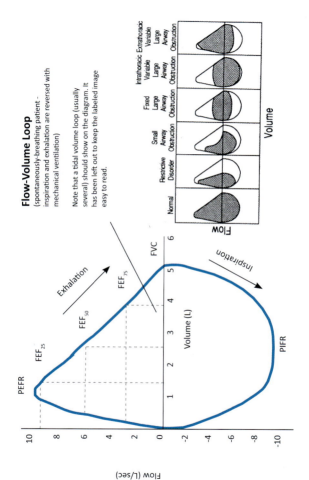

PFT 6-11

Other Volumes/Capacities (measures RV and its derivatives: TLC, FRC)

PFT Measure	Description
Body Plethysmography (Body Box)	- Use of gas law (Boyle's) to measure the gas volume in the lungs. - Any other trapped air may alter results (pneumothorax, air in abdomen, etc.) - Patient performs normal tidal volume breathing, once near FRC the shutter is closed for 2-3 seconds. Patient holds cheeks and pants at a rate of 1/second.

Helium Dilution	- A closed-rebreathing circuit is used. The patient breathes a known concentration of helium-air mixture. Exhaled CO_2 is absorbed, O_2 is added at a rate equal to the patient's consumption.
	- Test is run until equilibrium of helium concentration
	  • Normal patient takes 3-5 minutes
	  • Obstructive disorders can take 20 mins (due to gas-mixing)
	- Note that BTPS-corrected volume has to be subtracted (30 mL/min) to compensate for helium crossing the A/C membrane.

Nitrogen Washout	- The patient breathes 100% oxygen which washes out the 78% nitrogen normally present until exhaled nitrogen is less than 1.5%.
	  • Normal patient takes 2-5 minutes to drop to < 1.5%
	  • Obstructive disorders take an increased amount of time to drop
	- Note that a correction factor (automatically) based on patient weight and time it takes to compensate for plasma/tissue excretion of N.

Diffusion across the Alveolar-Capillary Membrane

PFT Measure	Description	Values*	
Diffusing Capacity of Lung for Carbon Monoxide **DLCO** (mL/min/mm Hg) **TLCO (outside of US)** **(Transfer Factor)** (mmol/min/kPa)	Measure of how well gases diffuse across the alveolar-capillary membrane **Single-Breath DLCO:** Carbon monoxide is used as the test gas, and a tracer gas is added (helium, methane). The patient should fully exhale (to RV), then rapidly inhale to TLC in under 4-seconds, performing a 10-second breath hold. The patient finally exhales fully again (to RV). Note that two other methods: Intra-breath (calculated during exhalation) and rebreathing technique (usually during exercise) are used, though less frequently.	Normal	75-140% of predicted
		Mild	60-75% of predicted
		Moderate	40-60% of predicted
		Severe	< 40% of predicted
		*These are estimated values. Lower Limit of Normal (LLN) should be used. There is greater value in trending DLCO. **Indications for testing include:** • Measure of anatomic emphysema • Differentiation of interstitial lung diseases • Diagnosis of pulmonary vascular disease • Pre-op screening for lung resection • Supplemental O_2 qualification for patients with dyspnea on exertion	

Compliance and Resistance (see also chapter 13 for a more in-depth exploration)

Test	Description	Interpretation
Static Compliance (C_{stat})	Change in lung volume per unit change in pressure with **no flow** (static = no movement) How much will the lungs expand for each unit increase in pressure?	**Normal:** 200 mL/cm H$_2$O = 0.2 L/cm H$_2$O A combination of chest wall and lung tissue compliance Represents elasticity of lungs and thoracic recoil ↓C_{stat} = ↑ elastic recoil (so ↑C_{stat} = ↓ elastic recoil)
Dynamic Compliance (C_{dyn})	Change in lung volume per unit change in pressure **measured in the presence of gas flow** (dynamic = movement)	**Normal:** ~40-70* mL/cm H$_2$O A combination of chest wall and lung tissue compliance, **as well as airway resistance.**
Airway Resistance (R_{aw})	Ratio of alveolar pressure to airflow	**Normal:** 0.6 - 2.4 cm H$_2$O/L/sec Measurement of the flow-resistive properties of the airways. Varies inversely with lung volume

* There is a fair amount of variation in reported normals

Respiratory Parameters

Often performed to determine therapeutic interventions (such as intubation) in neuromuscular disorders (Myasthenia Gravis, Guillain-Barré Syndrome, etc.)

Test	Description	Interpretation
(Forced) Vital Capacity (FVC)	The most powerful number associated with monitoring. A spirometer is not critical to this—a respirometer that measures volume with good coaching will work. 3-5 attempts with 1 minute break in between each	A low FVC indicates potential for respiratory failure (note: values vary by disease/study, but somewhere around < 12-15 mL/kg should be considered respiratory failure)
Maximal Inspiratory Pressure (MIP) **Negative Inspiratory Force (NIF)** **(P_{IMAX})**	There is some debate about the use of this as a predictive value. Measured at RV. Pressure is measured as the patient inhales forcefully through a mouthpiece (or airway) while the therapist occludes the inspiratory valve. Pressure should be maintained for about 1.5 sec, 3-5 attempts with 1 min break in between each	**Normal varies widely-consider using LLN** **Normal:** More negative than -80 cm H_2O **Concern:** More positive than -20 cm H_2O (-19, -18, -17) is considered concerning. ATS: -80 cm H_2O usually excludes clinically important inspiratory muscle weakness. Estimation of ability to take sufficiently deep breaths (inspiratory muscle strength)

Test	Description	Interpretation
Maximal Expiratory Pressure (MEP) (PE_{MAX})	Measured at TLC. Pressure is measured as the patient exhales forcefully through a mouthpiece (or airway) while the therapist occludes the expiratory valve. Pressure should be maintained for about 1 sec, 3-5 attempts with 1 min break in between each.	**Normal varies widely - consider using LLN** **Normal:** ~120 cm H_2O Estimation of ability to exhale forcefully, or clinically, this is an estimation of ability to cough effectively.

Other values used for determining respiratory muscle strength include tidal volume, respiratory rate (tachypnea), arterial blood gases, capnography, and others. No one value is likely to be a determinant-utilize multiple values and systematic assessment. Use of noninvasive or invasive ventilation may become necessary depending on the underlying disease.

Basic Pulmonary Function Interpretation Using Lower Limits of Normal (LLN)

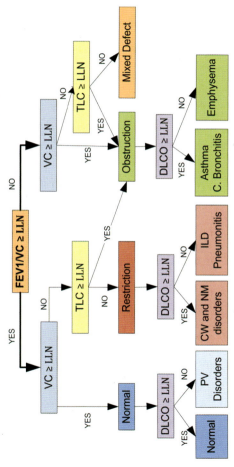

LLN: lower limits of normal; PV: pulmonary vascular; CW: chest wall; NM: neuromuscular; ILD: interstitial lung disease

Adapted with permission ATS/ERS Task Force-Standardization of Lung Volume Testing (2005)

*Note:
In general, Lower Limits of Normal (LLN) is a value determined in part by a patient's sex, age, and height and takes into account population studies from which a reference equation has been developed/based.

The American Thoracic Society has recommended the use of LLN instead of a percentage of predicted (which can be easily influenced by anatomic differences resulting from age/height/sex/race.

Fixed percentages to determine PFT abnormalities can result in false negatives at a young age or false positives at an older age. LLN adjusts for these disparities.

Overview Of Patterns Of Abnormal Pulmonary Functions

	Obstructive				Restrictive
	Asthma	Emphysema	Chronic Bronchitis	Small Airway Disease	
Lung Volumes					
SVC	N▼	N▼	N▼	N	▼
RV	▲	▲	▲	N▲	N▼
FRC	▲	▲	▲	N	N▼
TLC	N▲	▲	N▲	N	▼
RV/TLC	▲	▲	▲	N▲	N▲
Mechanics					
FVC	▼	▼	N▼	N	▼
FEV_1	▼	▼	▼	N	N
$FEF_{200-1200}$	N▼	N▼	▼	N	N▼
FEF_{25-75}	▼	▼	▼	▼	N▼
PEF	▼	▼	▼	N	N▼
MVV	▼	▼	▼	N	N▼
Cstat	N	▲	N	N	▼
Cdyn	▼	▼	▼	N▼	▼
Raw	▲	N▼	▲	N	N
CV	▲	▲	▲	N▲	N▲
V/Q Relationships					
A-a Gradient	▲	▲	▲	▲	N▲
$\dot{Q}_S/\dot{Q}_T$	▲	▲	▲	▲	N▲
V_D/V_T	▲	▲	▲	N▲	▲
D_LCO	N	▼	N	N	N▼

N = Normal, ▲ = Increased, ▼ = Decreased

General Guidelines for Assignment of Severity of Lung Volume Disorders

This is one general approach to severity of lung volume disorders (restrictive disorders vs. obstructive disorders), but there are other approaches as well.

Volume (Normal)	Disorder	Severity (%)		
		Mild	Moderate	Severe
TLC (80-120% Pred)	Restrictive	70-80	60-70	< 60
	Obstructive	120-130	130-150	> 150
VC (> 90% Pred)	Restrictive	70-90	50-70	< 50
	Obstructive	70-90	50-70	< 50
FRC (65-135% Pred)	Restrictive	55-65	45-55	< 45
	Obstructive	135-150	150-200	> 200
RV (65-135% Pred)	Restrictive	55-65	45-55	< 45
	Obstructive	135-150	150-250	> 250

Adapted originally from Madama, V. Pulmonary Function Testing and Cardiopulmonary Stress Testing. 1993, Delmar Publishers.

Obstructive Disorders
Majority of volumes are increased (esp. with air-trapping), while flows (and vital capacity) are decreased.

Restrictive Disorders
Most values are decreased proportionally (esp. TLC, VC), while flows are normal.

7 Hemodynamics

Hemodynamic Parameters	7-2
Oxygen Delivery	7-4
Blood Flow Through the Heart	7-5
Catheters/Lines Overview	7-6
Disease Entities (Pressure)	7-7
Right vs Left Heart Failure	7-8
Hemodynamic Presentation (Diseases)	7-9

HEMO

Hemodynamic Values

1. This chapter is intended to provide a very basic overview. See Oakes' Hemodynamic Monitoring Pocket Guide for detailed content.
2. As with so many other areas, values vary greatly between one resource and another. We have presented wide ranges to account for these various sources.
3. Check with your facility to determine acceptable normal ranges.

Hemodynamic Parameters

Measured Value		Abbreviation	Normal Value
Measured Values			
Heart Rate		HR	60-100 beats/min
Arterial Blood Pressure	BP to remember		120/80 mm Hg
	Systolic	BPsys	90-140 mm Hg
	Diastolic	BPdia	60-90 mm Hg
	Mean*	$\overline{BP}$ or $\overline{MAP}$	65-105 mm Hg
	Pulse Pressure	PP	20-80 mm Hg
Central Venous Pressure		CVP	0-8 mm Hg
Pulmonary Artery Pressures (PAP)	PAP to remember:		25/10 mm Hg
	Systolic	PASP	15-35 mm Hg
	Diastolic	PADP	5-15 mm Hg
	Mean	PAMP or $\overline{PAP}$	10-20 mm Hg
	End Diastolic	PAEDP	0-12 mm Hg
	Wedge	PAOP or PCWP	6-15 mm Hg
Right Atrial Pressure		RAP or $\overline{RAP}$	0-8 mm Hg
Right Ventricular End Diastolic Pressure		RVEDP	0-8 mm Hg
Right Ventricular End Systolic Pressure		RVESP	15-25 mm Hg

*Sometimes MAP (no line over top) is used to refer to mean arterial pressure. This is also very commonly used to refer to mean airway pressure with mechanical ventilation.

Measured Value	Abbreviation	Normal Value
Derived Values		
Body Surface Area	BSA	See pg 13-26
Cardiac Output	CO	4-8 L/min
Cardiac Index*	CI	2.5 - 4.0 L/min/m²
Left Atrial Pressure	LAP	4-12 mm Hg
Left Ventricular End Diastolic Pressure	LVEDP	4-12 mm Hg
Left Ventricular End Systolic Pressure	LVESP	100-140 mm Hg
Left Ventricular Stroke Work	LVSW	60-80 gm/m/beat
Left Ventricular Stroke Work Index*	LVSWI	40-60 gm/m/beat/m²
Pulmonary Vascular Resistance	PVR	< 250 dynes•sec•cm⁻⁵
Pulmonary Vascular Resistance Index*	PVRI	255-285 dynes•sec•cm⁻⁵
Right Ventricular Stroke Work	RVSW	10-15 gm/m/beat
Right Ventricular Stroke Work Index*	RVSWI	7-12 gm/m/beat/m²
Stroke Volume	SV	60-100 mL
Stroke Volume Index*	SVI	35-65 mL/beat/m²
Systemic Vascular Resistance	SVR	800-1600 dynes•sec•cm⁻⁵
Systemic Vascular Resistance Index*	SVRI	1400-2600 dynes•sec•cm⁻⁵

*The index values (PVRI, for example) typically take the absolute value (PVR, for example) and relates it to the patient's body surface area (BSA) to account for the effect of body size on blood flow

Oxygen Delivery

Parameters measured are below each item. See Pg 7-2 to 7-3 for explanations of abbreviations

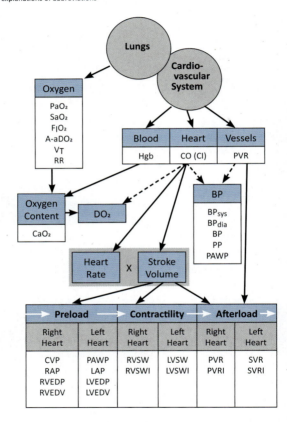

Blood Flow through the Heart

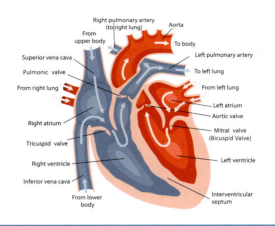

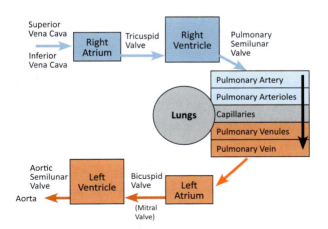

Hemodynamics 7-5

Catheters

Catheters	Placement	Key Values	Sample Type and Clinical Value	
Arterial Line Catheter (A-Line, ABP)	**Arteries:** Radial, Dorsalis Pedis, Femoral	BP, MAP	**Arterial Sample** <ul><li>Direct/continuous blood pressure measurements</li><li>Facilitates ABG draws</li><li>Transducer should be horizontal/at level of the right atrium</li><li>ABP systolic is slightly higher than noninvasive BP</li><li>ABP diastolic is slightly lower than noninvasive BP</li><li>MAP < 60 indicates a lack of perfusion to vital organs</li></ul>	
Central Line Catheter (CVP)	**Veins:** Subclavian, Jugular, Femoral, Antecubital	CVP	**Venous Sample** <ul><li>Catheter tip: superior vena cava, outside right atrium</li><li>Direct measurement of the pressure in the right atrium</li><li>Assesses right heart function and volume status</li><li>Provides central IV access for drug admin/blood samples</li></ul>	
Pulmonary Artery (PA) Catheter (Swan Ganz)	**Veins:** Subclavian, Jugular, Femoral, Antecubital (advanced further)	CVP, RAP, RVEDP, LVEDP, CO, CI, PAP, PCWP (PAOP), PVR, CvO₂, SvO₂	**Proximal = Venous**	**Distal = Mixed Venous** <ul><li>Catheter tip: pulmonary artery</li><li>Directly measures right-sided heart pressures, PA pressures</li><li>Indirectly measures left-sided heart pressures, cardiac output, when in wedge position</li><li>Indexed values take BSA into account</li><li>A cardiac ultrasound may approximate PA pressures</li></ul>

Select Causes of Abnormal Hemodynamic Values

	BP	CVP	PAP*	PCWP (PAOP)
Increased	Aortic Insufficiency Arteriosclerosis Drugs (inotropes, vasopressors) Essential Hypertension	↑Preload: Hypervolemia ↑Afterload: COPD, Cor Pulmonale Hypoxemia Ventilator (w/ PEEP) PVR ↑ (emboli, HTN) Cardiac Tamponade Cardiomyopathy Left Ventricular Failure (CHF, MI) Right Ventricular Failure Shock Myocardial Infarction	Cardiac Tamponade Hypervolemia L-R shunt (ASD, VSD) LVF (CHF, MI, shock) Mitral/Aortic Valve dis. ↑ PVR: Acidosis Thromboembolism Pulm. Hypertension, Hypoxemia Vasopressors * If > 50 (mean), acute cause is less likely	Cardiac Tamponade Hypervolemia R-L shunt LVF (CHF, MI, shock) Mitral/Aortic Valve dis. Pneumothorax Ventilator (w/ PEEP)
Decreased	Aortic/Mitral Stenosis Arrhythmias Cardiac Tamponade LVF (CHF, MI, shock) Shock	Hypovolemia: Absolute (loss) Relative (shock, drugs)	Hypovolemia: Absolute (loss) Relative (shock, drugs)	Hypovolemia: Absolute (loss) Relative (shock, drugs) Pulmonary Embolism

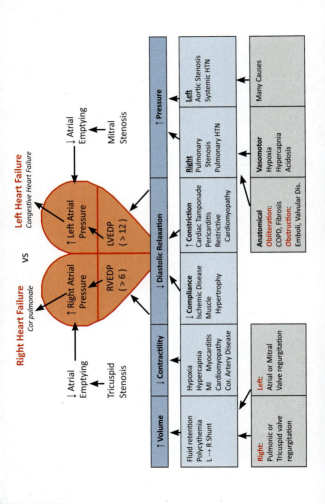

7-8 Hemodynamics

Overview of Hemodynamic Presentation in Various Disease Entities

Disease/Disorder	RR	HR	BP	PP	CO	CVP	PAP	PAWP	SVR	PVR	SvO₂
ARDS	↑	↑	↑↓	↑↓	N	N	↑	N	N	↑	↓
Heart Failure: Left-Sided	↑	↑	↑↓	↓	↓	N↑	↑	↑	↑	↑	↓
Heart Failure: Right-Sided	↑	↑	↑↓	↓	↓	↑	N	N	↑	N	↓
Cardiac Tamponade	↑	↑	N↓	↓	N↓	↑	↑	↑	↑	N↑	N↓
Cardiomyopathy	↑	↑	N↓	↓	N↓	N↑	↑	N↑	↑	N↑	N↓
COPD	↑	↑	N	N	N↓	N↑	↑	N	N↑	↑	↓
Myocardial Infarction	N↑	↑	↑↓	↓	N↓	N↑	N↑	N↑	N↑	N↑	N↓
Pulmonary Edema	↑	↑	N	N	N	N	↑	↑	↑	↑	↓
Pulmonary Embolism	↑	↑	N	N	N	N	↑	N	N	↑	N↓

Disease/Disorder	RR	HR	BP	PP	CO	CVP	PAP	PAWP	SVR	PVR	S$\bar{\text{v}}$O$_2$
Shock:											
Anaphylactic	↑	↑	↓	↓	↓	↑	↑	↑	↓	N	↓
Cardiogenic	↑	↑	↓	↓	↓	N	↑	↑	↑	N	↓
Hypovolemic (compensated)	↑	↑	N↓	N↓	↓	↓	↓	↓	↑	N	↓
Decompensated	↑	↑	↓	↓	↓	↓	↓	↓	↑	N	↓
Neurogenic	↑↓	↓	N↓	↓	N↓	↓	↓	↓	↓	N	↓↑
Septic (Warm)	↑	↑	↓	↑	N↑	↓	↓	↓	↓	N	↑
Septic (Cold)	↑	↑	↓	↓	↓	↑	↑	↑	↑↓	N	↓↑
Valvular:											
Aortic Stenosis	↓	↓	↓	↓	↓	N↓	↑	↑	↑	↓	↓
Aortic Regurgitation	↓	↓	↑	↑	↑	↓	↑	↓	N↓	↓	↓
Mitral Stenosis	N↓	N↓	N↓	↓	N↓	N↓	↑	↑	N↓	N↓	N↓
Mitral Regurgitation	↓	N↓	N↓	↑	↓	↑	↑	↑	N↓	N↓	↓

Oakes' Hemodynamic Monitoring Pocket Guide covers diseases/disorders in much greater detail (an entire chapter) - this is meant to be a summary resource.

8 Cardiac Monitoring

Standard ECG Leads 8-2
   12-Lead 8-3
   15-Lead 8-3
ECG (Labeled) 8-4
Interpretation
   Basic Steps to Interpret 8-6
   ECG Paper 8-7
   Measuring Ventricular Rate 8-7
      By Rate 8-8
      By P Wave 8-8
      By PR Interval 8-8
   Summary of Basic Arrhythmias 8-9
   Interpreting ECG Abnormalities 8-14
   Cardiac Ischemia 8-15

Standard ECG Leads

Limb		Chest (Precordial)	
Positive Electrode			
I	Left arm	V1	R of sternum in 4th ICS
II	Left leg	V2	L of sternum in 4th ICS
III	Left leg	V3	Midway between V2 and V4
aVR	Right arm	V4	Midclavicular line in 5th ICS
aVL	Left arm	V5	Anterior axillary, same level as V4
aVF	Left leg	V6	Midaxillary line, same level as V4

Negative Electrode	
I	Right arm
II	Right arm
III	Left arm

TROUBLESHOOTING

Problem in:	Check Leads:
V1-V6	Chest lead that corresponds to tracing
Lead I	LA, RA
Lead II	LL, RA
Lead III	LL, LA
aVR	RA, LA, LL
aVL	LA, RA, LL
aVF	LL, RA, LA

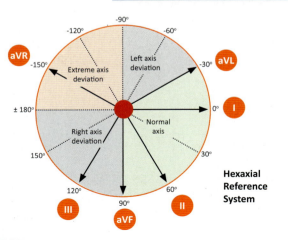

Hexaxial Reference System

12-Lead ECG Placement

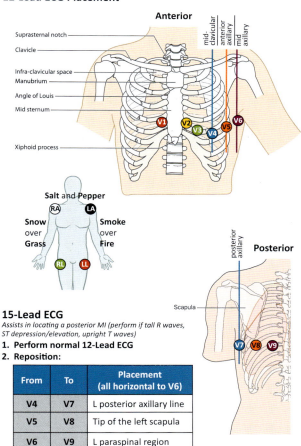

15-Lead ECG
Assists in locating a posterior MI (perform if tall R waves, ST depression/elevation, upright T waves)

1. **Perform normal 12-Lead ECG**
2. **Reposition:**

From	To	Placement (all horizontal to V6)
V4	V7	L posterior axillary line
V5	V8	Tip of the left scapula
V6	V9	L paraspinal region

3. **Clearly mark on ECG that leads have been repositioned**

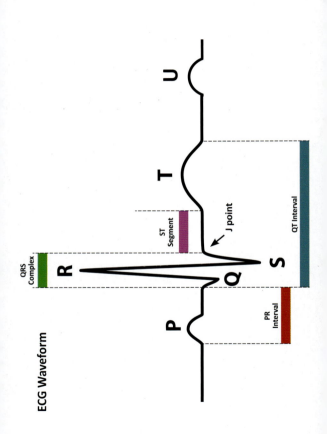

	P wave	PR Interval	QRS complex	ST segment	T wave	QT interval	U wave
Major Events	atrial depolarization		ventricular depolarization (+ atrial repolarization, hidden)		ventricular repolarization		
Description	Positive in most leads, notched in limb leads, biphasic in V1	Beginning of P wave to 1st part of QRS (atrial depolarization through AV node + His-Purkinje)	1st negative deflection = Q (if present) positive deflection = R	ECG silence	Slow upstroke, rapid downstroke, irregularity = probable P wave superimposed	QRS complex, ST segment + T wave (primarily a measure of ventricular repolarization)	seen in some leads (V2-V4), actual cause unknown
Duration	< 0.12 sec (3 small boxes)	0.12 - 0.20 sec (3-5 small boxes)	0.06 - 0.10 sec (1.5-2.5 small boxes)	--	--	0.40 sec or less	--
Amplitude	< 0.25 mV (2.5 small boxes)	Variable	Variable	Flat or no more than 1 mm above or below baseline. > 1-2 is consistent with a STEMI	at least 0.2 mV (leads V3, V4) at least 0.1 mV (leads V5, V6)	--	1/3 T wave (same lead)

Cardiac

Basic Interpretation of an ECG (Adult)

1. Verify	• Patient name, MRN, DOB, etc. • ECG speed/calibration (see next page)
2. Regular	Is there ventricular regularity? • Verify R-R distance (mm) is consistent (should not vary by more than 0.12 sec)
3. Rate 60-100/min	• **Ventricular Rate**: Count the number of R waves over 6 seconds (30 large squares) and multiply by 10. **R Waves for 6 sec x 10** See also Rule of 300, bottom next page • **Atrial Rate:** Count the number of P waves (see next page) over 6-seconds and multiply by 10. **P waves for 6 sec x 10** *If the rhythm is regular these numbers should be the same.*
4. P wave Dur: < 0.12 Amp: < 0.25	What is the shape and rhythm (position) of the P wave? Calculate amplitude and duration.

5. PR Interval
 	
Dur: 0.12-0.20
	What is the PR Interval?
	  Short = Wolff-Parkinson-White Syndrome?
	  Long = 1st degree AV Block?

6. QRS complex
 	
Dur: 0.06-0.10
	What is the shape and interval of the QRS?
	  Wide = bundle branch block?
	  Increased voltage = ventricular hypertrophy?
	  Q waves = infarction?

7. ST segment
 	
< 1 mm above/
below baseline
	What is the position of the ST segment?
	  Depression or Elevation =
	    myocardial infarction or ischemia?

7. Final	Complete Final Interpretation

ECG Standard Paper Speed = 25 mm/sec*
This ECG paper diagram has been enlarged to make it easier to understand.

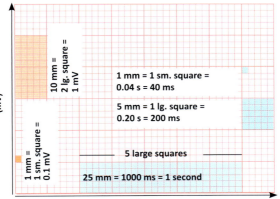

* **Paper Speed can be changed. For example, 50 mm/sec:**
  Doubling the rate may help reveal more subtle ECG findings (waveforms)
  1 mm = 1 sm. square = 0.02 s = 20 ms
  5 mm = 1 lg. square = 0.1 sec = 100 ms

Measuring Ventricular Rate

1. **Irregular rhythms (or slow)**: Count # R waves (in 6 seconds; i.e., two 3 sec intervals or 2 boxes) X 10 = rate/min

2. **Regular Rhythms**: "Rule of 300": Count # of large boxes between R waves (start with 1 on a red line). Divide 300 by the # of boxes.

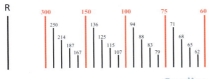

Cardiac 8-7

Interpreting ECGs: According to Rate

Normal	Slow	Fast
Sinus rhythm	Sinus bradycardia	Sinus tachycardia
Sinus arrhythmia	(< 60/min)	(>100/min)
SA block	AV nodal rhythm	PAT (150-250)
Wandering	(40-60/min)	Atrial flutter
pacemaker	2nd ° AV block	(250-350)
PAC	(1/2 to 1/3 atrial rate)	Atrial fib (350-450)
PNC	3rd ° AV block	AV nodal tach
1st ° AV block	(< 40/min)	(150-250)
PVC	V-fib / V standstill (0/min)	V-tach (150-250)

According to P Wave

	Absent	Buried	Abnormal	Inverted
Wandering pacemaker		X	X	
PAC			X	X
PAT		X	X	
Atrial flutter			X	
A-fib	X		X	
PNC		X		X
AV nodal tachycardia		X		X
AV nodal rhythm		X		X
PVC	X			
Vent. tachycardia	X			

According to Prolonged PR Intervals

P with every QRS	1st ° Heart Block
Progressive PR prolongation	2nd ° Heart Block (Type I)
Constant PR with dropped beats	2nd ° Heart Block (Type II)
No relationship between P and QRS	3rd ° Heart Block

Cardiac

Summary of Basic Arrhythmias (according to site of origin)

Type	Identifying Features	Appearance (Lead II)	Causes/Notes
SA Node (default pacemaker)			
Normal Sinus Rhythm	Rate: 60-100/min, P waves regular, P-R Interval (0.12-0.20), QRS regular (< 0.12), R-R regular, T wave upright and round, ST segment is flat		Normal rhythm (see pg 8-4 for a labeled diagram)
Sinus Arrhythmia	Variation in P-P interval by 0.12 sec or more (normal P waves, P-R intervals)		Many causes, including heart failure, CHD, K+, drugs (digoxin, morphine), diabetes. Usually asymptomatic: no treatment
Sinus Tachycardia	Regular Rhythm Rate > 100/min		Fever, hypoxemia, ↓BP, hypovolemia, pain, sepsis, heart failure, bronchodilators. May lead to ischemia.
Sinus Bradycardia	Regular rhythm Rate < 60/min		Carotid massage, hypothermia, Valsalva, tracheal suction. May lead to ↓BP/CO, syncope, CHF, shock. Some athletes have a resting HR < 60

Type	Identifying Features	Appearance (Lead II)	Causes/Notes
Sinoatrial Exit Block	Entire beat absent		Vagal stimulation, inferior MI, myocarditis, drugs (digoxin, beta-blockers, calcium channel blockers, amiodarone)
Wandering Atrial Pacemaker	Rate varies, **P waves vary in shape and position**, P-R interval varies, Rate is < 100/min		Not considered abnormal, many athletes exhibit, may be found with COPD and digitalis toxicity. Asymptomatic: no treatment indicated
Atrial			
Premature Atrial Contractions (PAC)	Premature P waves **(abnormal or inverted)**, short T-P interval before beat, long T-P after beat, may occur in repeating patterns		Not considered abnormal for most, anxiety, beta-agonists, hypokalemia, hypomagnesemia, digoxin toxicity, MI. If frequent may cause palpitations
Premature Atrial Tachycardia (PAT, PSVT)	Rate 150-250/min, P waves abnormal or buried. Called supraventricular tach (SVT) and may be paroxysmal.		Sudden onset and termination. Patients may experience light-headedness or palpitations. May lead to ↓BP/CO, myocardial ischemia, CHF.

Cardiac

Type	Identifying Features	Appearance (Lead II)	Causes/Notes
Atrial Flutter	Atrial rate 250-350/min, ventricular rate normal, sawtooth P waves, 2:1, 3:1, 4:1 block of QRS		Commonly associated with pulmonary disease. May return to normal or deteriorate to A-fib. ↑ risk for embolism
Atrial Fibrillation (A-fib)	No clear P waves, atrial rate 350-450/min, irregular ventricular rhythm		Often asymptomatic, except ↓ cardiac reserve. ↑ risk for embolism.
Nodal			
Premature Nodal Contractions	P wave absent or inverted after the QRS		PJC (or PNC) = Premature junctional complex. May confuse with PAC
Paroxysmal Junctional (A-V nodal) Tachycardia	Rate 150-250/min, P wave variable		
A-V Nodal (Junctional) Rhythm	Rate 40-60/min, P waves absent or inverted		Also called junctional escape or idiojunctional rhythm

Cardiac

Type	Identifying Features	Appearance (Lead II)	Causes/Notes
1st° A-V Heart Block	Constant, prolonged P-R interval (> 0.2 sec)		Often asymptomatic. May be misread as a normal sinus rhythm
2nd° A-V Heart Block (Type I, Wenckebach)	Progressively longer P-R interval until a beat is dropped		Often asymptomatic
2nd° A-V Heart Block (Type II)	Some non-conducted P waves (no QRS), constant P-R intervals, slow ventricular rate		May lead to ↓ BP/CO, weakness, and fainting. Also called Mobitz II
3rd° A-V Heart Block (Complete)	No relationship between P waves and QRS, atrial rate normal		Atria and ventricles beat independently (A-V dissociation). Rate 40 – 60/min = Junctional rhythm Rate < 40/min = Ventricular rhythm
Bundle Branch Block (R or L)	QRS widened (>/= 0.12) with rabbit-ear feature		Appearance highly variable Cause: underlying heart disease
Ventricular			
Premature Ventricular Contractions (PVC)	Premature, wide (> 0.12), distorted QRS with no P wave, T wave opposite, full compensatory pause		> 6/min is pathological. Most common cause is myocardial ischemia. May be caused by anxiety, ↓K+, excessive caffeine, or medications. The appearance of R-on-T may lead to V-tach.

Cardiac

Type	Identifying Features	Appearance (Lead II)	Causes/Notes
Ventricular Tachycardia (V-Tach*)	Series of PVCs (> 3 in row), rate 150-250/min		May quickly lead to ↓BP/CO, V-fib, loss of consciousness, and death.
Ventricular Flutter	Series of smooth sine waves, rate 250-350/min		May quickly lead to ↓BP/CO, V-fib, loss of consciousness, and death
Torsades de Pointes	a form of VTach where QRS complex varies beat-to-beat, ventricular rate 150-250.		May return to NSR or become more serious. Treat with ACLS algorithm for V-Tach. May change from + to - axis.
Ventricular Fibrillation (V-fib)	No well-defined, erratic QRS, rate 350-450/min		Rhythm may be mistaken for either V-Tach or asystole. Immediate ↓CO →coma. Treat with defibrillation.
Ventricular Standstill (Asystole)	Cardiac standstill (known as a flat-line though often not completely flat)		Caution: a simple disconnect of ECG lead can resemble asystole. Check for immediate pulselessness, ↓ BP, and loss of consciousness.
Pulseless Electrical Activity (PEA)	Any heart rhythm (except VF or VT) that should be producing a palpable pulse but is not.	Appearance Varies, Treat underlying cause: Most Common: resp. failure due to hypoxia	

Interpreting ECG Abnormalities

Pulmonary	
COPD	Low voltage in all leads Right axis deviation Multifocal atrial tachycardia
Pulmonary Embolism	Wide S in V1 Large Q in VIII Inverted T in III and V1-V4

Cardiac Enlargement (Hypertrophy)	
Right Atrial	II: P wave > 2.5 mm amplitude V1: QRS voltage < 5 mm
Left Atrial	II: P wave is 0.12 or greater duration V1: Notched P wave
Right Ventricular	Slight ↑ in QRS duration R wave progressively smaller Right axis deviation
Left Ventricular	Wide QRS with ↑ amplitude (tall R) T wave slants down slowly, then returns rapidly (inverted) in V5 or V6 Left axis deviation

Electrolytes	
Hyperkalemia	P waves: widened, low amplitude QRS: widened, loss of ST segment T waves: peaked/tall
Hypokalemia	ST: depressed T waves: flattened U wave: may be visible
Hypercalcemia	P waves: disappeared (if severe) T waves: peaked/tall QRS: very wide (if severe)
Hypocalcemia	PR: reduced QRS: narrowed T waves: flattened/inverted U wave: prominent

Cardiac Ischemia, Injury or Infarction

Acute

Ischemia = Inverted T Wave

Inverted T wave is symmetrical
(V2-V6)
Signifies an acute process and usually
  lasts only a few hours

Injury = ST segment elevation

Signifies an acute process and usually
lasts only a few hours. If T wave is
also elevated off baseline, suspect
pericarditis. Location of injury may
be determined like infarct location.
ST depression = digitalis, subendocar-
  dial infarct or exercise stress test.

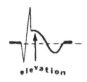

elevation

Acute or Chronic

Infarction = Q Wave

Insignificant (small) Q waves may be
normal (esp. V5 and V6).
Significant (abnormal) Q waves must
be > one small square (0.04 sec) wide
or > 1/3 QRS height in lead III.

Q

Location of Infarct (or injury)

Anterior	Q wave in V1,V2,V3 or V4 (ST elevation)
Inferior	Q in II, III, and aVF
Lateral	Q in I and aVL
Posterior	Large R in V1 and V2 (ST depression) Mirror test

Respiratory Therapies

Aerosol Therapy
- Types of 9-4
- Bland Aerosol Administration 9-5
- Aerosol Delivery Devices 9-6
- Selection and Overview 9-8
- Recommended Particle Sizes 9-9
- Nebulizers 9-10
  - Small Volume Jet 9-10
  - Mesh or Ultrasonic 9-10
  - Continuous Bronchodilator Therapy 9-11
- Metered-Dose Inhalers 9-12
- Dry Powder Inhalers 9-13

Airway Management
- Bag-Valve-Mask (BVM) Ventilation 9-14
- Airway Adjuncts 9-15
- Endotracheal Tubes 9-16
- Mallampati Scoring 9-16
- Intubation 9-17
  - Confirmation Checklist 9-18
  - End-tidal CO_2 9-19
- Tracheostomy Tubes 9-20
  - Indications, Care, Monitoring 9-21
  - Speaking Valves 9-21
  - Troubleshooting 9-22
  - Replacing 9-24
  - Stoma Care 9-26
  - Capping and Decannulation 9-26

Airway Clearance
- Overview 9-27
- Selecting 9-28

Suctioning	9-29
Pressures	9-30
Sizing	9-31
Procedure	9-31
Nasotracheal Suctioning (AARC)	9-32
Directed or Therapeutic Coughing	9-33
Active Cycle of Breathing	9-34
Autogenic Drainage	9-35
Diaphragmatic Exercises	9-36
Diaphragmatic Strengthening	9-37
Pursed-Lip Breathing	9-37
Chest Physiotherapy	9-38
Postural Drainage	9-38
Percussion and Vibration	9-39
Modified CFF Positions	9-41
Traditional Postural Drainage Positions	9-44
Effects and Considerations	9-45
AARC: Nonpharmacologic AW Clearance	9-46
AARC: Pharmacologic AW Clearance	9-47
Assistive Mechanical Devices	9-48
Positive Expiratory Pressure (PEP)	9-49
High-Frequency Oscillations	9-50
Acapella	9-51
Flutter Valve	9-51
Intrapulmonary Percussive Ventilation	9-52
Percussive Vests/Wraps	9-53
Selection Algorithm	9-54
ACCP Summary Recommendations	9-55

Humidity Therapy

Overview	9-56
Devices	9-57
AARC Expert Guidelines	9-58

Lung Expansion Therapy

Overview and Selection	9-59
Incentive Spirometry	9-60
AARC Expert Guidelines	9-61
Intermittent Positive Pressure Breathing	9-63
AARC Expert Guidelines	9-64

Medical Gases

Cylinders
- Cylinder Color Standards 9-66
- Cylinder Duration Charts 9-67

Oxygen/Oxygenation
- Monitoring Oxygenation Status 9-68
  - Troubleshooting the Pulse Oximeter 9-69
  - Transcutaneous Monitoring 9-71
  - Lung Adequacy 9-72
  - Oxyhemoglobin Dissociation Curve 9-73
  - Oxygen and Carbon Dioxide Cascade 9-74
- Assessment of Oxygenation 9-75
  - Hypoxemia 9-76
  - Versus Hypoxia 9-76
  - Signs and Symptoms 9-77
  - Types and Causes 9-78
  - Diagnostic Algorithm 9-80
- Oxygen Therapy 9-81
  - AARC Expert Guidelines 9-82
  - Oxygen Delivery Devices 9-83

Gases Measured/Used 9-89
- Heliox 9-90

Aerosol Therapy

Types of Aerosol Therapy	**Bland Aerosol Delivery** *(see AARC CPG, Next Page)* Delivering a non-medicated liquid to a patient with therapeutic goals. May include: • Isotonic (0.9%) solution: generally used to humidify inspired air (see also humidification, may include heat) or as a way of decreasing upper airway edema (without heat) • Hypertonic (> 0.9%) or Hypotonic (< 0.9%) solution*: used to induce cough and aid in airway clearance
	Medicated Aerosol Delivery *(See Also Chapter 11)* delivering a drug via aerosol (nebulizer, MDI, DPI) for therapeutic effect

The physiological salinity of the airways is 0.9%. Using a hypo- or hypertonic solution is irritating to the airways, a therapeutic method (with debate) used to produce a cough. Note: sterile water is hypotonic (0.0%)

Potential Hazards of Aerosol Therapy
- Adverse reaction to drug
- Airway obstruction
- Caregiver exposure to airborne contagion
- Bronchospasm
- Drug reconcentration (dosage increases over time of nebulization)
- Infection
- Overhydration (hypernatremia)
- Overmobilization of secretions
- Systemic effects

Bland Aerosol Administration [1]

Indications
A bypassed upper airway (heated bland aerosol, MMAD 2-10 μ) [2]
Mobilization of secretions
Sputum induction (hypo or hypertonic saline, MMAD 1-5 μ)
Upper airway edema – (cool bland aerosol, MMAD ≥ 5μ):
  Laryngotracheobronchitis
  Subglottic edema
  Post extubation edema
  Post-op management

Assessment of Need
One or more: stridor, croupy cough, hoarseness following extubation, Hx of upper airway irritation with ↑ WOB, LTB or croup, bypassed airway, or patient discomfort.

Hazards/Complications
Bronchoconstriction or wheezing: artificial airway or hypertonic induction (in COPD, asthma, CF, other)
Caregiver exposure to airborne contagion
Edema of airway wall or assoc. with ↓C + ↑Raw
Infection
Overhydration
Patient discomfort

Contraindications
Bronchoconstriction
History of airway hyper-responsiveness

Monitoring
Patient:
Respiratory: rate, pattern, mechanics, accessory muscle use, BS.
CV: rate, rhythm, BP
Response: pain, dyspnea, discomfort, restlessness.
Sputum: quantity, color, consistency, odor
Skin color
Pulse oximetry (if hypoxemia suspected)
Equipment: Spirometry if concern of adverse reaction.

Frequency
Post extubation – 4-8 hrs
Subglottic edema – until edema subsides
Bypassed upper airway – as long as bypassed
Sputum induction – prn

Clinical Goals
Water, hypo- or isotonic saline: ↓ dyspnea, stridor, or WOB, Improved ABGs, O_2 Sat, or VS
Hypertonic saline: sputum sample

---

1 Adapted from the AARC Clinical Practice Guideline: Bland Aerosol Administration, 2003 Revision and Update, **Respiratory Care**, Vol. 48, #5, 2003.
2 Not as effective as heated water nebulizers or HME.

Overview of Aerosol Delivery Devices (see following pages for more information on each type)

Type	Overview	Considerations
Dry Powder Inhaler (DPI)	Very fine powder form of drug breathed into lungs using patient's own inspiratory flow	• 10-25% of drug deposits into the lungs • Higher Inspiratory flows usually required (> 60 L/min): assess ability (age, etc.) • Patient technique is critical (education is key)
Metered Dose Inhaler (MDI, pMDI)	• Liquid dose of drug (with propellant and suspension agents) actuated from a canister into an aerosolized form • Use of a holding chamber or spacer is preferred with most drugs	• 1-40% of drug deposits into the lungs (varies by size, age, etc.) • Inspiratory flow rates should be ≤ 30 L/min • At least some hand-breath coordination required • Patient technique is critical (education is key)
Soft Mist Inhaler (SMI)	• Propellant-free device that mechanically releases a slow-moving fine mist	• May allow for lower doses than typical • Increased lung deposition due to slower speed of drug

*The AARC Clinical Practice Guideline, "Aerosol Delivery Device Selection for Spontaneously Breathing Patients: 2012," has been summarized in part in the above tables and the following pages. See also: "A Guide to Aerosol Delivery Devices for Respiratory Therapists" (Gardenhire, et al, 4th edition)

Type	Overview	Considerations
Small Particle Aerosol Generator (SPAG)	Specific large-volume nebulizer for the drug ribavirin that has a drying chamber to reduce MMAD	Scavenging system is recommended (ribavirin is known to have teratogenic properties)
Small Volume Nebulizer (SVN) *Jet Nebulizer* *Ultrasonic Nebulizer* *Vibrating-Mesh Nebulizer*	A liquid solution of drug + diluent (normal saline) is turned into an aerosol to be inhaled • Intended for single treatments (intermittent therapy) • Multiple interfaces: mouthpiece, masks (face, tracheostomy, etc.), T-piece (including vent circuit)	• <15% of drug deposits into the lungs (varies by brand) • Solution concentrates during treatment • Breath-actuated (only delivers on inspiration + vents exhalation) and Breath-enhanced (vents exhalation) may improve percentage of drug delivered. • Be aware of impact on ventilator exhaled volumes and flow sensor function
Large Volume Nebulizer (LVN)	• Intended for bland aerosol/humidity or continual drug delivery (albuterol, etc.) • Use with a mask or T-piece	• Each device (HEART, HOPE, etc.) has specific flow output, so drugs should be mixed per manufacturer • Patient should be closely monitored during treatment (critical care preferred)

Selection and Overview

- The CDC recommends that nebulizers be filled with sterile fluids (do not use tap/distilled), and be changed or replaced every 24 hrs (bottle should be labeled with time/date)
- The efficacy of drugs can be affected by the device, the inhalation technique, severity of disease, and patient age
- Cost, convenience, and the ease-of-use may affect compliance
- Unit dose (vs. multi dose bottled) drugs are preferred

General Steps for Respiratory Drug Administration*
1. Review patient chart, including verifying physicians' orders and appropriateness of treatment ordered (notify physician or follow protocol if not clinically indicated, if a contraindication exists, etc.)
2. Gather equipment and drug(s)
3. Verify patient using name and other identifier(s) (MRN, etc.) and explain procedure
4. Ensure appropriate patient position (sitting upright), when possible
5. Assess patient (vital signs, auscultation, appearance, and peak flow if treating reactive airways)
6. Give treatment (see following pages for specific devices). During treatment, monitor patient closely, assess vital signs, auscultate, observe general appearance.
7. Once treatment is finished, place back on any supplemental oxygen if necessary, then re-assess (see #5)
8. Document administration in a timely and objective manner (document return to supplemental O$_2$), and communicate with MD/RN as indicated

*Always perform appropriate infection control, including hand-washing, adhering to isolation guidelines, etc.

Recommended particle sizes:

1-5 μ	sputum induction
2-5 μ	pharmacologically active aerosols
2-10 μ	bypassed upper airway
> 5 μ	upper airway administration

MMAD = mass medium aerodynamic diameter (μ)

It is important to again remember that MMAD can be affected by improper patient technique, resulting in inertial impaction, and ultimately less therapeutic deposition

Effective aerosol therapy requires the correct matching of an appropriate device with the patient's ability to use it effectively

Nebulizers

- Nebulizers should be cleaned and changed periodically according to manufacturer recommendations
- Small volume jet nebulizers should be shaken, rinsed with sterile water (avoid tap or distilled water), and left to air dry after each use. Drying may be enhanced by gas flow through the device after rinsing.
- Heated nebs require sterile solution and sterile immersion heaters, if used.

Small Volume Jet Nebulizer Administration
(see General Steps, pg 9-7)

1. Assemble and verify operation of nebulizer with appropriate patient interface (mouthpiece, mask, etc.)
2. Place drug aseptically into drug chamber
3. Nebulize drug at appropriate setting (flow, frequency) ~8 L/min for jet nebulizer
4. Verify output (aerosolization)
5. Verify appropriate technique, mouth seal if mouthpiece. Encourage periodic breath holds (2-3 sec) to improve drug distribution/deposition

Mesh or Ultrasonic Nebulizer Administration
(see General Steps, pg 9-7)

1. These are specialty nebulizers - be familiar with individual manufacturer instructions
2. Place drug aseptically into reservoir (do not overfill)
3. Coach patient on proper use (actual instruction varies by device/manufacturer)
4. Turn off nebulizer for any interruptions
5. Disassemble/clean per manufacturer (do not touch mesh during cleaning if mesh nebulizer)

Continuous Bronchodilator Therapy (CBT)
(see General Steps, pg 9-7)

1. Assemble and verify operation of nebulizer with appropriate patient interface (mouthpiece, mask, etc.)
2. Prepare drug with diluent aseptically into drug chamber
3. Nebulize drug at appropriate setting (flow, frequency). With some jet nebulizers (HEART, HOPE), be aware of output rate and drug concentrations.
4. Verify output (aerosolization)

HEART large volume nebulizer
Gas flow: 10-15 L/min
Aerosol output: 30-50 mL/min

HOPE large volume nebulizer
Gas flow: 10-15 L/min
Aerosol output: 25 mL/min

Continuous Bronchodilator Therapy (CBT) Procedure

1. **Determine number of hours nebulizer should run**
   typically not more than 3-4 hours because dosage can change

2. **Place desired amount of albuterol (5 mg/mL) in large volume nebulizer cup**

   Amount of albuterol (mL)=
   $$\left(\frac{\text{Desired mg/hr}}{5 \text{ mg}}\right) \times \text{Desired \# hours}$$

3. **ADD saline up to desired total output**
   the aerosol output/hr must be known to do this, which is usually secondarily dependent on gas flow to the nebulizer. This is found in the manufacturer's literature.

   Amount of saline (mL) =
   [(LVN Output (mL/min) x 60) x (Desired # hours)] - [albuterol added (mL)]

Metered Dose Inhalers (MDIs)

- Assessing patient for appropriate technique is critical to effective lung deposition. Every patient interaction should include observation/education.
- Consider use, as appropriate, of:
  - Spacer: device that extends space between MDI outlet and patient's mouth, allows for less impaction (loss)
  - Valved Holding Chamber: device that both extends space and vents exhalation outside of the device (allowing patient to take several breaths to take the drug)
- Counting: for MDIs without a built-in counter, patients should be instructed to keep a tally of actuations, including wasted ones, NOT by placing in a bowl of water
- Mouthpieces should be washed with mild soap/water (or vinegar/water if sensitive) every few days

MDIs Steps to Administration *(see General Steps, pg 9-6)*
1. Assemble MDI. Be aware of individual instructions for each MDI but in general: • Inspect mouthpiece • Shake vigorously per manufacturer (3-4 times) • Prime (1-2 sprays into air) if 1+ day since use or new • Attach spacer/holding chamber
2. Instruct patient to exhale normally
3. Instruct patient to immediately place mouthpiece ~4cm (about 2 finger-widths) from mouth (spacer: place mouth on mouthpiece, breath-actuated: place mouth on mouthpiece
4. Instruct patient to inhale slowly to TLC while depressing MDI cannister at same time (inspiratory flow rate < 30 L/min, unless breath-actuated: then > 30 L/min) *If whistle, inspiration is too fast*
5. Encourage breath hold (4-10 seconds)
6. Instruct to pause between actuations (15-60 sec)
7. Instruct to rinse mouth (corticosteroids)

Dry Powder Inhalers (DPIs)

- Assessing patient for appropriate technique is critical to effective lung deposition. Every patient interaction should include observation/education.
- The drugs in DPIs may have no taste or texture. Some patients mistake this for no drug delivered. Ensure adequate education.
- Ensure adequate inspiratory flow ability (> 60 L/min usually)
- Humidity may affect the drug (exhaled + ambient humidity)

DPI Steps to Administration *(see General Steps, pg 9-6)*
1. Assemble DPI. Be aware of individual instructions for each DPI but in general: • Inspect mouthpiece • Load drug (per manufacturer)
2. Instruct patient to exhale normally
3. Instruct patient to immediately place mouthpiece into mouth with tight seal and inhale per manufacturer directions (some devices require short, quick inhalation, while others require gradual inhalation)
4. Encourage breath hold (4-10 seconds)
5. Instruct to rinse mouth after use (corticosteroids)

Airway Management
Bag-Valve-Mask (BVM) Ventilation

Variable	Considerations	
Rates	**General**	ADULT: 10-12 breaths/min (every 5-6 sec) PEDIATRIC: 20-30/min (every 2-3 sec)
	COPD **Raw ↑** **Hypovolemia**	6-8 breaths/min (every 7-10 sec) *minimizes Auto-PEEP*
	Adult CPR	No Airway: 30:2 ratio Airway: 10/min (every 6 sec) *allows venous return*
Volumes	Estimated (deliver enough for visible chest rise):	
	Adult	Visible chest rise 500-600 mL (6-7 mL/kg) 1 L Adult Bag: 1/2 - 2/3 volume 2 L Adult Bag: 1/3 volume
	Infant/Child	Visible Chest Rise Bag size should be < 450-500 mL
Gas Source	Usually connected to oxygen (commonly 15 L/min). Verify flow is from Oxygen outlet/tank, verify tubing is connected	
Personnel	1 Person: Ensure adequate airway position Use good C:E technique Most effective with 2 Rescuers - 1 opens airway/seals mask, 2nd squeezes bag while both observe chest rise	
Risks	• Avoid high rates: higher rates may decrease venous return to the heart, decreasing coronary/cerebral perfusion • Avoid large volumes: risk of gastric insufflation (mask) or lung injury (mask or artificial airway)	
Inadequate Ventilation	• General deterioration (SpO$_2$, ETCO$_2$, HR, BP) • Decreased (or absent) breath sounds, chest rise	

Airway Adjuncts

Adjunct	Indications/Complications	Procedure
Nasopharyngeal Airway (NPA, Nasal Trumpet)	• Facilitates (nasotracheal) suctioning when required frequently (helps prevent trauma to the nares) • Assists in relieving upper airway obstruction in a conscious or unconscious patient (esp. tongue against posterior pharyngeal wall) Complications: Epistaxis, sinusitis	1. Determine correct size* (tip of nose to tragus of the ear) 2. Lubricate NPA (water soluble lubricant) 3. Inspect nares, use widest 4. Insert NPA with bevel towards septum, following the curvature of the nasal cavity floor, twisting gently to advance through the turbinates. If obstructed, try other naris. 5. If left in place, monitor skin integrity, switch nares every 8-12 hrs
Oropharyngeal Airway (OPA)	• Assists in relieving upper airway obstructions in an **unconscious** patient (often to facilitate bag-valve-mask ventilation) • Bite block with ET tube** Complications: gag/vomit	1. Note: patient must be unconscious/no gag reflex noted 2. Determine correct size* (corner of mouth to earlobe) 3. Insert with curve upward or lateral, then gently rotate curve to be towards the tongue 4. Should be used short-term, monitor skin integrity closely

*Too small: will not prevent obstructing; Too large: may occlude the airway, cause gastric distension
** If used as a bite block, use very temporarily due to higher risk of skin breakdown than with commercial bite block designs

Therapies

Endotracheal Tubes (ET Tubes)

Types:
- Regular (with Murphy Eye), usually slightly curved, pliable
- Subglottic tubes (allow for suction above the cuff)
- Anti-Aspiration Designs (microcuff, silver-coated, etc.)
- Reinforced with metal coiling (if kinked, must replace)

Typical Sizing

	ET Tube I.D.(mm)	Avg Depth	Blade	Mask	Suction Catheter*(Fr)
Adult Male	6.5-9.5	21-23	3-4	4	8-14
Adult Female	6.0-8.5	19-21	3	4	8-12

* While suction catheter size should be determined by patient response, a starting point can be calculated using the formula: **[(ET Tube Size in mm) x 3] / 2**, then choose closest even number (at or below)

1 FR = 3 mm.

Modified Mallampati Scoring for Predicting a Difficult Airway

I	II	III	IV
Soft palate visible	Soft palate visible	Soft palate visible	Soft palate NOT visible
Uvula visible Pillars visible	Uvula visible	Base of uvula visible	Uvula NOT visible
Generally uncomplicated airway management		Potentially difficult airway management (including intubation)	

Intubation

Equipment
Prepare and check all equipment
- Bag and valve mask ventilation (BVM)
  - connected/running on oxygen (12-15 L/min)
- Laryngoscope
  - check function of light/video
- Laryngoscope blades (Miller or MacIntosh)
- Endotracheal Tube (several sizes) with stylet
  - check cuff patency
  - use new endotracheal tube on each Intubation attempt
  - place stylet in endotracheal tube, if using
  - Lubricate the ET tube using water-soluble lubricant
- 10-cc Syringe
- Suction (rigid tonsillar suction connected and running)
- Waveform capnography running and ready
  - If unavailable, consider qualitative (e.g. Easy Cap) or Esophageal Detector Device (EDD)

Procedure
1. Ensure equipment is setup and checked
2. Position patient in sniffing position
3. Assess for difficult airway (see previous page)
4. Open mouth of patient (thumb-index-finger technique)
5. Insert laryngoscope blade, pulling upward and outward (keep wrist straight/rigid; do not pivot wrist)
6. Suction as needed
7. Insert the ET tube, watching specifically for indicator marks to go through the vocal cords
8. Inflate ET tube cuff with 10-cc syringe
9. Hold tube while removing laryngoscope and pulling stylet out
10. Attach BVM to tube
11. Verify tube placement (see checklist, next page)
12. Verify tube position (insertion distance from teeth should be around 19-21 cm female, 21-23 cm male)
13. Secure ET tube using commercial holder or tape

Confirmation of Tracheal Intubation Checklist:

Visualize Vocal Cords as Tube Passes Through	The best indicator of successful placement is visualization of tube going through vocal cords (preferably by 2 people)
Continuous Quantitative Waveform Capnography	Assumes adequate perfusion • This is the preferred method for verification (AHA) • Normal waveform/number should be present to confirm presence of CO_2
Qualitative Capnography (See next page)	Assumes adequate perfusion • The use of a device that changes color with CO_2 (yellow indicates CO_2 in most)
Esophageal Detector Device (See next page)	Less reliable than capnography but may be considered per ACLS guidelines
Upper Airway Ultrasonography	Consider instead of capnography if inadequate perfusion (shock, cardiac arrest) • Enables visualization of upper airway structures to identify tube placement
Note Chest Rise	Should be bilateral, adequate rise *If R > L, suspect right mainstem intubation*
Vitals and Patient Color	Should be normal to ethnicity; pallor/cyanosis can be indicators of tube not in place
Auscultate over Chest Wall	Should be equal and bilateral breath sounds *If R > L suspect right mainstem intubation* *If both R + L ↓ suspect ET tube not in trachea*
Auscultate Epigastrium	Should be absence of breath sounds/gurgling over the abdomen
ET Tube	Note warm air flowing on exhalation from tube, condensate in tube, appropriate depth marking (at teeth)
Chest Radiograph (CXR)	A chest radiograph is a follow-up step for verifying tube proper position (see pg 3-10)

End-tidal CO₂ Detector (P$_{ET}$CO$_2$) for Verification

CO$_2$ Detected	
Tube likely in Trachea	Initial confirmation - verify w/ other methods. Most turn YELLOW.
CO$_2$ Not Detected	
Tube is in Esophagus	• Absent Chest Rise • Absent Breath Sounds • Stomach gurgling and distension
Tube is in Trachea *Verify with several other methods*	*Decreased CO$_2$ IN Lungs:* • Poor blood flow to lungs • Cardiac Arrest • Pulmonary Embolus • IV Bolus of Epinephrine *Decreased CO$_2$ FROM Lungs:* • Airway Obstruct (Status Asthmaticus, etc.) • Pulmonary Edema • Mucus Plugging
Unclear Where Tube Is	Detector contaminated with gastric contents or acidic drug
ETCO$_2$ device applied incorrectly, Time	Many disposable devices require "activation" (such as by pulling of paper tab), and may req. a few ventilations to change color

Esophageal Detector Device for Verification

Syringe-Type plunger is attached to ET Tube.	
Able to Pull Back on Plunger	ET Tube likely in trachea (rigid structure of trachea allows for air passage)
Unable to Pull Back on Plunger	ET Tube likely in esophagus (floppy structure of esophagus collapses over end of ET tube)

Caution: May be misleading in morbid obesity, late pregnancy, status asthmaticus, or with copious secretions. Use in children only if > 20 kg with perfusing rhythm.

Tracheostomy Tubes
Types:

Characteristics	Typical Variations Available
Material	Metal (Jackson) Plastic (Shiley, Portex, Bivona, etc.)
Presence of Cuff	Cuffed or Uncuffed
Type of Cuff	Air, Fluid, or Foam Filled
Shape	Normal versus Specialty (extra-long: distal or proximal; custom)
Fenestrations	Fenestrated or Non-fenestrated
Inner Cannula	None or Removable (Non-disposable, Disposable)
Adjuncts	Speaking Valves (see next page)
Sizes	Vary, Adult usually 4-9

Indications for Tracheostomy Placement
- Patients unable to protect their airways
- Excessive secretions or can't maintain otherwise
- Swallowing or cough impairment with chronic aspiration
- Requiring invasive ventilation for a prolonged period
- Contraindications to, failed, or cannot tolerate NPPV
- Need to reduce anatomical dead space

Tracheostomy Care and Monitoring
- See pg 9-24 for daily care and trach changes
- Basic vitals should be monitored (HR, RR, SpO2)
- Humidity is usually required (upper airway is bypassed)
- Active humidity is recommended for new tracheostomies
- HMEs (passive humidity) are acceptable unless thick secretions, high minute ventilation, etc. (see Humidity, page 9-56)
- Suctioning is preferably done when indicated (only): ensure trach-length in-line suction catheter is used
- There is evidence to support the use of trach bundles, protocol-directed care, and dedicated tracheostomy teams (*AARC Clinical Practice Guideline, 2021*)

Speaking Valves

Description	• A one-way valve placed on the trach tube • Inhale: air comes in through valve • Exhale: air is blocked from trach, goes through upper airway around trach
Purposes	• Enables verbal communication • Facilitates swallowing (eating/drinking) • Improves secretion clearance (cough secretions to upper airway)
Procedure	• **DEFLATE TRACH CUFF*** • Attach speaking valve to tracheostomy • If needed, increase V$_T$ on vent-dependent pts (leak has been created) • On initial placement, monitor for tolerance: vital signs, dyspnea, work of breathing • If indicated provide oxygen (over stoma)
Problems	• Air-trapping • Fatigue and/or intolerance • Mucus can occlude one-way valve

*Failing to deflate the cuff will result in the patient being able to inhale through the valve, but will have no way to exhale.

Tracheostomy Troubleshooting

Guiding Principles:
- Newly placed tracheostomies should be considered critical airways. If the trach comes out, it may be difficult to place back (or is more likely to go into a false tract)
- If the patient is in distress and the cause is the airway, remove the inner cannula. If no improvement, remove airway.
- To verify patency: run a suction catheter gently into the trach. If resistance is met, trach is either occluded (mucus, etc.) or is in soft tissue. Remove and check inner cannula.
- If unable to reinsert a trach, multiple options are available:
  - Cover stoma with gloved hand and use upper airway for BVM or intubation (if complete laryngectomy, do not use upper airway as there is no anatomical connection between upper and lower airways)
  - If stoma is patent, use a #6.0 ET tube (or smaller), insert several centimeters beyond stoma, then inflate cuff

Complications and Possible Actions

Complication	Possible Causes	Possible Actions
Cuff won't stay inflated	Cuff not patent (cuff leak evident)	Consider trach change, clamp pilot balloon line
Bleeding (from trach)	Suction trauma Blood from procedure Other causes	If small amount: monitor If new/large amount: notify physician
Chest pain	Cardiac Malpositioned trach Occluded trach Respiratory failure	Perform ECG (rule out cardiac) Verify placement (run suction catheter into tracheostomy to ensure no occlusion) Discontinue capping trial
Crackling/edema around stoma	Trach in soft tissue (crepitus)	Verify placement Consider trach change

Complication	Possible Causes	Possible Actions
High cuff pressures to seal Should be 20-25 mm Hg	Incorrect size	Consider trach change (Note: increasing trach size is challenging, ensure adequate support)
Difficulty passing suction catheter	Suction catheter too large Malpositioned trach Occluded trach	**Consider lavage. If still unable to pass suction catheter, and/or patient distress, remove and inspect inner cannula. If still unable to pass catheter, likely need to remove the trach.**
Excessive secretions, Change in secretions	Infection Humidity (excess) Humidity (insufficient)	Send sputum culture Check labs See pg 4-16 for secretions Consider humidity setting (heat may liquefy secretions, turn down temp if clinically appropriate) If thick secretions, consider change from HME (if used) to active humidity
Skin redness Drainage (Pus)	Infection Pressure wound	Culture if infection suspected Consider cleaning with 1:1 mixture of Hydrogen Peroxide with NS*
Granulation Tissue (immature blood vessels, may cause bleeding to occur easily)	Extended placement	Consider regular trach changes (every 1-2 weeks)
Excessive coughing or gagging, dyspnea, feeling of choking	Excessive secretions Tolerance of trach	Non-pharmacological or pharmacological airway clearance Anxiety interventions

*Hydrogen peroxide may be irritating and is not recommended for routine cleaning, but may help with infected skin/stoma

Tracheostomy Daily Care

1. Explain procedure to patient
2. Position patient supine or head slightly elevated
3. Stand to side of patient (pt is likely to cough)
4. Perform hand hygiene, don gloves, face shield/mask
5. Gently clean stoma with normal saline, noting skin integrity and secretions
6. Replace inner cannula, trach tie, gauze/dressing, taking care to secure the tracheostomy tube at all times

Performing a Tracheostomy Change
A second skilled person should be at the bedside to assist with the trach change

1. Explain procedure to patient
2. Position patient supine (sniffing position) or slightly elevated
3. Perform hand hygiene, don gloves, face shield/mask
4. Clean stoma from inner to outer rim (use normal saline or sterile water), then dry
5. Remove inner cannula of new tube (if present), insert obturator. Check new cuff for leaks (if cuffed).
6. Lubricate outside of tube with water-soluble lubricant
7. Stand on side of pt to avoid exposure to body fluids from trach (patient is likely to cough)
8. Oxygenate, suction trach and airway, re-oxygenate
9. Remove holder/tie, have patient take a deep breath (or give deep breath with resuscitation bag), <u>deflate cuff</u>, then remove old trach tube gently
10. Quickly, but gently, insert new tube (sideways, then gently downward) (do not force), hold tube in place and immediately remove obturator
11. Insert inner cannula and lock in place (if present), inflate cuff, if present
12. **Verify placement ($ETCO_2$, pass suction catheter, auscultate, feel for air flow). Remove tube if cannot be placed properly or airflow is inadequate; ventilate as needed and attempt to reinsert tube.**
13. Hold tube in place until urge to cough subsides
14. Secure trach holder/ties (leave one finger width loose)
15. Suction and oxygenate if needed. Re-auscultate/assess.

Non-disposable Tracheostomy Tube/Inner Cannula

1. Perform hand hygiene, don gloves, face shield/mask
2. Open all packages
3. Suction tracheostomy tube before removing
4. Remove inner cannula by unlocking/gently pulling outward or remove single tube or outer cannula by cutting ties, holding tube in place with finger, deflate cuff, pull gently outward and downward
5. Soak tube in cleaning solution for indicated time
6. Clean skin/stoma with cotton dipped in solution and pat dry with gauze
7. Brush inside of tube with cleaning solution
8. Rinse tube thoroughly with sterile water
9. Pat dry with clean gauze and replace

Considerations for Trach Changes

Variable	Considerations
Equipment	Always have a BVM ready and connected to O_2 with appropriate flow running. Intubation equip. should be easily accessible.
People at Bedside	Minimum of 2 qualified people
Age of Trach	Fresh tracheostomies (< 1 week old) should be changed only if emergent, and by MD. Risk of loss of patent airway if pulled. Intubation equipment should be present.
Anatomical	**Caution Should be Used in:** • Obese Patients • Abnormal neck anatomy • Any trach placed for patency
Size	Downsizing is generally easier than replacing same size, and extreme caution in upsizing.
Verification	Always verify correct placement following a trach change. Use auscultation, $ETCO_2$, chest rise, return volumes if on vent, SpO_2, WOB, ability to pass sx catheter and/or able to "bag" patient effectively

Tracheostomy Capping and Decannulation Trials[1]

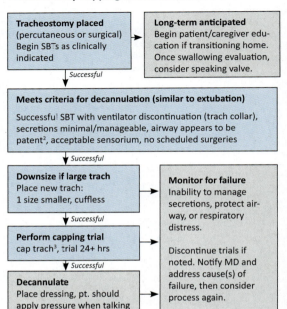

[1] Consistent with AAO-HNS Consensus Guidelines
[2] Swallow evaluation and/or endoscopic assessment if concerns
[3] If cuffed trach, ensure it is deflated for capping trial

Airway Clearance

Variable	Considerations
Indications	**Prevent Secretion Retention** Acute respiratory failure, atelectasis, immobile patients, lung disease (COPD, etc.), neuromuscular disorders, post op **Remove Copious Secretions** Allergens/irritants, asthma, bronchiectasis, bronchitis, cystic fibrosis, infection Copious Secretions = 25-30 mL/day (1oz/shot glass)
Signs & Symptoms	**Symptoms** ↑ Chest congestion, ↑ cough (or ineffective), ↑ SOB or WOB, ↑ wheezing, ↑ or ↓ sputum **Signs** BS – abnormal, audible or ↓, ↑ RR, ↑ HR, ↑ respiratory tract infections and fever, ↓ SpO2 or worsening ABG's, ↓ expiratory flow rates, secretions (↓ or ↑, thick, or discolored), CXR changes **Note**: The effectiveness of bronchial hygiene therapy is commonly determined by improvement of the above signs & symptoms
Factors Affecting Secretion Clearance	**Impaired mucociliary transport**
	Analgesics, anesthetics, cigarette smoking, cuffed ET or trach tube, dehydration (dry gases > 4 L/m, bypass of upper airway), electrolyte imbalance, hypoxia or hypercapnia, loss of cilia (COPD, infection), pollutants
	Impaired cough strength
	Abdominal restriction, surgery, pain, air trapping (emphysema), airway collapse, constriction, inflammation, obstruction (allergens, asthma, CF, COPD, infection, irritants, tumors), artificial airway, CNS depression, drugs (analgesics/narcotics), neuromuscular weakness, fatigue, paralysis
	Excessive or thick secretions
	Allergens/irritants, asthma, bronchiectasis, bronchitis, cystic fibrosis, infection

Therapies

Selecting an Airway Clearance Technique

Patient Concerns	Technique Factors
• Ability to self administer is an important factor • Disease type and severity • Fatigue or work required • Pt's age and ability to learn • Patient's pref. and goals	• Clinician skill in teaching the technique • Cost (direct and indirect) • Equipment required • Physician/caregiver goals • Therapy effectiveness

See Bronchial Hygiene Selection Algorithm (pg 9-54) and ACCP Recommendations (pg 9-55)

Make choices based upon the above factors/concerns, but as with most therapies you should consider least intense options first, moving to more intense options as a therapy is not effective, or not appropriate for patient's clinical condition/ability

Suggested Order of Therapy Implementation

Least Intense (Self)	• Directed cough *+ • Diaphragmatic exercises *+ • Pursed lip breathing • Autogenic drainage/ACBT
(Device)	• Acapella device • Flutter valve
Intense (Device + Time)	• Postural drainage, percussion, vibration*+ • Percussive therapies (vest/wrap) *+ • In-exsufflator (Cough Assist) * • Intrapulmonary percussive ventil. (IPV)*+ • Nasotracheal suctioning (NTS)
Most Intense	• Therapeutic bronchoscopy *+ • Intubation (short-term) • Tracheostomy (longer-term)

* Options for patients who are non-vented w/ artificial airways
+ Options for patients who are mechanically ventilated

Suctioning

Guiding principles of suctioning:
- Perform when indicated, not as a scheduled procedure
- Attempts should be kept to a duration of 15 seconds or less
- Due to its invasive nature, this is a preferred sterile procedure, minimally a "clean" procedure
- Use the lowest effective pressure (see next page for suction pressures)
- Types of Suction
  - Open: advancing a suction catheter into the airway (natural or artificial)
  - Closed (also called in-line): a suction catheter within a sheath keeps a circuit "closed" (if on a ventilator), goal is to minimize risk of ventilator-associated pneumonia (VAP)

Indications/Need

Evidence of Secretions	• Visible secretions in artificial airway • Auscultation: coarse crackles, decreased • Palpation: coarse vibrations

Alterations in Patient/ Ventilator Interaction	• Patient: ↑ agitation, irritability, restlessness
	• Ventilator: ↑ Raw
	  Volume Mode: ↑ PIP, High Pressure alarm
	  Pressure Mode: ↓ V$_T$

Alterations in Vital Signs	• Change in respiratory pattern:
	  ↑ WOB, tachypnea, retractions
	• Change in cardiac pattern:
	  ↑ or ↓ HR

Alterations in O$_2$ and Ventilation	• ↓ SpO$_2$: often trends steadily but may drop quickly, particularly if a mucous plug • Skin color: pale, dusky, or cyanotic • ABG: ↓ PaO$_2$, respiratory acidosis

Suction Pressures for Airways

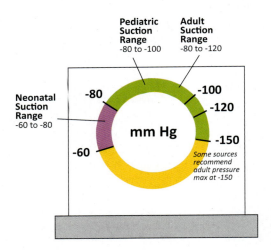

Suction Catheter Sizing

Suction catheter should be < 50% of the internal diameter of the ET Tube (but large enough to suction thicker sputum, mucous plugs, etc.).

Suction Catheter Size (FR) = (ET Tube Size x 3) / 2
(if not an even number, drop to next smallest even number)

Example:
Pt with a size 7.5 cm ET Tube
= (7.5 x 3) / 2
= 22.5/2
= 11.25
Next Smallest = 10 FR

Nasotracheal Suctioning Procedure
Equipment
- Portable or wall suction source/regulator
- Suction catheter (see previous page)
- Normal saline or sterile water (for flushing catheter)
- Water-soluble lubricant

Procedure (Gray boxes are suggested sterile technique)

Step	Tips
1. Assess indications/need	Avoid scheduled suctioning
2. Explain procedure to patient	Use pt-appropriate terms
3. Pre-oxygenate as indicated	100% O_2 for 30+ sec
4. Position in semi-Fowlers, neck slightly hyper-extended	Check for contraindications
5. Monitor vital signs and pt. response before, during, and after	If any adverse effect, STOP and assess
6. Test Suction Pressure	See previous page
7. Wash and glove (sterile or clean technique)	Keep dominant hand sterile/clean for duration
8. Coat distal end of catheter with lubricant, attach to suction	
9. Insert catheter tip into naris (no suction applied), gently twisting as catheter is advanced	Do not advance through nasal turbinates if any resistance. Advancing during cough or inhalation may help catheter enter trachea
10. Apply intermittent suction while steadily withdrawing, using a slightly circular motion	Do not re-advance once withdrawing. Withdraw completely within 15 sec.
11. Clear suction catheter with sterile water.	Max 2-3 attempts (only if needed) with 60 sec break in between each attempt
12. Return to previous O_2, document procedure (include patient tolerance, sputum amount/color/consistency)	

Nasotracheal Suctioning
(AARC Expert Panel Reference-Based Guideline)

Indications
Patient's cough unable to clear secretions or foreign material in the large central airways.
Evidenced by:
  Audible or visible secretions in airway
  Chest x-ray (retained secretions → atelectasis or consolidation)
  Coarse, gurgling BS or ↓ BS
  Hypoxemia or hypercarbia
  Suspected aspiration
  Tactile fremitus
  ↑WOB
To stimulate cough or for un-relieved coughing
To obtain sputum sample

Contraindications
Croup, eppiglottis
Relative: Acute facial, head or neck injury, bronchospasm, coagulopathy or bleeding disorder, high gastric surgery, irritable airway, laryngospasm, MI, nasal bleeding, occluded nasal passages, tracheal surgery, URI.

Recommended Pressures
Adult   -100 to -150 mm Hg
Child   -100 to -120 mm Hg
Infant   -80 to -100 mm Hg
Neonate -60 to -80 mm Hg

Suction time should be < 15 sec.

Frequency
Only when indicated and other measures have failed.

Monitoring
(before, during, and after) BS, cough, CV parameters (HR, BP, EKG), ICP, laryngospasm, oxygen saturation, RR, pattern, SpO_2, skin color, sputum (color, volume, consistency, odor), subjective response (pain), trauma, bleeding.

Hazards/Complications
Atelectasis, bronchospasm, CV changes (↓ HR,↑↓BP, arrhythmia, arrest), gagging, vomiting, hypoxia, hypoxemia,↑ ICP (IVH, cerebral edema), laryngospasm, mechanical trauma (bleeding, irritation, laceration, perforation, tracheitis), misdirection of catheter, nosocomial infection, pain, pneumothorax, respiratory arrest, uncontrolled coughing.

Assessment of Outcome
Improved BS, improved ABGs or SpO_2, secretions removed, ↓WOB (↓RR or dyspnea)

Adapted from the AARC Clinical Practice Guideline: Nasotracheal Suctioning, *Respiratory Care*, Volume 37, #8, 1992 and 2004 update.

Directed or Therapeutic Cough

Indications	May assist in pts with limited cough ability, who are weak/deconditioned, but with adequate neurological function to follow/learn instructions	
Techniques	**Controlled Cough**	Three deep breaths, exhaling normally after the first two and then coughing firmly on the third
	Double Cough	A deep breath followed by two coughs with the second cough more forceful
	Three Coughs	A small breath and a fair cough, then a bigger breath and a harder cough, and finally a deep breath with a forceful cough
	Pump Coughing	A deep breath followed by three short easy coughs, then three huffs
	Huff Cough (Forced Expiratory Technique [FET])	A slow, deep breath (mid-lung) followed by a 1-3 sec hold, then a series of short, quick, forceful exhalations or "huffs" with the mouth and glottis kept open
	Manually-Assisted Cough	A deep breath followed by a forceful exhalation, plus an assistant quickly and firmly pushing the abdomen (or lateral costal margins of chest) up against the diaphragm during exhalation
Contra-indications	Pregnant women, abdominal pathologies, (e.g., aortic aneurysm, hiatal hernia), and/or unconscious patient with unprotected airways. Lateral costal margin pressure is contraindicated with osteoporosis or flail chest. ACCP does not recommend for patients with airflow obstruction, like COPD.	

Active Cycle of Breathing

Indications	Primarily used as part of the therapy regimen for cystic fibrosis in some patients
Technique	1. Gentle diaphragmatic breathing at normal V$_T$ with relaxation of upper chest and shoulders. 2. Four thoracic expansion exercises (TEE) - deep inspirations and relaxed expiration 3. Repeat #1 4. Forced Expiration Technique (FET) consists of one or two huffs at appropriate lung volume, dependent on location of secretions, followed ALWAYS by breathing control #1 (e.g. one or two mid- to low-lung volume huffs, if secretions located in more peripheral airways, one or two high lung volume huffs or cough, if secretions located in larger more central airways followed by #1. 5. Repeat cycle until chest is as clear as possible.
Note	• Avoid cough until secretions for expectoration in upper airways • Intersperse with #1 at any stage if patient becomes breathless or wheezy

Autogenic Drainage

Indications	Primarily used for cystic fibrosis, though may assist with others with thick secretions. Because of technique required, patient should be > 8 yrs old.
Techniques	• Requires several sessions to learn technique, but is then a self-directed (no equipment) therapy: • Instruct pt to sit or recline, with neck slightly extended. • Three Phases:

	Phase 1 (Unstick)	• Inhale small lung volume with a 1-3 sec breath hold • Exhale actively, but not forcefully • Repeat 1-3 minutes until secretions mobilized and heard/felt in larger middle sized airways (ie, crackles - coarse and loud)
	Phase 2 (Collect)	• Inhale medium lung volume with a 1-3 sec breath hold • Exhale actively, but not forcefully • Repeat 1-3 minutes until secretions mobilized and heard/felt in largest proximal airways (ie crackles - coarser and louder)
	Phase 3 (Evacuate)	• Inhale, slow, deep breaths (large lung volumes), with a 1-3 sec breath hold • Exhale actively, more forcefully • Repeat until secretions expectorated with huff or controlled cough • Follow with #1. • Repeat cycle until chest is as clear as possible.

Diaphragmatic Exercises

Indications	• Alleviate dyspnea, improve oxygenation • Increase ventilation • Reduce post-op complications
Technique	• Have pt assume comfortable position (sitting supported, semi-Fowlers, or supine with hip and knees flexed). • Explain purpose, goals, demonstrate desired result. • Place hand on epigastric area, asking them to breathe slowly and comfortably; follow patient's breathing with hand. • Pursed-lip breathing (as described later in this chapter) is often performed with diaphragmatic breathing. • After several breathing cycles, as the pt completes an exhalation, apply a firm counter-pressure with the hand and ask the patient to inhale and to "fill my hand with air"; observe the expansion under your hand, then instruct patient to exhale normally. • Continue practicing, then have the patient place his or her own hand on their epigastric area and repeat the procedure. • Continue practicing until patient can perform the exercise properly with no verbal cues or having hand on their epigastrium. • As an aid to teaching, the patient may place his other hand over the sternum and instruct the patient to keep that hand from moving up and down. • Advance teaching can be done by having the patient perform the exercise while sitting unsupported, standing, and walking.

Diaphragmatic Strengthening	
Indications	Patients with less than normal diaphragmatic strength
Technique	• The application of progressively increasing manual resistance or weights applied over the epigastric area with the patient in the supine position. • The patient should perform several series of three to five slow sustained deep diaphragmatic breaths with interposed rest periods. • Proper starting weight or pressure should permit full epigastric rise for 15 minutes with no signs of accessory muscle contraction. • Additional weight is added as strength improves. • Inspiratory muscle trainers may be beneficial to some patients
Note	Positioning the patient in a Trendelenburg position, using the force of abdominal contents to resist the diaphragm, can accomplish the same results. A 15° head down tilt results in approximately 10 lbs. of force against the diaphragm (caution when using head-down position, see pg 9-45).

Pursed-Lip Breathing	
Indications	To improve ventilation and oxygenation in patients with air-trapping (COPD, bronchiectasis, etc.)
Technique	• Instruct patient to inhale slowly through the nose • Patient is then told to exhale gently through pursed lips (as though whistling) without any use of abdominal muscles. One part of the breathing cycle should be for inspiration and two parts for exhalation (e.g., 2 sec for TI and 4 sec for TE). • If performed while walking; 2 steps as the patient breathes in and 4 steps as the patient breathes out. Expiration must always be longer than inspiration.

Chest Physiotherapy (CPT)
Consists of postural drainage, percussion, and vibration

Postural Drainage (See diagrams following pages)	
Indications	Particularly beneficial in cystic fibrosis. May benefit patients with thick secretions
Technique	• Perform a min. of 1 hr before/2 hrs after meals • Prescribed bronchodilator therapy should be given 15 min before therapy • Loosen any tight or binding clothing • Drainage should begin with superior segments and progress downward. Lung Segment to be drained should be placed such that main bronchus is pointing ↓ (use of pillows/blankets may assist in positioning) • Maintain position for 3-20 min, depending on quantity and tenacity of secretions and patient tolerance. Limit total to 30-40 min. • Apply Percussion and Vibration (see next page) • Have patient cough every 5 min during each position and after therapy (use FET in head down positions). There will be less of a rise in intracranial pressure if the patient is in an upright position during cough.

Monitoring	• Watch for signs of patient intolerance and monitor heart rate, BP, and SpO_2 during treatment
	• Signs of respiratory compromise:
	  • ↓ diaphragm excursion with head-down
	  • Airway obstruction from secretions/collapse
	• Therapy should be adjusted based upon the patient's clinical response and overall tolerance.

Clinical Notes	• Oxygen requirements may increase during CPT, but should decrease following. Positional changes will alter V/Q and may be either beneficial or detrimental to oxygenation/ventilation • **Debate exists about head-down position, particularly in Neo/Peds** (CF Foundation and various CPGs in Australia, Canada, and Europe).

Percussion and Vibration	
Indications	Particularly beneficial in cystic fibrosis. May benefit patients with thick secretions (debate exists on this)
Technique	• Percussion is applied to various lung segments either manually (with cupped hands) or mechanically with a motorized percussor/vibrator type unit (electric or pneumatic). • Chest percussion or clapping and vibration are often used in conjunction with postural drainage. • Percussion or clapping is usually applied for several minutes or as tolerated by the patient. • The therapist should remove rings/jewelry on hands/wrist. • Percussion is followed by vibration on exhalation. • Vibration is applied to the chest area with hands tensing at 6-8 vibrations per second for 4-6 exhalations. • The procedure concludes with a deep cough (several techniques are described in this chapter) and expulsion of secretions. • Patients should be allowed to rest as each lung segment is drained and cleared. • Should not be performed on a bare chest, over heart, stomach, spine, kidneys, women's breasts, chest tubes, incisions, wounds, fractures.

External Anatomy of Lungs

Used with Permission.
An introduction to postural drainage and percussion. In (2012). Cystic Fibrosis Foundation.

9-40   Therapies

Postural Drainage Modified Positions (CFF)

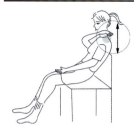

Upper Lobes
(Self Percussion)

Patient should sit upright. Instruct pt to percuss area between collarbone and top of shoulder blade, being careful to avoid bony structures.

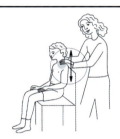

Upper Front Chest

Patient should sit upright. Percuss area between collarbone and top of shoulder blade, being careful to avoid bony structures.

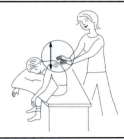

Upper Back Chest

Pt should sit upright, leaning forward at about 30 degrees. Stand behind pt and percuss both sides of upper back, being careful to avoid bony structures.

Used with Permission. Text adapted.

An introduction to postural drainage and percussion. In (2012). Cystic Fibrosis Foundation.

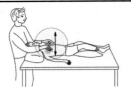

Upper Front Chest

Patient should be supine, with arms to sides. Percuss bilaterally between collarbone and nipple line.

Avoid bony structures and breasts on females.

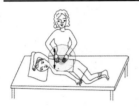

Left Side Front Chest

Patient should be on right side, with left arm over head if able. Percuss over lower ribs, just below nipple line on front of chest.

Avoid abdomen and breasts on females.

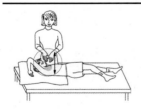

Right Side Front Chest

Patient should be on left side, with right arm over head if able. Percuss over lower ribs, just below nipple line on front of chest.

Avoid abdomen and breasts on females

Used with Permission. Text adapted.

An introduction to postural drainage and percussion. In (2012). Cystic Fibrosis Foundation.

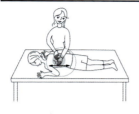

Lower Back Chest

Patient should be proned. Percuss bilaterally at bottom of chest wall (use bottom edge of rib cage as a guide)

Avoid bony structures (lower rib cage and vertebral column)

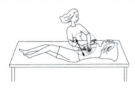

Left Lower Side Back Chest

Pt should be positioned on right side, rolled forward 1/4 turn. Percuss lower left side of chest above bottom edge or ribs

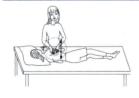

Right Lower Side Back

Patient should be positioned on left side, rolled forward 1/4 turn. Percuss lower right side of chest above bottom edge of ribs

---

Used with Permission. Text adapted.

An introduction to postural drainage and percussion. In (2012). Cystic Fibrosis Foundation.

Traditional Postural Drainage Positions

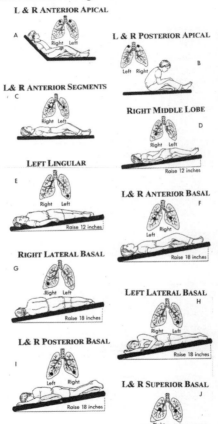

Adapted from Hirsch, J. and Hannock, L. *Mosby's Manual of Clinical Nursing Practice.* Copyright 1985 by Mosby.

Potential Effects of a Head-Down Position
Check with patient frequently, monitor vital signs and appearance, STOP treatment if negative effect, assess, modify position if necessary.

- Aspiration risk (GERD, gastric tube, etc.)
- Bronchospasm
- Cardiovascular changes/hypotension
- Discomfort or pain, general anxiety
- Dyspnea
- Intracranial pressures increased (CPP)
- Oxygenation decreased (SpO_2)
- Vital capacity decreased
  (abdomen pushes on diaphragm, ↓ lung expansion)
- V/Q changes (may be benefit or risk)

General Considerations for Airway Clearance Techniques

- Carefully and frequently assess patient for effectiveness and tolerance. Consider modifications as necessary.
- Effective pain control can be an important aspect of airway clearance
- Most patients breathe and cough better when sitting upright, leaning slightly forward (head and neck upright, not bent over)
- A pillow held firmly against the abdomen (splinting) may permit a stronger cough
- Patients should be encouraged to drink more water when secretions are extremely thick (unless on fluid restrictions)
- Consider pharmacologic interventions as needed
- Quadriplegics can use glossopharyngeal breathing or "frog breathing" to improve cough and usually cough better with head of bed flat and often in a side-lying position

Effectiveness of Nonpharmacologic Airway Clearance Therapies in Hospitalized Patients[1,2]
AARC Clinical Practice Guideline Summary

Hospitalized Patients without Cystic Fibrosis

1. Chest physiotherapy is not recommended for the routine treatment of uncomplicated pneumonia.
2. Airway clearance techniques are not recommended for routine use in patients with COPD.
3. Airway clearance techniques may be considered in patients with COPD with symptomatic secretion retention, guided by patient preference, toleration, and effectiveness of therapy.
4. Airway clearance techniques are not recommended if the patient is able to mobilize secretions with cough, but instruction in effective cough technique (FET) may be useful.

Neuromuscular Disease, Respiratory Muscle Weakness, or Impaired Cough

1. Cough assist techniques should be used in patients with neuromuscular disease, particularly when peak cough flow is < 270 L/min.
2. CPT, PEP, IPV, and HFCWC is not recommended.

Postoperative

1. Incentive spirometry is not recommended for routine, prophylactic use in postoperative patients.
2. Early mobility and ambulation is recommended to reduce post-op complications and promote airway clearance.
3. Airway Clearance Techniques are not recommended for routine postoperative care.

---

[1]*Adapted from AARC Clinical Practice Guideline: Effectiveness of Nonpharmacologic Airway Clearance Therapies in Hospitalized Patients, Respiratory Care, Dec 2013, Vol 58, #12.*
[2]*Guidelines are appropriate for adult and pediatric populations*

Effectiveness of Pharmacologic Airway Clearance Therapies in Hospitalized Patients[1,2]
AARC Clinical Practice Guideline Summary

Hospitalized Patients without Cystic Fibrosis

1. Recombinant human dornase alfa should not be used in patients with non-cystic fibrosis bronchiectasis.
2. Routine use of bronchodilators to aid in secretion clearance is not recommended.
3. Routine use of aerosolized N-acetylcysteine to improve airway clearance is not recommended.

Neuromuscular Disease, Respiratory Muscle Weakness, or Impaired Cough

The use of aerosolized agents to change sputum physical properties or improve airway clearance are not recommended.

Postoperative

1. Mucolytics are not recommended for use in the treatment of atelectasis.
2. Routine administration of bronchodilators is not recommended.

[1]Adapted from AARC Clinical Practice Guideline: Effectiveness of Pharmacologic Airway Clearance Therapies in Hospitalized Patients, Respiratory Care, July 2015, Vol 60, #7.
[2]Guidelines are appropriate for adult and pediatric populations

Assistive Mechanical Devices

In-Exsufflator (Cof-flator™ or Cough Assist™)	
Description	Applies a positive pressure to the airway (mask or tube) and then rapidly shifts to a negative pressure producing a high expiratory flow rate from the lungs stimulating a cough.
Indications	The inability to effectively cough or clear secretions as a result of reduced peak expiratory flow rates (< 5-6 L/s) as seen in high spinal cord injuries, neuromuscular conditions, or fatigue associated with intrinsic lung disorders.
Contra-indications	• Bullous emphysema, recent barotrauma, or patients prone to pneumothorax or pneumomediastinum. • Patients with cardiovascular instability should be monitored for SpO_2 and HR.

Directions for use	• Patients usually given 4-5 coughing cycles in succession, followed by a 30 second rest period.
	• There are usually 6-10 cycles for a full treatment
	• A typical cycle consists of the following:
	  • The unit slowly builds up positive pressure in the chest over 1-3 sec period to about + 40 mm Hg
	  • Rapidly switch to "exhale" mode with a drop in pressure to − 40 mm Hg in 0.02 seconds (total drop of 80 mm Hg)
	  • Exhalation pressure is held for 2-3 sec
	  • Result: cough/expectoration of secretions
	• The device can be titrated to maximum insufflation by chest wall excursion, bs, and patient comfort
	• Some models allow for "Manual" versus "Automatic" modes. In automatic mode, inspiratory and expiratory times and pressures are set as well as a pause in between breaths. In manual mode, pressures are set, manually switching from Inspiration to Expiration - Breathing at the same rate with the patient can be helpful in synchronizing.
	• May be used by mouthpiece or mask, as well as by tracheostomy
	• Suction should be available to clear the airway during therapy

Positive Expiratory Pressure (PEP) Therapy	
Description	Positive expiratory pressure (PEP Therapy) is the active exhalation against a variable flow resistor reaching pressures of ~ 10-20 cm H_2O.
Indications	PEP Therapy enhances bronchial hygiene therapy by improving airway patency and airflow through airways that are partially obstructed by stenting the airways and/or increasing intrathoracic pressure distal to retained secretions, which: • Reduces air-trapping in susceptible patients • Promotes secretion mobilization and clearance • Enhances collateral ventilation, opens airways behind mucus obstructions, improving pulmonary mechanics + facilitating gas exchange Secondarily, it may help prevent or reverse atelectasis, prevent recurrent infection, and slow disease progression.
Devices	Often a disposable, single-patient use device that is self-administered. It is less time-consuming and does not require the precise positioning of chest physical therapy. Used with FET ("huff coughing").
Procedure	1. Instruct to sit upright with a tight seal around mouthpiece/mask, then inhale, using the diaphragm, to a volume > V_T (but not TLC). 2. Instruct to exhale actively, but not forcefully, to FRC, achieving an airway pressure of 10-20 cm H_2O*. I:E ratio 1:3, 1:4 3. Perform 10-20 breaths through the device, then 2-5 huff coughs. 4. Repeat cycle 5-10 times (15-20 minutes) or until secretions are cleared. *The amount of PEP varies with the size of the adjustable orifice and the level of expiratory pressure generated by the patient. Adjust to meet patient's need.
Oscillatory PEP	The combination of PEP therapy with airway vibrations or oscillations. See *High Frequency Oscillations* on following pages.

Therapies

High Frequency Oscillations (HFO) Summary

See following pages for detailed information on devices

Airway Oscillations

Patient Generated	**Oscillatory PEP Therapy**	The patient's active exhalation through a device performs the work of creating oscillations which are transferred to the patient's airway.
	Ex: Acapella, Flutter, Lung Flute, Quake	
Device Generated	**Intrapulmonary Percussive Ventilation (IPV)**	A device which creates short, rapid inspiratory flow pulses into the airway. Expiration is passive from chest wall elastic recoil.
	Ex: MetaNeb, Percussionator, PercussiveNeb, IMP2	

Chest Wall Oscillations

Device Generated	**High Frequency Chest Wall Compression (HFCWC)** **Vest/Cuirass**	A device which creates short, rapid expiratory flow pulses in the airway by compressing the chest wall externally. Chest wall elastic recoil returns lung to FRC.
	Ex: The Vest, SmartVest, InCourage	
	High Frequency Chest Wall Oscillation (HFCWO)	A device which creates short, rapid biphasic (positive & negative) pressure changes (oscillations) on the chest wall externally, which is transferred to the airway.
	Ex: Hayek Oscillator	

Acapella™	
Description	A disposable, single-patient use device (self-administered) that delivers positive expiratory pressure with high frequency oscillations. Vibratory positive expiratory pressure therapy
Directions	Pt exhales air through an opening that is periodically closed by a pivoting cone. As air passes through the opening, the cone will open and close the airflow path. This produces a vibratory pressure waveform, allowing secretions to be mobilized and expectorated.
Settings	Dial on end of the device sets vibration/oscillation frequency (6-20 Hz). Device is available in three flow rate ranges.

Flutter Device	
Description	A device which produces oscillations in expiratory pressure and airflow. The resultant vibration of the airways loosens mucus from the airway walls.
Contra-indications	Patients with pneumothorax or right-sided heart failure
Directions	• Patient seated with back straight, head tilted slightly back, head tilted slightly back. • Initially, stem is positioned horizontally. Then adjusted up or down to get the maximum "fluttering" effect within the patient's chest (Vibrations can be felt by placing one hand on back and the other on the front of chest). • Patient takes a deep breath (but not to TLC), holds for 2-3 seconds, then exhales actively (but not forcefully) as long as possible while keeping cheeks as hard and flat as possible. • Exhale repeatedly through the device until coughing is stimulated. • Continue for approx. 15 minutes or until patient feels no additional mucus can be raised. • Perform procedure 2-4 times/day or as directed.

Intrapulmonary Percussive Ventilation (IPV)	
Description	The delivery of high-frequency percussive breaths (sub-tidal volume) into the patient's airways by a pneumatic device.
Indications	The inability to effectively cough or clear secretions as a result of reduced peak expiratory flow rates.
Contra-indications	Bronchospasm, lung contusion, pneumothorax, pulmonary hemorrhage, subcutaneous emphysema, TB, vomiting and aspiration.
Directions	• Pt breathes through a mouthpiece or artificial airway and the unit delivers high flow rate bursts of gas into the lungs from 100-300/min. Continuous positive pressure is maintained (typically 15-40 cm H_2O) while the pulses dilate the airways. At the end of the percussive inspiratory cycle (5-10 sec), a deep exhalation is performed with expectoration of secretions. • Normal treatment time is 20 min. Aerosols (bland or medicated) may also be delivered via the attached nebulizer.
Settings	• Pressure is set via a manometer with optimum range being 30-40 cm H_2O (less for ↑ Compliance, more for ↓ Compliance). This is equivalent to setting a "mean airway pressure" • Difficulty knob changes the frequency of the oscillations which may improve clearance and recruitment. It is recommended that this knob be turned back and forth every few minutes during treatment.
Notes	• Can be performed with mechanical ventilation • Circuit configurations are different for ventilator versus non-vented, and should be assembled carefully • When effective, several breaks may need to be taken in order to get pt to cough or suction. • Many clinicians recommend utilizing an in-line suction catheter when used in conjunction with an artificial airway to facilitate suctioning. • Cuffed artificial airways: Suction above cuff, and then at least partially deflate cuff during treatment to facilitate secretion clearance.

Percussive vests/wraps	
Description	• The system includes an air pulse generator, inflatable vest, and connecting tube. • It provides high frequency chest wall compressions which help mobilize secretions.
Indications	• Cystic fibrosis, bronchiectasis, or conditions where the patient is unable to effectively mobilize and expectorate secretions.
Contra-indications	Active hemorrhage, cardiac instability, chest wall pain, lung contusion, recent thoracic skin grafts, recently placed pacemaker, subcutaneous emphysema, suspected tuberculosis, unstable head and/or neck injury.
Directions	• As the patient wears the inflatable vest, small gas volumes alternately flow into and out of the unit – rapidly inflating and deflating (compressing and releasing) the chest wall to create air flow and cough-like shear forces to move secretions. • Timing of the pulse is manually controlled by the patient or clinician • The intensity (25-40 mm Hg) and frequency (5-25 Hz) of the pulses can also be adjusted by the patient or clinician • Vests come in various styles (full chest vest down to simple wrap around chest), disposable/nondisposable, and sizes. Ensuring a proper fit and style helps ensure better pt compliance with therapy.

Airway Clearance Selection Algorithm

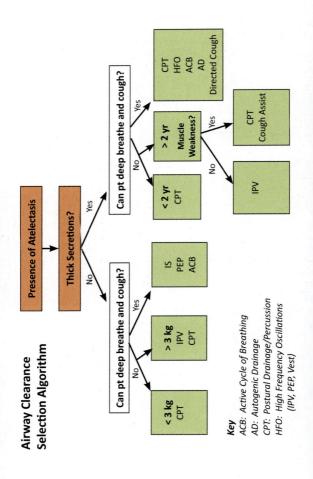

Key
ACB: Active Cycle of Breathing
AD: Autogenic Drainage
CPT: Postural Drainage/Percussion
HFO: High Frequency Oscillations
(IPV, PEP, Vest)

Summary Recommendations for Airway Management by the American College of Chest Physicians*

Recommendations are based upon 2006 Guidelines which remain active. Recommendations in general support teaching airway clearance techniques to patients, the specific technique determined by disease severity and secretion characteristics using an individualized approach.

Autogenic Drainage
Should be taught as an adjunct to postural drainage for patients with CF as it can be performed without assistance and in one position.
Chest Physical Therapy
Recommended in CF patients as an effective technique to increase mucus clearance. Long-term benefits are unproven.
Cough Assist
Mechanical cough assist devices are recommended in patients with neuromuscular disease with an impaired cough
Expiratory Muscle Training
Recommended in patients with neuromuscular weakness and impaired cough to improve peak expiratory pressures
High Frequency Techniques
Consider as an alternative to chest physiotherapy for patients with CF
Huff Cough
Consider in addition to other methods of clearance in COPD/CF
Manually-Assisted Cough
Should be considered in patients with expiratory muscle weakness to reduce the incidence of respiratory complications. Avoid use with obstructive disorders (COPD, etc.)
Positive Expiratory Pressure Therapy
Recommended in patients with CF over conventional chest physiotherapy, because it is approximately as effective as chest physiotherapy, and is inexpensive, safe, and can be self-administered.

* Nonpharmacologic Airway Clearance Therapies: ACCP Evidence-Based Clinical Practice Guidelines, ***Chest***. 2006; 129:250S-259S. See also Chestnet.org.

Humidity Therapy

Variable	Considerations
Indications	**Primary Indications** • Humidify dry medical gases (> 4 L/min) • Overcome humidity deficit when upper airway is bypassed **Secondary Indications** • Treat bronchospasm due to cold air • Treat hypothermia • Thickened secretions
Therapeutic Modalities	Used specifically with the following modalities: • Oxygen therapy with higher flow rates • Non-invasive positive pressure ventilation (CPAP and NPPV ventilation) • Invasive positive pressure ventilation • Artificial airways via collar or T-Piece
Under-Humidification	• Atelectasis (mucus plugging) • Dry, nonproductive cough • Substernal pain • Thick, dehydrated secretions • Hypoxemia • ↑ Airway Resistance • ↑ Infection • ↑ WOB
Over-Humidification	• Fluid overload • Pulmonary edema • Surfactant alteration • Thermal damage to mucosa • ↑ Airway secretions (↑ airway resistance) • Atelectasis • Hypoxemia
Heat	• Heated humidification is recommended for artificial airways, thick secretions, and/or patient comfort

Humidification Devices

Type	Use	Comments
Low Flow		
Bubble Diffuser	Used with low flow devices (>4 L/min) and air entrainment masks (> 50%)	Provides only 20% to 40% of body humidity, may be heated to deliver 100% humidity (and with low-flow devices), should not be used for patients with ET tube or tracheostomy. If whistle is heard, bubble humidifier is building up with pressure.
High Flow		
Cascade Humidifier	Mainstream "bubble" humidifier for patients with ET tube or tracheostomy.	100% humidity and body temperature. Correct water level is required
Passover Humidifier	Used for either low or high flow devices (CPAP/ NPPV) and ventilators.	Effective humidity only when heated to body temperature
Wick Humidifier	Mainstream "passover" using a porous hygroscopic "wick" to ↑ surface area.	100% humidity and body temperature
Heat/Moisture Exchanger (HME) (Hygroscopic condenser humidifier [HCH] or artificial nose)	Mainstream "passover" reservoir containing hygroscopic material. Short-term use with mechanical ventilation (≤ 5 days)	Condenses and "traps" exhaled heat and moisture and then evaporates, warms, and humidifies the inhaled gas. (= 70% body humidity) Exchange daily or per manufacturer
Room Humidifier (cool mist, steam vaporizer, centrifugal)	Used to humidify the room.	Produces 100% humidity at room temperature when in a closed area. Should not be used with ET tube or trach.

Therapies

Notes (from opposite page):
Sterile water should be used in bubble humidifiers.
Monitor patient's quantity and quality of airway secretions.

HME: Inspect regularly for partial or complete obstruction by secretions

Heated Humidity
- Close monitoring of operating and output temperatures, adequate water supply/proper level, and condensation buildup is required
- Prevent inadvertent tracheal lavage from the condensate
- Check that alarms are set and working properly

Humidification During Invasive and Noninvasive Mechanical Ventilation[1] (AARC Expert Reference-Based Guideline)

Indication
Mandatory with ET tube or Trach Tube.
Optional with NIV (use HH if humidifying)

Contraindication
None except **HME** when: Body temperature < 32°C, low V_T strategies, expired V_T < 70% of delivered V_T, spont $\dot{V}_E$ > 10 L/min, thick, copious, or bloody secretions.

Monitoring
Check: alarm settings (30 – 41°C) (HH), humidifier temp setting (HH), inspired gas temp (34-40°C) (HH), water level and feed system (HH), sputum quantity and consistency
Remove condensate in circuit, Replace HMEs contaminated with secretions

Frequency:
Continuous during gas therapy

Hazards/Complications
Burns (patient or caregiver)(HH)
Electrical shock (HH)
Hypo/hyperthermia
Hypoventilation (HME → ↑VD)
↑ Resistive WOB through humidifier
Infection (nosocomial)
Tracheal lavage (pooled condensate or overfilling) (HH)
Underhydration (mucous impaction or plugging of airways → air-trapping, hypoventilation, ↑ WOB)
Ventilator malperformance: pooled condensate → ↑ airway pressures or asynchrony with patient (HH)
HME → ineffective low pressure alarm during disconnection

Clinical Goal
Humidified and warmed inspired gases without hazards or complications.

1) Adapted from AARC Clinical Practice Guideline: Humidification During Invasive and Noninvasive Mechanical Ventilation, ***Respiratory Care*** Vol. 57, #5, 2012.
HH = heated humidity, HME = heat moisture exchanger

Lung Expansion Therapy

Variable	Considerations
Indications	Risk for, or evidence of atelectasis (usually secondary to pt either not taking deep breaths, or unable to) See *types of atelectasis, page 10-19*

Clinical Signs	• **History:**
	  • Recent abdominal or thoracic surgery
	  • COPD or cigarette smoking
	  • Prolonged bed rest
	  • Morbid obesity
	• **↑ RR, ↑ HR**
	• **Auscultation:**
	  • Crackles (fine)
	  • Bronchial (consolidation)
	  • ↓ BS (blocked airways)
	• **CXR:**
	  • ↓ volumes (tracheal shift if severe)
	  • Opacity
	  • Air bronchograms
	  • Elevated diaphragm

Minimally Intensive (Self)	• Encourage deep breaths
(Device)	• Incentive spirometry • PEP therapies (Acapella, Flutter) - *see airway clearance, 9-27*
Intensive (Device + Time)	• Intermittent Positive Pressure Breathing (IPPB) • Intrapercussive Ventilation (IPV) - *see airway clearance, 9-27* • Continuous Positive Airway Pressure (CPAP)
Most Intensive	• Therapeutic bronchoscopy (resorptive)

Incentive Spirometry (IS)	
Description	• Device which encourages deep breathing, usually with measurement (mL) of breath size, as well as indicator of speed (slow is more effective)
Technique	• Designed to mimic natural sigh breaths, by encouraging patients to take slow, deep diaphragmatic inspirations (performing an IC from FRC to near TLC), followed by 5-10 sec breath hold. • Pt should be sitting upright to be most effective. • Directions should be intentionally worded (put the mouthpiece in your mouth, and then take a slow deep breath in like you're drinking a milkshake from a straw). Demonstration may assist in learning. • Set realistic goals, but ones that encourage pt to keep pushing further. • Patient should exhale normally and then rest as long as necessary between maneuvers (prevents respiratory alkalosis) • Each session should contain a minimum of 5-10 breaths, generally with a minimum of 10 breaths/hour.
Notes	• For post-surgical use, it is best to teach technique prior to surgery and have pt practice (it is more difficult to teach a new skill with pain medication interfering). • Device should be placed in plain sight and reach of pt. Instruct family and/or other available staff to assist in encouraging compliance. • For pts that struggle with technique/coordination, consider instead on focusing on key elements without device - deep, slow breaths with 5-10 second hold.

Incentive Spirometry [1,2]
(AARC Expert Panel Reference-Based Guideline)

Indications
Screen at-risk patients for post-op complications:
  Pre-op screening to obtain baseline
Atelectasis or predisp. for:
  Surgery (upper/lower abdom, thoracic, COPD, prolonged bedrest, lack of pain control, restrictive lung defect (dysfunctional diaphragm or muscles, NM disease, SCI), sickle cell, CABG

Contraindications
Patient unable or unwilling to use device appropriately (including young pts, delirium, heavy sedation)
Patient unable to take deep breath (VC < 10 mL/kg or IC < 1/3 predicted)

Hazards/Complications
Fatigue
Hyperventilation
Inappropriate (as sole tx for major collapse/consolidat)
Ineffective (if used incorrectly)
Hypoxemia (O2 therapy interrupt)
Pain

Monitoring
Initial instruction and observation of proper performance.
Periodic observation for:
  compliance, frequency, number of breaths/session, volume or flow goals (improvement), effort, motivation, device availability,

Suggested Frequencies
10x every 1-2 hr while awake
10 breaths - 5x/day
15x every 4 hrs

Outcome Assessment
Decreased atelectasis –
Breath sounds improved, fever resolved, ↑oxygenation, reduced FIO_2 requirement, improved chest x-ray, pulse rate normal, respiratory rate ↓

See Next Page for Evidence-Based Recommendations
(based on GRADE scoring system)

---

1) IS is a component of bronchial hygiene therapy designed to encourage spontaneously breathing patients to take long, slow, deep breaths and hold them for ≥3 seconds (sustained maximal inspiration, SMI). The primary purpose is to maintain airway patency and prevent/reverse atelectasis.

2) Adapted from the AARC Clinical Practice Guideline: Incentive Spirometry, ***Respiratory Care***, Volume 56, #10, 2011.

AARC Evidence-Based Recommendations: IS
(based on GRADE system)

- Incentive spirometry alone is **not** recommended for routine use in the preoperative and postoperative setting to prevent postoperative pulmonary complications.
- It **is** recommended that incentive spirometry be used with deep breathing techniques, directed coughing, early mobilization, and optimal analgesia to prevent postoperative pulmonary complications.
- It **is** suggested that deep breathing exercises provide the same benefit as incentive spirometry in the preoperative and postoperative setting to prevent postoperative complications
- Routine use of incentive spirometry to prevent atelectasis in patients after upper-abdominal surgery is **not** recommended
- Routine use of incentive spirometry to prevent atelectasis after coronary artery bypass graft surgery is **not** recommended.
- It **is** suggested that a volume-oriented device be selected as an incentive spirometry device.

Intermittent Positive Pressure Breathing (IPPB)

Goal	• An augmented V_T, achieved with minimal effort
Technique	• Semi-Fowler's position is preferred; supine is acceptable when an upright position is contraindicated. • Effectiveness is usually dependent on proper patient instruction and demonstration. • Use mouthpiece/noseclips - mask as last resort. • Optimal breathing pattern is slow, deep breaths held at end-inspiration. • Resulting volumes should be measured and pressure adjusted according to needs and response. • Note: To be effective, Deliver VT > Pt spont efforts • Bland aerosols (NSS) can be delivered via IPPB, but more often, medicated aerosols consisting of a bronchodilator, mucoactive or combination are used. • Treatments usually last 15 - 20 minutes.

Common Goals and Settings

Parameter	Suggested Goal/Setting
Sensitivity	1-2 cmH$_2$O (easy trigger, but no autocycle)
Pressure	Initial: 10-15 cm H$_2$O Goal: set to Target V_T (see below)
Target Vol.	10-15 cc/kg PBW (30% pred. IC)
Rate	6 breaths/min
I:E Ratio	1:3 to 1:4

Troubleshooting

Large negative Pressure swings	Incorrect sensitivity: set to autotrigger, then decrease sens until pt able to trigger easily
↓ Press after insp. begins; failure to rise until breath's end	Inspiratory flow too low
Premature cycle off	Insp flow too high or airflow obstructed (kinked tubing, occluded mouthpiece, active resistance to inhalation)
Failure to cycle off	Leak (neb, exhalation, pt interface, nose)

IPPB[1,2]
(AARC Expert Panel Reference-Based Guideline)

Indications

Lung expansion –
Atelectasis (when not responsive to other therapies or patient can't/won't cooperate)
Secretions (inability to clear)

Short-term ventilation (alternative form of MV for hypoventilating patients, consider NPPV)

Delivery of aerosolized medication [3] –
Used when other aerosol techniques have been unsuccessful. [4]
Patients with fatigue, severe hyperinflation or during short-term ventilation.

Assessment of Need

Acute, severe, unresponsive bronchospasm/ COPD exac.
Impending respiratory failure
NM disorders
PFT (FEV1 < 65% pred, FVC < 70% pred, MVV < 50% pred, VC < 10 mL/kg) w/o eff cough
Significant atelectasis

Contraindications

Absolute – untreated tension pneumothorax
Relative – active hemoptysis, active untreated TB, air swallowing, bleb, hemo instability, hiccups, ICP > 15 mm Hg, nausea, recent oral, facial, esophageal or skull surgery, TE fistula.

Monitoring

Patient: RR, V_T, HR, rhythm, BP, BS, response (mental function, pain, discomfort, dyspnea), skin color, O_2 Sat, sputum, ICP, chest x-ray.
Machine: f, V_T peak, plateau, PEEP pressures, sensitivity, flow, FIO_2, T_I, T_E.

Clinical Goals

For lung expansion: a V_T of at least 33% of IC predicted
↑ FEV_1 or PF
More effective cough, enhanced secretion clearance, improved chest x-ray and BS, good patient response.

Hazards/Complications

Air trapping (auto PEEP), barotrauma, ↓ venous return, exacerbation of hypoxemia, gastric distention, hemoptysis, hyperoxia (with O_2), hypocarbia, hypo / hyperventilation, ↑Raw, V/Q mismatch, infection, psychological dependence, secretion impaction.

Frequency

Critical care: q 1-6 hrs as tolerated, re-evaluate daily

Acute care: bid to 4 times per day per patient response, re-evaluate q 24 hrs

SEE NOTES NEXT PAGE

NOTES (from Previous Page)
1) Intermittent positive pressure breathing (IPPB) is intermittent, or short-term mechanical ventilation for the purpose of augmenting lung expansion, assisting ventilation, and/or delivering an aerosolized medication (not the therapy of first choice) (Does not include NPPV).
2) Adapted from the AARC Clinical Practice Guideline: IPPB, 2003 Revision + Update, ***Respiratory Care***, Volume 48, #5, 2003.
3) Efficacy is technique dependent (coordination, breathing pattern, VI, PIP, inspiratory hold), device design, and patient instruction.
4) MDI or nebs are devices of choice for aerosol therapy to COPD or stable asthma patients.

Medical Gases

Cylinder Color Standards, by Gas
This is provided as a reference. Never administer a gas solely based upon the color of the canister, wall plate, or gas adapter. Confirm by label and if any doubt analyze the gas prior to administering to a patient.

Gas	USA	ISO*
Air (Medical) Pin Position: 1-5	Yellow/Silver	White/Black
Carbogen (CO_2 + O_2)	Gray/Green	Grey/White
Carbon Dioxide (CO_2)	Gray	Grey
Cyclopropane (C_3H_6)	Orange	Orange
Ethylene (C_2H_4)	Red	Violet
Heliox (He and O_2)	Brown/Green	Brown/White
Helium** (He)	Brown	Brown
Nitrogen (N_2)	Black	Black
Nitrous Oxide (N_2O)	Blue	Blue
Oxygen (O_2) Pin Position: 2-5	Green	White

*ISO: International Standards Organization

**Never administer helium in its pure form to a patient. It must be mixed with oxygen prior to administration.

E-Cylinder (O₂) Estimated Tank Duration in Minutes *(no reserve)*
(0.28 x PSIG / Liters per Minute)

L/min	Pressure (PSIG)							
	500 (reserve)	750	1,000	1,250	1,500	1,750	2,000	2,200
1	140	210	280	350	420	490	560	616
2	70	105	140	175	210	245	280	308
3	46	70	93	116	140	163	186	205
4	35	52	70	87	105	122	140	154
5	28	42	56	70	84	98	112	123
6	23	35	46	58	70	81	93	102
10	14	21	28	35	42	49	56	61
12	11	17	23	29	35	40	46	51
15	09	14	18	23	28	32	37	41

H-Cylinder (O₂) Estimated Tank Duration in Minutes *(no reserve)*
(3.14 x PSIG / Liters per Minute)

L/min	Pressure (PSIG)							
	500 (reserve)	750	1,000	1,250	1,500	1,750	2,000	2,200
1	1570	2355	3140	3925	4710	5495	6280	6908
2	785	1177	1570	1962	2355	2747	3140	3454
3	523	785	1046	1308	1570	1831	2093	2302
4	392	588	785	981	1177	1373	1570	1727
5	314	471	628	785	942	1099	1256	1381
6	261	392	523	654	785	915	1046	1151
10	157	235	314	392	471	549	628	690
12	130	196	261	327	392	457	523	575
15	104	157	209	261	314	366	418	460

*****These charts represent total duration with no Reserve.** Best Clinical practice dictates not including the last 500 PSI in your calculation (this is emergency reserve).

See Chapter 13 for Detailed Oxygen Duration Equations

Monitoring Oxygenation Status

Measures of Oxygenation
(see also pg 9-75)

Method	Normal Values	Description
Noninvasive		
SpO_2	> 95%	Peripheral O_2 saturation (measured hemoglobin saturation by a pulse oximeter)
TCOM	~80-100 mm Hg	Transcutaneous monitoring estimates PaO_2 by inducing hyperperfusion (via heating) of skin site; measures electrochemically
Invasive		
PaO_2	80-100 mm Hg	Partial pressure of oxygen molecules within blood from ABG (not those bound to hemoglobin)
SaO_2	> 93%	Calculated oxygen saturation from PaO_2 (if an analyzer) or actual measured value (co-oximeter)

Notes:
- Trends are more important than single measures
- SpO_2 may be a poor indicator of SaO_2
- Periodic baseline correlations should be made with PaO_2 and/or SaO_2 (Co-oximetry).
- Pulse oximetry alone can not indicate hyperoxemia (maximum is 100%).
- SpO_2 values may vary between various models of oximeters, so caution in interchanging oximeters on same pt

Troubleshooting the Pulse Oximeter

Problem	Possible Cause(s)	Interventions
Inaccurate SpO$_2$ (does not correlate with SaO$_2$ from ABG) *New pulse oximeters are less likely to cause these problems	**Patient** • Movement* • Poor perfusion (cool skin, PVD, etc.) • Skin pigment (darker)* • High carboxyhemoglobin or methemoglobin • Reduced arterial blood flow	• Encourage pt to be still, if possible or able • Check sensor site - consider moving from one finger to another, earlobe, toe, forehead, naris (correlate w/ ABG) • Consider replacing sensor • Use other forms of measure if needed to confirm (ABG, TCM, etc.) • Warm site with approved warming device
	Environment • Cool Room* • Ambient Light* • BP Cuff Placement	• Warm site with approved warming device • Cover sensor to block ambient light • Ensure sensor is not distal to BP cuff
	Equipment • Blood Pressure • Sensor not adhering well	• Ensure sensor is placed securely; replace if necessary. • Check sensor site - consider moving from one finger to another, earlobe, toe, forehead, nare • Consider different type of sensor (neonatal, etc.) • Use ECG signal synchronization. • Select a longer (10-15 sec) averaging time, if possible.

Therapies

Problem	Possible Cause(s)	Interventions
Loss of Pulse Signal, Poor Waveform *New pulse oximeters are less likely to cause these problems	**Patient** • Reduced arterial blood flow • Anemia • Hypothermia • Shock (hypotension, vasocon) • Nail polish*	• Confirm or follow with ABG • Check Hemoglobin level • Consider warming site, replace sensor • Always check pt's condition, vitals • More likely to interfere if contains metallic flakes, remove
	Environment • Excessive ambient light*	• Cover sensor to block ambient light
	Equipment • Constriction by sensor • Sensor is not on patient	• Check sensor • Move to a different site or change type of sensor used • Confirm sensor is on patient
Inaccurate Pulse Rate	**Patient** • Excessive patient motion	• Encourage pt to be still if possible, or able
	Equipment • Pronounced dicrotic notch on art. waveform • Poor quality ECG signal • Electrocautery interference	• Move sensor to a different site • Check ECG leads; replace if necessary. • Same as above.

Transcutaneous Monitoring

Oxygen ($PtcO_2$) and Carbon Dioxide ($PtcCO_2$) can both be monitored.

Indications:
- Diagnosis, clinical management, and early identification of cardiac and respiratory problems
- Prevention of hyperoxia/hypoxia, hypercapnia/hypocapnia
- Evaluate response to therapeutic interventions, including noninvasive and invasive therapies
- Monitor effects of apnea, right-to-left shunts, crying, and breath-holding ($PtcO_2$)

Technique:
A heated electrode (*Clark* for Oxygen, *Severinghaus* for Carbon Dioxide) is placed on the skin surface (the heat arterializes the site and increases permeability to gas diffusion)

Preferred Sites *(Avoid bony areas and extremities)*:

- Anterior chest
- Abdomen
- Back
- Inner thigh

Hazards:
- Burns (rotate site every 2-6 hours)
- Values are dependent on barometric pressure
- May underestimate PaO_2 in children with chronic conditions (BPD)

Interpretation

$PtcO_2$	reads lower than actual PaO_2 (dependent on dissociation curve)
$PtcCO_2$	reads higher than actual $PaCO_2$ (by 2-20 mm Hg)

- Transcutaneous measures must be correlated with appropriate blood gas values. Draw an ABG, being sure to record transcutaneous values <u>at the time of the blood draw</u>, then correlate.
- Note that $PtcO_2$ is a crude but accurate estimate of PaO_2. $PtcCO_2$ is less reliable

Therapies

Lung Adequacy

Relationship of SpO₂ to PaO₂

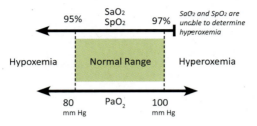

SaO₂ and SpO₂ are unable to determine hyperoxemia

PaO₂ (mm Hg)	SaO₂* (%)
150	100
100	97
80	95
60	90
55	88
40	75

* varies with shifts in oxyhemoglobin curve

! Always Check for proper correlation between the PaO₂/SaO₂ calculated values and the measured SpO₂ value.

Oxyhemoglobin Dissociation Curve

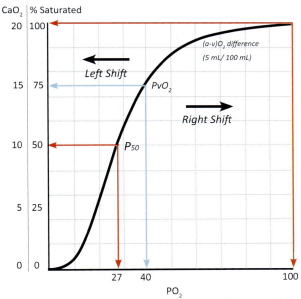

- The graph above is the normal curve. A shift to the right or left will affect the affinity of hemoglobin for oxygen (see table below)
- P_{50} (labeled above) is the PaO_2 when hemoglobin is 50% saturated. This is normally 27 mm Hg.

Left Shift (↑ Hgb-O_2 affinity; ↓ P_{50})	Right Shift (↓ Hgb-O_2 affinity; ↑ P_{50})

Alkalosis
Decreased:
  temp, PCO_2, PO^4, 2,3 DPG
Polycythemia
Abnormal Hgb
  (Fetal Hgb, HgbCo, metHgb)
	Acidosis
	Increased:
	  temp, PCO_2, PO^4, 2,3 DPG
	Anemias (sickle cell)
	Chronic hypoxemia (high altitude)

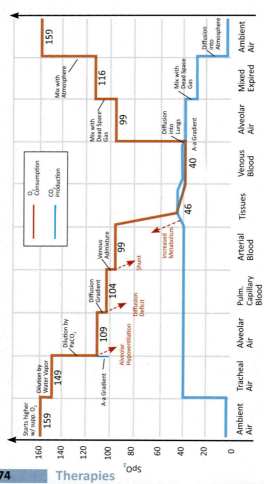

Assessment of Oxygenation

Oxygenation at the Lungs (external respiration)			Oxygenation at the Tissues (internal respiration)		
Value	Normal	Abnorm	Value	Normal	Abnorm
Adequacy					
PaO_2*	80-100 mm Hg	< 80 mm Hg	$P\bar{v}O_2$	35-42 mm Hg	< 35 or > 45 mm Hg
CaO_2	15-24 mL/dL	↑↓	$C\bar{v}O_2$	12-15 mL/dL	↑↓
SaO_2**	> 95%	< 95%	$S\bar{v}O_2$	60-80%	< 60%
SpO_2	> 95%	< 95%	$C(a-\bar{v})O_2$	4.5-5.0 mL/dL	↑↓
Efficiency					
$P(A-a)O_2$	10-25 mm Hg (room air) 30-50 mm Hg (100%)	>25 mm Hg	O_2ER	25%	↑↓
			$\dot{V}O_2$	200 - 250 mL/min	↑↓
			$\dot{D}O_2$	750 - 1000 mL/min	↑↓
PaO_2/PAO_2	0.8-0.9	<0.6	VQI	0.8	↑↓
PaO_2/FIO_2	> 300	< 300			
$P(A-a)O_2/PaO_2$	< 1.0	> 1.0			
$\dot{Q}_S/\dot{Q}_T$ phys	2-5%	> 20%			

*Normal Variations: Due to age, FIO_2, or barometric pressure
Age: $PaO_2 \approx 110 - 1/2$ patient's age
**SaO_2: Calculated O_2 saturation from PaO_2
SpO_2: Peripheral O_2 saturation: measured value of Hgb saturation with a pulse oximeter.

Hypoxemia
Levels of Hypoxemia

	PaO₂	SpO₂ %	Clinical Notes
Mild Hypoxemia	60-79 mm Hg	90-94%	
Moderate Hypoxemia	40-59 mm Hg	75-89%	
Severe Hypoxemia	< 40 mm Hg	< 75%	30 mm Hg: loss of consciousness 20 mm Hg: anoxic brain injury likely

Hypoxemia is considered **responsive** if there is an expected increase in PaO₂ with delivery of supplemental O₂ (PaO₂ should increase by at least 5 torr for every 10% increase in O₂)

Hypoxemia is considered **refractory** if there is little (< 5 torr) or no response of PaO₂ to an increase in supplemental O₂

See Diseases (page 10-63) for details on Hypercapnic vs. Hypoxemic Respiratory Failure

Hypoxemia vs Hypoxia

Hypoxemia	Oxygenation below normal (abnormally low PaO₂, SaO₂, SpO₂, etc.)
Hypoxia	Failure of oxygenation at the tissue level (insufficient O₂ to meet metabolic demands of the tissues)

The presence of hypoxemia suggests hypoxia, but:
- Hypoxemia without hypoxia: compensation for low PaO₂ by increasing O₂ delivery
- Hypoxia without hypoxemia: tissues unable to use oxygen effectively, or if oxygen delivery to the tissues in general is impaired

Signs and Symptoms of Hypoxemia/Hypoxia*

In general, hypoxemia leads to hypoxia. Once hypoxia occurs, cells are robbed of the oxygen they need to function aerobically. Some tissue recovers from periods of hypoxia (skeletal muscle, for example), while others may have irreparable damage (brain, etc.)

Mild *Body compensates*	Tachypnea Tachycardia Dyspnea Pallor Increased BP Diaphoresis
Moderate *Transition as effects become more apparent*	Headache Anxiety Cyanosis Arrhythmias Vision changes Confusion
Severe *Body unable to compensate (tiring)* *Cell death becomes apparent (due to lack of needed O_2)*	Bradycardia Hypotension Nausea/vomiting Lethargy Tremors Stupor/Coma Loss of pupillary response Death
Chronic *Range of symptoms vary by underlying disease severity*	Arrhythmias Decreased cardiac output Digital clubbing Dyspnea/dyspnea on exertion Irritability Fatigue Polycythemia Pulmonary hypertension Myoclonic jerking/tremors Vision issues (papilledema)

* The time between changes in symptom severity (for example: from confusion to lethargy to stupor/death) may vary. Hypoxia, especially moderate or severe signs, should be treated as a medical emergency

Types & Causes of Hypoxemia/Hypoxia

Types	Causes		Examples
Hypoxic Hypoxia (Alveolar)	**Dead Space (alveolar)** (wasted ventilation; ventilation without perfusion) (V/Q)		• Complete block: Pulmonary embolism (air, blood, fat, tumor) • ↓ Blood Flow: Shock, cardiac arrest, ↑ PVR • ↑V/↓Q: ↑ VT and/or PEEP (↑ lung zones 1+2 from ↑ Palv)
	Shunt		**Anatomical shunts:** Pleural, bronchial, Thebesian veins, anatomical defects **Capillary shunts and/or shunt effect:** • Alveoli collapsed, fluid filled or blocked (complete or partial): ARDS, atelectasis (most common), cystic fibrosis, pneumonia, pneumothorax, pulmonary edema • ↓ or no alveolar ventilation: Airway obstruction, asthma, COPD, position changes, secretions, etc.
		Absolute (True) $0/\dot{Q}$*	Perfusion without ventilation
		Relative ↓V/Q	Perfusion with ↓ ventilation (V/Q mismatch, shunt effect, venous admixture)
	The 0 indicates NO ventilation		
	Diffusion Defect (↑ a-c membrane thickness)		Alveolar and/or interstitial inflammation/fibrosis: pulmonary fibrosis, interstitial lung disease, ARDS

Types	Causes	Examples
Hypoxic Hypoxia (Atmospheric)	**Primary Cause: Lungs** (or supply) Reduction of PAO_2 - a lack of available oxygen	↓ FIO_2:: Drowning (no O_2), O_2 therapy error (unintentionally leaving a patient off necessary oxygen) ↓ PAO_2: High altitude (PaO_2 ↓ as altitude ↑), Hypoventilation
Anemic Hypoxia (Hemoglobic)	**Primary Cause: Hemoglobin** Decrease in oxygen content (CaO_2)	Decreased hemoglobin (anemia, hemorrhage), abnormal hemoglobins (carboxyhemoglobinemia, methemoglobinemia, etc.)
Histotoxic Hypoxia	**Primary Cause: Tissues** Lungs and circulatory system are working, but the tissues are unable to use the oxygen	Cyanide poisoning, sepsis (NO overproduction, antioxidant depletion)
Circulatory Hypoxia (Stagnant)	**Primary Cause: Cardiovascular** Stagnant or hypoperfusion (blood flow to cells is inadequate) = pump issue	Cardiovascular failure, ↓ cardiac output, hemorrhage, arrhythmias

Hypoxemia Diagnostic Algorithm

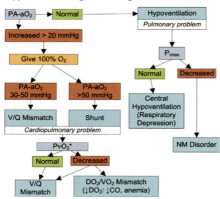

* $P\bar{v}O_2$ is obtained from a CVP line or PA catheter

Types of Hypoxemia/Hypoxia, by Abnormal Values

Types		PAO_2	PaO_2	$P(A-a)O_2$	$P(a-v)O_2$	$PaCO_2$	$PACO_2$	$P(a-A)CO_2$
Atmospheric		↓	↓	N	N	↓	↓	N
Tidal (Hypoventilation)		↓	↓	N ↑	N	↑	↑	N
ALVEOLAR	Dead Space	N ↓	N ↓	N ↕	N ↕	N ↕	↓	↑
	Absolute Shunt	N ↑	↓	↑	↑	N ↕	N ↕	N ↕
	V/Q Mismatch	N	↓	↑	↑	N ↕	N ↕	N ↕
	Diffusion defect	N	N ↓	↑	N	N ↓	N ↓	N
Hemoglobic		N	N	N	N	N ↓	N ↓	N
Circulatory (stagnant)		N	↓	↑	↑↑	N ↕	N ↕	N ↕
Histotoxic		N	N	N	↓	N	N	N
Demand		Any of the above						

Oxygen Therapy

Goals should balance the need to avoid tissue hypoxia (thought to be < 55-60 mm Hg) with the need to avoid hyperoxemia (no defined limit, but the goal should be to deliver the least amount of supplemental oxygen to maintain adequate oxygenation)

Suggested Oxygenation Targets in Adults*

Patient	PaO_2** (mm Hg)	SpO_2 (%)	Rationale
Acute Infection/Process	80-90	95-97	No chronic lung disease, maintain adequate O_2 tension
Coronary Artery Disease	80-90	95-97	May not clinically tolerate hypoxemia
Pulmonary Hypertension (severe ↓ DLCO)	80-90	95-97	May not clinically tolerate hypoxemia
Chronic Lung Disease***	60-65	90-92	Maintain reasonable oxygenation goals, COPD-GOLD guidelines
ARDS	55-80	88-95	ARDSnet guidelines

*Both lower limits (to avoid tissue hypoxia) and upper limits (to avoid hyperoxia/oxygen toxicity) should be established. Hyperoxia is known to cause lung injury (parenchymal, airway, extrapulmonary) and clinically should be actively avoided.

**It is important to remember that treating to achieve a PaO_2 of > 90 mm Hg has minimal additional effect (see pg 9-73 Oxygen Dissociation Curve)

***Withholding oxygen from a patient with COPD due to fear of hypoxic drive is contraindicated. Instead, establish reasonable oxygenation goals (such as those listed above) and do not allow oxygenation to drop below that (as tissue hypoxia will occur, leading to cell death). Goals provided are from GOLD (see Disease Ch)

Oxygen Therapy for Adults in the Acute Care Facility[1]
(AARC Expert Panel Evidence-Based Guideline)

Indications
Acute MI
Hypoxemia (actual or suspected)
  PaO_2 < 60 mm Hg
  SaO_2 < 90%
  (or below desired) in adults, children, infants > 28 days in room air.
Severe trauma
Short-term therapy or postop

Precautions/Complications
Ventilatory depression: patients on an O_2 drive with elevated $PaCO_2$ and $PaO_2 \geq$ 60 mm Hg.
F_IO_2 > 0.5: absorption atelectasis, ↓ciliary function, ↓leukocyte function, fire hazard, bacterial contamination (humidification system), caution in patients with paraquat poisoning or receiving bleomycin, O_2 toxicity.

Contraindications
none

Monitoring
Patient:
Clinical assessment (pulm, CV, neuro status)
PaO_2 and/or SaO_2:
Upon initiation of therapy or within –
  2 hours (COPD)
  8 hours (FIO_2 > 0.4)
  12 hours (FIO_2 < 0.4)
  72 hours (acute MI)

Equipment:
every day or more frequent when: FIO_2 > 0.5, clinically unstable, heated gas mixture, artificial airway, blending systems.

Frequency
Continuous or intermittent (exercise, sleep)

---

1) Adapted from the AARC Clinical Practice Guidelines: Oxygen Therapy for Adults in the Acute Care Facility, 2002 Revision & Update ***Respiratory Care***, Volume 47, #6, 2002.

Oxygen Delivery Devices

Delivery System	Liter flow	O2% delivered	Clinical Considerations	Hazards (strategies to address)
Low Flow Devices: Actual oxygen % delivered varies with the patient's inspiratory needs (may deliver 100% if flow > patient's inspiratory demand; otherwise room air is entrained to meet total flow need)				
Nasal Cannula	1-6 L/min	24-44% (~21% + 4% per set liter)	**Standard for lower oxygen needs** Many benefits: inexpensive, usually well-tolerated as patient can eat, talk, and sleep. Risk of dislodging	Dry nose, dry throat, nosebleed (humidify at 4+ L/min or per patient comfort) Skin breakdown (monitor, pad contact areas when possible Deviated septum may block flow (use other method)
Nasal Catheter	2-5 L/min	24-45%	*Uncommonly used* Soft catheter with multiple holes at tip, inserted through nare to sit at oropharynx (distance = length of nose to tragus) Usually secured to bridge of nose. Must be changed every 8 hours.	May cause dry throat (humidify) May become clogged (change every 8-hours, monitor)

Delivery System	Liter flow	O2% delivered	Clinical Considerations	Hazards (strategies to address)
Simple Mask	5-10 L/min	35-50%	**Primarily used for procedures or short-term transport** It can not be humidified without altering flow/delivered O2%	CO_2 build-up (keep minimum flow of 5 L/min to wash out) Uncomfortable, interferes with eating/talking (use for short-term, procedures only)
Partial Re-breathing Mask (PRB)	10+ L/min	40-70%	**Used for emergency situations** Flow needs to be set so that reservoir bag is 1/3 to 1/2 full on inspiration **Partial Rebreather**: Mask with 300-500 mL reservoir bag, ~1/3 of exhalation mixes with O2 in reservoir bag, rebreathed	CO_2 build-up (keep minimum flow of ~ 10 L/min to ensure adequate wash-out, if reservoir bag empties on inspiration flow is too low; do NOT wean device when FiO_2 needs decrease)
Non-Rebreathing Mask (NRB) (Nonrebreather)	10+ L/min	60-80% with 1 exhalation port open (close to 100% if both ports closed*)	**Non-Rebreather**: One-way valve between mask and reservoir and on one or both of the exhalation ports in the mask which prevents rebreathing of CO_2 Can not be humidified without altering flow/delivered O2%	Asphyxiation concern if no oxygen flow to device (*leave 1 exhalation port on mask open for safety) NRB: valves on PRB: valves off

Delivery System	Liter flow	O2% delivered	Clinical Considerations	Hazards (strategies to address)
High Flow Devices: Oxygen % delivered is stable, meeting or exceeding the patient's inspiratory needs					
Air Entrainment Mask (AEM) (Venturi)	Variable (see device)	24–50%	Used for delivering consistent oxygen %	Entrainment ports may become occluded, ↓ total flow while ↑ delivered FiO2. Airway dryness (rare, but device can be humidified) Note: when higher FiO2 and high minute ventilation, total flow may be inadequate
Air Entrainment Nebulizer		24–100%	Same as air entrainment mask, but entrainment is usually on an aerosol bottle, can technically be set to O2 of 100% (see note)	

Air Entrainment Ratios					
See Equations (pg 13-30) for details on calculating air-entrainment ratios and total flow	Oxygen %	Air:O2 Ratio		Oxygen %	Air:O2 Ratio
	24	25:1		50	1.7:1
	28	10:1		60	1:1
	30	8:1		70	0.6:1
	35	5:1		80	0.3:1
	40	3:1			

Delivery System	Liter flow	O2% delivered	Clinical Considerations	Hazards (strategies to address)
High-flow Nasal Cannula	Adult: 20-60 L/min	21%-100%	**Bridge therapy for less stable patients** (may help prevent intubation): delivers a high-flow of gas through a larger bore nasal cannula. Flow is set separately from O2%. Used for both O2 delivery and for a "PEEP-like" effect (estimated to be about 1 cm H2O PEEP for each 10 L/min flow) Must be humidified to minimize humidity deficit	Aspiration risk (use caution with eating/drinking with high flow) Skin breakdown (monitor closely, consider use of skin barrier devices at points of contact)
CPAP or NPPV	**	21%-100%	Used with various patient interfaces (masks, etc.) to provide a positive pressure with a desired % of oxygen. See Oakes' *Ventilator Management Pocket Guide* for complete details	

Delivery System	Liter flow	O2% delivered	Clinical Considerations	Hazards (strategies to address)
Oxygen Conserving Devices: Devices that decrease the necessary flow rate of delivered oxygen, either by incorporating a reservoir, delivering oxygen when most needed, or by decreasing anatomical dead space					
Reservoir Cannula	Less flow to deliver similar FIO2		**Indicated for patients who require long-term oxygen on flow rates of 4+ L/min** Combines the design of a nasal cannula with an oxygen reservoir (mustache, pendant) to decrease the O2 flow required	Operation is similar to a nasal cannula in terms of hazards/concerns
Pulse-Dose or Demand-Flow	Less oxygen to deliver similar FIO2		**Indicated for patients who have increased O2 needs** (over Reservoir Cannula) - pulmonary hypertension, for example Pulse-dose provides a bolus of oxygen at a relatively high flow rate at the 1st part of inspiration Demand-flow provides a set flow throughout the inspiratory phase.	Battery operated (be sure to have back-ups available, or can transition to normal nasal cannula if needed)

Therapies

Delivery System	Liter flow	O2% delivered	Clinical Considerations	Hazards (strategies to address)
Transtracheal Oxygen (TTO)	1-15 L/min	Varies	**Primarily indicated for patients with chronic hypoxemia who require low O2 rates,** although flows of up to 15 L/min may be tolerated (for exercise, etc.) by some patients A catheter placed surgically directly into the trachea provides oxygen at lower flowrates than usually needed (due to bypassing anatomic dead space of upper airway) Reduces oxygen flow required by 55% (at rest), 30% (exertion)	Complications (extensive pt education required, trained TTO team should be in place) Mucus accumulation - mucous ball forms on distal tip (requires frequent cleaning, adequate humidity + hydration, mucokinetics) Loss of stoma/tract, especially if newly placed (backup O2 is necessary, lubricate catheter and attempt to gently reinsert, if no success the TTO team should be consulted, then consider guidewire placement. Multiple attempts may lead to a false tract) Pneumothorax (ensure placement, avoid reinsertions)

Gases Measured or Used in Respiratory Therapy (in addition to oxygen)

Gas	General Uses
Carbon Dioxide	Measured: exhaled CO_2 (capnography) as a measure of ventilation status. Critical to airway management (tube placement, ROSC), general monitoring
Carbogen	Administered: 5% CO_2 + 95% O_2 Historically used for severe singultus (hiccups), but may treat retinal artery occlusion related to anesthesia as well
Carbon Monoxide	Administered and Measured: Used as a tracer gas in some PFT testing (DLCO)
Heliox See Next Page	Administered: Helium + Oxygen Helps facilitate treatment for severe bronchospasm, obstructions, etc.
Nitric Oxide	Administered (inhaled nitric oxide, or iNO): works as a potent pulmonary vasodilator for pulmonary hypertension (including PPHN in neonates, ARDS in adults) Measured (fractional nitric oxide, or Fe_{NO}): Used in diagnosis of eosinophilic airway inflammation, and specifically provides data on the potential effectiveness of steroid responsiveness
Nitrous Oxide	Administered (N_2O): used as a mild sedative during procedures (conscious sedation)

Heliox Therapy (Helium - Oxygen)	
Function	Helium reduces the resistance of air/O2 flowing through narrowed airways. Treats airway obstruction by enhancing the delivery of oxygen and aerosol to the distal areas of the lung. Helium can be used as a temporizing agent to reduce WOB and allow time for the more standard forms of therapy to reach peak effect.
Indications	• Acute exacerbations of COPD or asthma • Post extubation stridor • Status asthmaticus • Tracheal stenosis • Upper airway obstruction (tumor, foreign body, etc.)

Benefits	• Improved homogeneity of gas distribution resulting in:
	    • ↑ alveolar ventilation, oxygenation and V_T
	    • ↓ WOB, $PaCO_2$, gas trapping, auto-PEEP, PIP and Pplat, barotrauma, I:E ratios, and shunting

Common Mixtures	• 80% He / 20% O_2 • 70% He / 30% O_2 * (* Used when O_2 therapy is indicated for hypoxemia. If FIO_2 > 0.6 is required, He/O_2 will have little effect)

Administration	**Spontaneous breathing**: Deliver via tight-fit nonrebreather mask. Some add O_2 nasal cannula to titrate to desired SpO_2.
	
	Intubated: Deliver as adjunct via ventilator
	
	Delivery using an oxygen flowmeter (vs one calibrated to Heliox) requires flow conversion:
	   70/30: set flow x 1.6 = total flow delivered
	   80/20: set flow x 1.8 = total flow delivered

Monitoring	ABG sampling / Heart rate Arrhythmia / Pulse oximetry Dyspnea (WOB & SOB) / Pulsus paradoxus
Hazards	Anoxia- analyze delivered gas Barotrauma- when using ventilators not designed for heliox Alterations in drugs delivered or flows used in delivery Hypothermia - via hood on infants

10 Diseases/Disorders

DISEASES

Acute Coronary Syndrome (ACS)	10-4
Acute Respiratory Distress Syndrome (ARDS)	10-5
Alveolar Hypoventilation Syndromes	10-8
Aspergillosis *(see Fungal Disorders)*	
Aspiration Pneumonia *(see Pneumonia)*	
Asthma	10-9
Atelectasis	10-18
Blastomycosis *(see Fungal Disorders)*	
Bronchiectasis	10-20
Carbon Monoxide Poisoning	10-21
Cardiac Tamponade	10-22
Chronic Bronchitis *(see COPD)*	
Chronic Obstructive Pulmonary Disease (COPD)	10-23
Coccidioidomycosis *(see Fungal Disorders)*	
Congestive Heart Failure *(see Heart Failure)*	
Coronavirus *(see Viral Infections)*	
Cor Pulmonale *(see Heart Failure)*	
Cryptococcus *(see Fungal Disorders)*	
Cystic Fibrosis	10-32
Diabetic Ketoacidosis	10-36
Drowning	10-37
Drug Overdose	10-38
Emphysema *(see COPD)*	
Fungal Disorders	10-39
Flail Chest	10-41
Guillain-Barré Syndrome *(see Neuromuscular Disorders)*	
Heart Failure	10-42
Left-Sided (LHF, CHF)	10-43
Right-Sided (RHF, Cor Pulmonale)	10-44
Histoplasmosis *(see Fungal Disorders)*	
Immunocompromised	10-45
Interstitial Lung Disease (ILD)	10-46
Kyphoscoliosis *(see Restrictive Lung Disease)*	
Lung Abscess	10-48
Myasthenia Gravis *(see Neuromuscular Disorders)*	

Myocardial Infarction *(see Acute Coronary Syndrome)*
Neuromuscular Disorders.. 10-49
Obesity *(see Alveolar Hypoventilation Syndromes)*
Obstructive Sleep Apnea *(see Sleep-Disordered Breathing)*
Oxygen Toxicity.. 10-52
Pleural Effusion.. 10-53
Pleuritis (Pleurisy)... 10-54
Pneumonia... 10-55
Pneumoconiosis *(see Interstitial Lung Disease)*
Pneumothorax (Air Leak Syndromes)............................ 10-58
Pulmonary Contusion *(see Trauma)*
Pulmonary Edema... 10-60
Pulmonary Embolism... 10-61
Pulmonary Hypertension.. 10-62
Respiratory Failure... 10-63
Restrictive Lung Disease... 10-64
Sarcoidosis *(see Interstitial Lung Disease)*
Shock... 10-65
Sleep-Disordered Breathing... 10-66
Smoke Inhalation/Thermal Burns................................. 10-67
Tracheoarterial Fistula.. 10-68
Tracheoesophageal Fistula... 10-69
Trauma... 10-70
   Traumatic Brain Injury.. 10-71
   Chest Trauma... 10-72
Tuberculosis.. 10-73
Viral Infections... 10-75

Important Chapter Considerations

- We have focused primarily on respiratory presentations of diseases. It is important to know that many diseases have extrapulmonary types and extrapulmonary considerations.

- Disease presentation is alphabetical, but some have been presented within other syndromes/diseases - using the index or table of contents will help locate these easily.

- Important aspects of each disease have been presented. Some items have been omitted (such as PFTs) when deemed to be less clinically relevant.

We also recommend:

Oakes' Neonatal/Pediatric Pocket Guide
A more complete coverage of neonatal and pediatric disorders can be found in this pocket guide, the most complete source of its type.

Oakes' Hemodynamic Monitoring Pocket Guide
For complete hemodynamic presentations of major respiratory diseases, including extensive information on shocks.

Oakes' Ventilator Management Pocket Guide
For complete disease-centered presentations of noninvasive and invasive management, initial ventilator settings, critical care strategies and management, weaning, etc.

The full table of contents for each can be found at
RespiratoryBooks.com

Acute Coronary Syndrome (ACS)
A group of conditions where the blood supply to the heart is suddenly impaired

Conditions that fall under ACS
ST-elevation Myocardial Infarction (STEMI)
non-ST-elevation Myocardial Infarction (NSTEMI)
Stable or Unstable Angina

Clinical Manifestations

Physical Exam	Chest pain (pressure/squeezing/burning), may radiate (abdomen, teeth, jaw, neck, shoulder, lower arm) Tachycardia, tachypnea Shortness of breath Dyspnea on exertion Diaphoresis Anxiety Nausea
ECG	Varies by exact cause: ST-segment elevation T-wave changes (inversions, etc.) ST-depression (junctional, downsloping)
Labs	Abnormal cardiac enzymes (esp for differentiating between NSTEMI and unstable angina)

Treatment
- Stabilize the patient, relieve ischemic pain, and provide anti thrombotic therapy to reduce further injury.
- Supplemental oxygen to maintain SpO_2 > 90%; oxygen for patients with normal oxygenation is debated: may be harmful, having a direct vasoconstrictive effect on coronary arteries
- Drugs (anti-platelet [aspirin], anticoagulants [heparin], anti-dysrhythmics, β-blockers, nitrates, morphine, ACE inhibitors, statin therapy)
- Stabilize hemodynamics (ensure adequate CO and perfusion)
- Coronary reperfusion may be indicated (PCI, CABG). The timing of this varies by institution and philosophy.

Acute Respiratory Distress Syndrome (ARDS)

An acute, diffuse inflammatory lung injury resulting in diminished functional residual capacity, severe shunting, alveolar transudates, atelectasis, decreased compliance, and refractory hypoxemia.

Pathophysiology
Three phases with some overlap and variation between them:
- **Phase 1: Exudative (first 7-10 days)**
  Intense inflammatory response, resulting in:
  - Alveolar and endothelial damage
  - Increased vascular permeability = pulmonary edema
  - Type II cell hyperplasia
  - Hyaline membrane formation

- **Phase 2 Proliferative (10+ days)**
  Repair and regeneration occur, resulting in:
  - Pulmonary edema resolves
  - Type II cells regenerate, replacing surfactant loss
  - Some level of fibrosis (collagen deposits, interstitial infiltration)

- **Phase 3: Fibrotic Phase**
  Varies, not apparent in all patients, severity varies widely:
  - Fibrosis
  - Damage/remodeling of lung structures

Etiology
There are many possible causes of ARDS, but some of the most common include:
- **Sepsis (most common)**
- Aspiration (~1/3 of pts who aspirate in hospital develop ARDS)
- Cardiopulmonary bypass (post-perfusion injury)
- Lung transplantation
- Pancreatitis
- Pneumonia: Community-acquired and Nosocomial
- Transfusions (massive)
- Trauma (severe, including lung contusions, fat emboli, tissue injury, drowning, burns)

Diagnosis
There are 4 clinical criteria for diagnosis (Berlin definition):
1. Acute Onset of Respiratory Distress
Must be within 7 days of a defined event (sepsis, trauma, pneumonia, etc.). Most cases occur within 72 hours.

2. Hypoxemia:

Severity of ARDS	PaO_2/FIO_2 ratio (P/F) (on PEEP ≥ 5 cm H_2O)
Mild	200 - 300
Moderate	100 - 200
Severe	< 100

3. Bilateral consolidation on CXR or CT
Bilateral infiltrates - diffuse or not (pulmonary edema)

4. Ruled out cardiac failure and fluid overload
Determined either by PCWP < 18 cm H_2O (noncardiogenic), <u>or by clinical examination</u> (because PA catheters are less common, examination techniques, such as echocardiography, are acceptable)

Clinical Manifestations
Significant hypoxemia in initial phase, usually refractory. May note a steady increase in need for supplemental O_2 (with minimal to no improvement in PaO_2). Symptoms often worsen to respiratory failure.

Physical Exam	Increasing respiratory distress: tachypnea, tachycardia, ↑ work of breathing, dull percussion
Auscultation	Coarse crackles (pulmonary edema) Bronchial breath sounds (consolidation)
ABGs	<table><tr><td>Early</td><td>Respiratory alkalosis* with hypoxemia</td></tr><tr><td>Later</td><td>Respiratory acidosis* with severe hypoxemia</td></tr></table>* If underlying cause of ARDS is metabolic, there will be a metabolic component to ABG

Imaging	Often "white out" of lungs (ground glass appearance): bilateral infiltrates (often diffuse), air bronchograms
Hemodynamics	PCWP Normal or ↓ CVP ↑ Hemodynamics may also be determined by underlying cause (such as septic shock)
Pulmonary Dynamics	Decreased compliance Increased PIP on ventilator V/Q mismatch

Treatment

The goal of treatment with ARDS is largely protective (protect the lungs from as much damage as possible), supportive (support failing systems), and treatment-based (treat underlying cause):

Lung Protection	Lung protective ventilator strategies (maintaining plateau pressures < 30 or driving pressure < 15 by keeping tidal volumes low, allowing permissive hypercapnia)
Supportive	**Support failing systems:** **Oxygenation** (refractory hypoxemia is likely): Optimize O₂: use of PEEP (vs FIO_2) or other recruitment strategies (mode, etc.), patient positioning - proning (improves V/Q), Decrease O₂ consumption: ensure synchrony on ventilator (mode, settings, sedation), treat pain and fever, etc. **Hemodynamics**: monitor closely (CVP, A-Line), maintain mean arterial pressure > 60 to ensure adequate perfusion
Treatment	Treat underlying causes when able (see etiologies for common causes)

See ***Oakes Ventilator Management Pocket Guide*** for critical care strategies, including lung protection, oxygenation optimization, ARDSnet guidelines, etc.

Alveolar Hypoventilation Syndromes

Insufficient ventilation, which can be either acute or chronic, which results in an increased $PaCO_2$ above normal (> 45 mm Hg)

Etiology

Central Alveolar Hypoventilation	Often caused as a result of severe trauma to the brain/brainstem, resulting in alveolar hypoventilation.
Chest Wall Deformity	Δ shape causes a physical restrictive disorder (kyphoscoliosis, pectus excavatum, etc.)
COPD	when FEV_1 < 1.0 L or < 35% predicted
Neuromuscular Disorder	Guillain-Barré Syndrome, Myasthenia Gravis, Muscular Dystrophy, ALS
Obesity Hypoventilation Syndrome	Multifactorial, but BMI in obese range results in a restrictive lung disorder resulting in alveolar hypoventilation (weight on chest, abdominal weight preventing adequate diaphragmatic function, etc.)

Clinical Manifestations

Usually non-specific, though sleep-disordered breathing is nearly always present. When chronic, expect to see symptoms consistent with chronic hypoxia (see pg 9-77)

Treatment/Strategies

Treatments vary and usually focus on treating the underlying cause (diaphragmatic pacing, weight loss, etc.) while supporting needs (CPAP/NPPV for OSA, PEEP if on a ventilator, respiratory stimulants, etc.)

Asthma

A disease of chronic airway inflammation with evidence of variable expiratory airflow limitation. Patients experience variable respiratory symptoms (wheeze, shortness of breath, chest tightness, and/or cough) consistent with airways that overrespond (hyperresponsiveness) to stimuli (allergens, etc.) by narrowing and producing mucus.

Pathophysiology

There is some variation based on phenotype (see below)

- **Inflammation of the airways**
  An overreaction to normal stimuli/allergens:
  - Antibodies develop after exposure to a stimulus
  - These stimuli "trigger" an overresponse
  - Mast cells, once triggered, degranulate and produce an inflammatory response

- **Bronchial hyperresponsiveness**
  Smooth muscles contract in an overreaction to normal stimuli

- **Airway remodeling**
  Permanent changes to the structure of the airways that result in irreversible obstruction in at least some patients
  - Increase in goblet cells (increasing mucus production)
  - Thickening of the bronchial walls
  - Change in smooth muscle function/structure resulting in air-trapping (dynamic hyperinflation)

Etiology/Risk Factors

There are many causes/risk factors. These can be loosely divided into clinical phenotypes:

- **Allergic asthma**: often starts in childhood, usually eosinophilic inflammation, often a genetic component
- **Non-allergic asthma**: not associated with an allergy, usually neutrophilic, but can be eosinophilic or nearly no inflammatory cells
- **Adult-onset asthma**: usually non-allergic, esp. in women (endometriosis, etc.)
- **Asthma with persistent airflow limitation**: a more chronic form of asthma, likely due to airway remodeling, persistent symptoms related to airflow limitation (not completely reversible)
- **Asthma with obesity**: strong respiratory symptoms, minimal evidence of eosinophilic involvement

Diagnosis[1]

1. History of variable respiratory symptoms

People with asthma have at least one (but usually more) of the following: wheeze, SOB, chest tightness, and cough.

- Symptoms vary in intensity and over time
- Symptoms are often worse at night/upon waking
- Symptoms are often triggered by a stimulus, and may worsen with viral infections

2. Proof of variable expiratory airflow limitation

At least one of the following should be abnormal at least once and be responsive to bronchodilator therapy. Repeat during symptoms or in AM as needed

Test	Adult	Pediatric
+ Bronchodilator Reversibility *Increase from baseline after administration of albuterol[2]*	FEV_1 > 12% and > 200 mL (↑ confidence if > 15%, > 400 mL)	FEV_1 > 12% predicted
Peak flow *Average daily diurnal peak flow variability over 2 weeks*	PEF > 10%	PEF > 13%
Anti-Inflammatory Lung Function Δ *Increase in lung function after 4-wks of treatment*	↑ FEV_1 by 12% and > 200 mL (or PEFR > 20%)	Not performed
+ Exercise Challenge *Decrease from baseline after exercise*	> 10% and > 200 mL	> 12% predicted (or PEF > 15%)
+ Bronchial Challenge *Fall in FEV_1 from baseline*	FEV_1 ↓ 20% (methacholine or histamine) FEV_1 ↓ 15% (hyperventilation, hypertonic saline, or mannitol)	Not performed
Lung Function between Visits	FEV_1 > 12% and 200 mL *outside of resp. infections*	FEV_1 > 12% (or PEF > 15%) *may include resp. infections*

[1] Adapted from GINA Guidelines 2020. See ginasthma.org for detailed information.
[2] Administer 200-400 mcg albuterol (or equivalent), then wait 10-15 min.

Clinical Manifestations

People with asthma may be asymptomatic when at baseline, unless lung remodeling due to chronic asthma. During an asthma exacerbation, symptoms are likely to develop/worsen.

Physical Exam	Early signs: tachypnea, tachycardia, hyperresonance, chest tightness/dyspnea/shortness of breath, diaphoresis Late Signs: Symptoms will worsen to bradypnea, bradycardia, hypotension, etc., as patient approaches respiratory arrest
Auscultation	Early: expiratory wheezes Late: decrease in lung sounds **Absence of wheezing (with decreased air movement and respiratory distress) may indicate respiratory failure**
Pulmonary Function Testing	See previous page for diagnostic criteria **Peak expiratory flow (PEF)** is recommended for patients with severe asthma (and all patients during an exacerbation). Two standards exist: Personal Best (esp used with pediatrics) and Predicted (nomogram-based) **Obstructive Pattern with reversibility** ↓ **FEV_1**: increased risk of exacerbations, decline (especially if < 60%) If normal or near-normal, consider other causes (GERD, post-nasal drip, cardiac, etc.) **Bronchodilator reversibility**: if significant reversibility (FEV_1 > 12% and > 200 mL from baseline) in a pt who has taken SABA (4-hrs) or LABA (12-24-hrs depending on drug), asthma is likely uncontrolled (not effective despite drug therapy) **General PFT Findings** ↑ **RV**: may indicate abnormal closure of airways ↑ **FRC**: may indicate presence of air-trapping **DLCO**: normal or high; if low consider other causes

ABGs	Early: Acute respiratory alkalosis with hypoxemia Late: Acute respiratory acidosis with severe hypoxemia A normal ABG with hypoxemia and respiratory distress indicates impending respiratory arrest *[Graph showing Arterial PCO₂ and PO₂ trends, with labels: Normal ABG, Normal appearing ABG but in respiratory late]*
Labs	Check Alpha-1 Antitrypsin level 1x to rule out deficiency CBC: ↑ eosinophils may indicate inflammation
Imaging	CXR: Signs consistent with hyperinflation: flattened hemidiaphragms, splayed ribs, radiolucent lung fields, narrow heart shadow

Management/Treatment

Management is centered on controlling symptoms, minimizing exacerbations, decreasing risk of chronic lung changes, and preventing asthma-related deaths. It is a continuous process of assessment, adjustment (modifiable risk factors, pharmacological and non-pharmacological strategies), and education.

Adapted from GINA 2020, Ginasthma.org

ICS: Inhaled Corticosteroid
LABA: Long-Acting Beta Agonist
LTRA: Leukotriene Receptor Antagonist
OCS: Oral Corticosteroid
SABA: Short-Acting Beta Agonist

Adjust as needed →

	Step 1	Step 2	Step 3	Step 4	Step 5
Symptoms	< 2x/mos	2x/mos or more but not daily	Most days OR wakes with asthma 1x/wk or more	Most days OR wakes with asthma 1x/wk or more OR low lung function	Persistent*
Controller	**Preferred:** PRN low-dose ICS-formoterol **Other Options:** Low-dose ICS whenever SABA taken	**Preferred:** Daily low-dose ICS OR PRN low-dose ICS-formoterol **Other Options:** Daily LTRA OR Low-dose ICS whenever SABA taken	**Preferred:** Low-dose ICS-LABA **Other Options:** Medium-dose ICS OR Low-dose ICS + LTRA	**Preferred:** Medium-dose ICS-LABA **Other Options:** High-dose ICS OR Tiotropium add-on OR LTRA add-on	**Preferred:** High-dose ICS-LABA Consider: • Phenotypic assessment • Add-on Therapy **Other Options:** Low-dose OCS (consider side-effects) *Persistent = uncontrolled symptoms and/or exacerbations despite Step 4 treatment
Reliever	1. PRN low-dose ICS-formoterol 2. PRN SABA		1. PRN low dose ICS-formoterol if prescribed maintenance/relievers 2. PRN SABA		

Step Treatment of Asthma (6-11 yrs)
Adapted from GINA 2020, Ginasthma.org

ICS: Inhaled Corticosteroid
LABA: Long-Acting Beta Agonist
LTRA: Leukotriene Receptor Antagonist
OCS: Oral Corticosteroid
SABA: Short-Acting Beta Agonist

Adjust as needed

	Step 1	Step 2	Step 3	Step 4	Step 5
Symptoms	< 2x/mos	2x/mos or more but not daily	Most days OR wakes with asthma 1x/wk or more	Most days OR wakes with asthma 1x/wk or more OR low lung function	Persistent* • Phenotypic assessment • Add-on Therapy
Controller	Other Options: Low-dose ICS whenever SABA taken OR Daily low-dose ICS	Preferred: Daily low-dose ICS Other Options: Daily LTRA OR Low-dose ICS whenever SABA taken	Preferred: Low-dose ICS-LABA OR Medium-dose ICS Other Options: Low-dose ICS + LTRA	Preferred: Medium-dose ICS-LABA Refer for expert advice Other Options: High-dose ICS-LABA OR Tiotropium add-on OR LTRA add-on	Other Options: Anti-IL5 OR Low-dose OCS *(consider side-effects)* *Persistent = uncontrolled symptoms and/or exacerbations despite Step 4 treatment

Assessing Asthma Control

Within the past 4 weeks patient has experienced:
1. Daytime asthma symptoms more than 2x/week
2. Nighttime waking due to asthma
3. SABA reliever for symptoms more than 2x/week
4. Activity limitation due to asthma

Well-controlled: None of the above
Partly-controlled: 1-2 of the above
Uncontrolled: 3-4 of the above

Assessing Asthma Severity

May be assessed once a patient has been on controller treatment for several months and clinically appropriate attempts have been made to establish minimum effective level of treatment. Note that severity may change over time.

Severity	Asthma is well-controlled when receiving treatment at the following step (assuming minimum effective level):
Mild	Step 1 or 2
Moderate	Step 3
Severe	Step 4 or 5

Differentiating Between Severe and Uncontrolled Asthma

Some patients remain symptomatic despite maximized therapies. Before determining severe asthma (harder to treat) rule out uncontrolled asthma first:
- Verify inhaler technique
- Verify compliance with treatment plan
- Explore the impact of comorbidities, especially if lifestyle
- Monitor controlled risk factors (avoiding allergens, for example)

Exacerbations

An exacerbation is a clinically significant change in symptoms/function from baseline

Self-Care of an Exacerbation

Use of an Asthma Action Plan can help guide the patient's treatment pathway, but in general:

Patient	Change in Plan
All patients	Closely self-monitor symptoms and lung function Increase reliever* Increase controller*
If PEF or FEV1 < 60% of best OR no improvement after 48-hrs	Continue reliever Continue controller Add prednisolone 40-50 mg/day Contact physician

*See ginasthma.org for specific recommendations

Acute Care of an Exacerbation

- Give inhaled SABA frequently (every 20 min x 3 initially). Consider pMDI with a spacer (preferred) or nebulizer; do not administer IV SABA.
- Systemic steroids may decrease the length of the exacerbation and risk of relapse. Goal is to administer within 1 hr (oral is preferred, but IV if unable to give oral due to dyspnea, vomiting, NPPV)
- Avoid sedation if possible
- Avoid routine (no specific indication) use of CXR, antibiotics
- Trial of NPPV may be attempted. Monitor closely, avoid in patients with agitation, do not sedate
- Once the need for intubation is identified, do not delay
- During BVM, be aware of high risk of air-trapping
- Continue administration of corticosteroids and high-dose bronchodilators when on ventilator

See next page for overview of Acute Care Management

Acute Care Management of Asthma Exacerbations*

1. Assess patient (Airway, Breathing, Circulation). If drowsiness, confusion, or silent chest, consider ICU, start SABA and O_2, prepare for intubation

2. Assess clinical status:

Parameter	Mild to Moderate	Severe
Talks in	Phrases	Words
Position Preference	Prefers sitting	Sitting, hunched forward
Agitation	No	Usually agitated
Respiratory Rate	Increased	Markedly increased (> 30/min)
Accessory Muscle Use	None	Usually
Heart Rate	100-120/min	> 120/min
SpO_2 (room air)	90-95%	< 90%
Peak Flow	> 50% predicted/best	≤ 50% predicted/best

3. Treat by clinical status (use the worst feature to determine severity)

SABA (inhaled)	Give	Give
SAMA	Consider	Give
SpO_2 Goal	Adult: 93-95% Peds: 94-98%	Adult: 93-95% Peds: 94-98%
Corticosteroids	Oral	Oral or IV Consider high dose ICS
IV Magnesium	No	Consider for persistent hypoxemia
Heliox	No	Consider if no response to other treatments

Assess Frequently (including 1-hr after initial treatment), including lung function. Once FEV_1 or PEF is at least 60-80% of predicted/best + symptoms improved, consider discharge. Otherwise, continue treatment.

* Adapted from GINA 2020 Guidelines. See Ginasthma.org for full explanations
SABA=Short-Acting Beta Agonist, SAMA=Short-Acting Muscarinic Antagonist

Atelectasis

A loss of lung volume as a result of the collapse of lung tissue. This can affect part or all of the lungs and results in impaired gas exchange.

Clinical Manifestations

Physical Exam	Dyspnea Increased work of breathing Decreased chest expansion Tracheal shift (same side, unless compressive) Fever Chest pain Refractory hypoxemia (leading to tachypnea, tachycardia, ↓ SpO_2)
Auscultation	Fine (late) crackles Decreased, if airway obstructed Bronchial, if airway patent Increased fremitus Dull percussion note
Chest Imaging	Opacifications (less aerated tissue) Air bronchograms Narrowing of rib spaces Elevation of diaphragm (on affected side) Tracheal/cardiac/mediastinal shift (same side, unless compressive)

Treatment/Strategies

- Lung expansion therapies (deep breathing, IS, PEP, etc.)
  When possible prevent atelectasis (teach IS before surgery)
- Airway clearance if secretions (IPV, etc.)
- CPAP (noninvasive) or optimal PEEP (invasive) to recruit (reinflate)
- Bronchoscopy if obstructive (secretions, etc.)

Types of Atelectasis

Type		Description	Clinical Examples
Obstructive (Resorptive)		Blockage of an airway- air distal to the blockage is resorbed, resulting in collapse.	Foreign body airway obstruction Mass/tumor (bronchial, etc.) Secretions (retained, mucus plug) High FiO₂ (occurs more rapidly)
Non-Obstructive Atelectasis	Adhesive	Collapse of alveoli as a result of an issue with surfactant (ARDS, RDS, pneumonitis)	Surfactant deficiency (ARDS, RDS) Radiation pneumonitis
	Compressive	Something physical pressing against the lung, causing lung volume to decrease	Tumor or mass (cancer, etc.) Elevated hemidiaphragm (ascites, pregnancy, morbid obesity, hepatosplenomegaly) Other (pleural effusion, pneumothorax)
	Hypoventilation	Low tidal volume results in hypoventilation, leading to collapse of alveoli	Post-operative patients Prolonged bed rest Chest pain/guarding Respiratory fatigue Central nervous system disorders
	Passive	Retraction of the lung when it separates from the chest wall	Diaphragmatic dysfunction Pleural effusion Pneumothorax

Bronchiectasis

Dilation and destruction of the larger bronchi as a result of repeated infections (and inflammation), characterized by a chronic cough with purulent secretions.

Types
Diffuse: affects most of the lungs
Focal: affects specific area(s) of the lungs

Etiology
- Aspirations (repeated)
- Autoimmune disorders (rheumatoid arthritis, Sjögren syndrome)
- Congenital defects
- Cystic fibrosis (common)
- Other diseases (COPD, Asthma)

Clinical Manifestations

Physical Exam	Chronic cough Mucopurulent, fetid sputum (may be layered) Hemoptysis Digital clubbing Hypoxemia leading to cor pulmonale
Auscultation	Wheezing
Chest Imaging	Thickening of airway walls/airway dilation Perihilar densities CT: signet ring sign (dilated airway adjacent to a smaller artery)
PFTs	Obstructive pattern (airflow limitation)

Treatment/Strategies
- Prevent exacerbations (vaccinations, smoking cessation)
- Airway clearance therapies
- Treat exacerbations with antibiotics, SABA, maybe corticosteroids

Carbon Monoxide (CO)

Inhalation of carbon monoxide (colorless, odorless) which attaches to hemoglobin (blocking oxygen from attaching), resulting in decreased oxygen content despite a normal-appearing SpO_2

Diagnosis
- Should be assumed and treated with any fire/smoke inhalation
- **Do not rely on SpO_2 or PaO_2 for oxygenation. Must perform co-oximetry to measure the abnormal hemoglobin**

Clinical Manifestations
Increasing in severity with exposure. Percentages listed below are carboxyhemoglobin levels.

Physical Exam	Patients do not typically appear "cherry red" ↑ Respiratory rate (↓ when severe) ↑ Heart rate (↓ when severe) Cardiac arrhythmias Headache Nausea/vomiting Change in level of consciousness confusion (~30%), syncope (~40%), coma (~60%), death (~70%)
ABGs	Metabolic acidosis (> 25%) + respiratory acidosis (> 60%) Oxygenation will appear normal but is not, must check co-oximetry for true oxygenation

Treatment/Strategies
- **Supplemental Oxygen**
  - COHb has a half-life of ~300 min with room air
  - **Give 100% oxygen to all patients regardless of SpO_2, SaO_2/PaO_2**
    Half-life decreases to ~90 mins
  - Consider high-flow oxygen or NIV (FiO_2 = 1.0)
    CPAP may decrease half-life more quickly than just giving 100% O_2
  - Consider hyperbaric chamber if available (COHb > 25%)
    Half-life decreases to ~30 mins (@ 2.5 ATA)
- Avoid hyperventilation and sodium bicarbonate (shifts oxyhemoglobin curve to the left)

Cardiac Tamponade

A medical emergency where there is an acute abnormal accumulation of fluid in the pericardial sac, resulting in heart compression and hemodynamic compromise

Diagnosis
ECHO for definitive diagnosis

Etiology
- Malignant disease (most common)
- Pericarditis (drugs, chest trauma, iatrogenic, uremia, etc.)

Clinical Manifestations
Symptoms reflect the severity of heart compression (from asymptomatic to cardiovascular failure)

Physical Exam	Tachypnea Dyspnea Hypotension (progressing to cardiogenic shock) Pulsus paradoxus Sinus tachycardia Beck's Triad (JVD or ↑CVP, ↓BP, muffled heart sounds) (often not all 3 will appear)
Chest Imaging	CXR: cardiac enlargement (water bottle shape) ECHO: assess size of pericardial effusion, chamber collapse

Treatment/Strategies
- Urgent ECHO for definitive diagnosis and to assess hemodynamic impact. This is a medical emergency requiring urgent intervention.
- Drainage of the pericardial fluid (pericardiocentesis). Check periodically for recurrent fluid accumulation.
- Maintain adequate cardiac output (volume expansion)
- Supplemental oxygen
- Avoid positive pressure ventilation (decreases venous return to the heart)
- Bed rest with leg elevation (increase venous return to the heart)

Chronic Obstructive Pulmonary Disease (COPD)

A preventable and treatable disease that is characterized by persistent airflow limitation that is not fully reversible and is usually progressive. It is associated with chronic inflammatory responses in the airways and the lungs to noxious particles or gases.

Pathophysiology
- Chronic inflammation including an increase in inflammatory cells throughout the lungs, but in particular in the peripheral airways, lung parenchyma, and pulmonary vessels
- Lung remodeling (structural changes) from repeated injury and repair
- These changes can result in airflow limitation, air-trapping, abnormal gas exchange (decreased ventilatory drive, increased dead space, etc.), mucus hypersecretion (increased number of goblet cells, enlarged submucosal glands), and pulmonary hypertension

Etiology
- Cigarette smoking (or exposure to cigarette smoking)
- Other types of smoke (marijuana, pipes, cigars, etc.)
- Exposure to chemicals, dusts and gases that are noxious to the lungs
- Genetic predisposition
- Early lung growth/development (factors that slow lung growth)
- History of asthma

Diagnosis
- A diagnosis of COPD should be considered in any patient who has dyspnea (persistent and progressive), chronic cough (may be intermittent, may be unproductive), or chronic sputum production (any pattern) and/or a history of exposure to risk factors, especially cigarette smoking, occupational dusts and chemicals, or indoor/outdoor pollution.
- The diagnosis should be confirmed by spirometry (FEV_1, FVC, FEV_1/FVC ratio < 70%)
- There may be a genetic component to COPD: Alpha-1 Antitrypsin Disorder (Alpha-1). The ATS, AARC, and ACCP all recommend routine, blood-based testing for Alpha-1 in all patients with suspected COPD.

COPD Severity

COPD GOLD Criteria[1]		COPD Foundation Criteria[2]
Severity	FEV$_1$ (% predicted)	
GOLD 1 Mild	80 or above	Uses a 7 Domain Approach: 1. Spirometry
GOLD 2 Moderate	50-79	
GOLD 3 Severe	30-49	2. Regular symptoms dyspnea, cough, sputum use mMRC or CAT 3. Exacerbations 2+ in last year = high risk 4. Oxygenation severe hypoxemia, SpO$_2$ rest < 89%
GOLD 4 Very Severe	less than 30	5. Emphysema (evidence of) 6. Chronic bronchitis (evidence of) 7. Comorbidities (define and treat)

Spirometry sub-table:

Grade	FEV$_1$/FVC Ratio	FEV$_1$
SG 0	Normal	
SG 1	< 0.7	60+
SG 2	< 0.7	< 60
SG 3	< 0.7	< 30
SG U	0.7+	< 80

[1] See goldcopd.org for more information
[2] See copdfoundation.org for more information

Clinical Manifestations (primary symptoms)

1. **Chronic and progressive dyspnea**
   - Sense of increased effort to breathe
   - Chest heaviness
   - Air hunger
   - Gasping
2. **Chronic cough**
   - Not always present
   - Productive or unproductive
   - Intermittent progressing to consistent (daily)
3. **Sputum production**
   - Small amounts of tenacious sputum is common
   - Varies - can be intermittent, worsens with infection

Differentiation

While COPD is the term used clinically, clinical manifestations can loosely be divided into chronic bronchitis and emphysema. Most patients with COPD have aspects of both, though may be predominantly one or the other (the diagram below illustrates this common overlap)

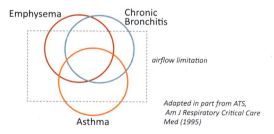

Adapted in part from ATS, Am J Respiratory Critical Care Med (1995)

Chronic Bronchitis: chronic productive cough for 3 months in each of two successive years in a patient in whom other causes of chronic cough have been ruled out

Emphysema: pathological term of structural changes including abnormal and permanent enlargement of the airspaces distal to the terminal bronchioles with destruction of airspace walls

Comparison of Clinical Manifestations

Emphysema and Chronic Bronchitis are both types of COPD. Patients may exhibit symptoms consistent with one, though many have both.

Characteristic	Emphysema	Chronic Bronchitis
General Appearance	Underweight Normal color	Overweight Evidence of cyanosis
Respiratory pattern	Hyperventilation Dyspnea (rest)	Hypoventilation
Barrel chest	Yes	No
Accessory muscles	Yes (exacerbations)	End-stage
Auscultation	Diminished ↑ Expiration	Coarse crackles Expiratory wheezes
Palpation	↓ Tactile fremitus ↓ Chest expansion	Normal
Percussion	Hyperresonance	Normal
Cough	Possible during severe stages	Productive, Severe (especially in AM)
Sputum	Minimal Mucoid	Copious Purulent
Cardiac	Less likely	Cor Pulmonale (JVD, pitting edema)
Chest Imaging	Hyperinflation Bullae/Blebs	Often normal until severe
ABG	Normal	Chronic Respiratory Acidosis with Hypoxemia
PFT	Obstructive ↓ DLCO	Obstructive
Hemoglobin/Hematocrit	Normal (until severe)	Polycythemia common

Stable COPD
See management algorithms: GOLD Guidelines (pg 10-28) and COPD Foundation Guidelines (pg 10-29)

The goal in Stable COPD is to reduce symptoms and reduce risk (prevent disease progression, prevent exacerbations, and reduce mortality)

- Provide interventions for smoking for all COPD patients
- Reduce exposure to other risk factors where possible
- Pharmacologic Treatment
    - Inhaled bronchodilators are preferred over oral forms
    - LABAs and LAMAs are preferred over SABAs and SAMAs (except if just occasional dyspnea, and for immediate relief for patients already on LABAs and/or LAMAs)
    - Inhaled corticosteroids can be used in addition to LABAs for patients with a history of exacerbations
    - Use of antibiotics should be limited to evidence of microbiological infection
    - Provide education at every interaction with a patient with COPD on appropriate use of all drugs, including technique (pMDI, DPI, Nebulizer, etc.)
- Pulmonary rehab should be encouraged in an individualized manner, but consider at diagnosis, after a hospitalized exacerbation, and when symptoms are progressively getting worse.

Chronic Hypoxemia
Treat with supplemental oxygen when:
- PaO_2 is 55 mm Hg or below (SaO_2 88%) confirmed twice over a 3-week period
- PaO_2 is 55-60 mm Hg (SaO_2 88%) if there is evidence of pulmonary hypertension, peripheral edema, or hematocrit > 55%
- Re-evaluate after 60-90 days and make adjustments as necessary
- Do not withhold oxygen from patients requiring oxygen based upon the above criteria

Chronic Hypercapnia
Consider long-term noninvasive ventilation when:
- Severe chronic hypercapnia + hospitalizations for acute respiratory failure

ABCD Approach to Stable Management

This has been adapted from GOLD 2020 Standards for Pharmacological Management as well as Non-Pharmacologic Management of COPD (see goldcopd.org for detailed information)

Groups can change over time and with treatment. A continual process of Review (symptoms, exacerbations), Assess (inhaler technique, non-pharmacology options like rehab), and Adjust (increasing or decreasing support) should occur.

mMRC[1]	0-1	2+
CAT[2]	< 10	10+
2+ moderate exacerbations OR 1+ leading to hospitalization	**Group C** LAMA	**Group D** LAMA LAMA + LABA (if many symptoms) ICS + LABA (eosinophils > 300)
	Smoking Cessation Pulmonary Rehab Physical Activity Flu + PNA vaccine	
0-1 moderate exacerbations (no hospitalization)	**Group A** Short-acting or Long-acting Bronchodilator	**Group B** LABA or LAMA 2 Bronchodilators (if severe breathlessness)
	Smoking Cessation	Smoking Cessation Pulmonary Rehab Physical Activity Flu + PNA vaccine

CAT: COPD Assessment Test
ICS: Inhaled Corticosteroid
LABA: Long-Acting Beta Agonist
LAMA: Long-Acting Muscarinic Antagonist
mMRC: modified Medical Research Council dyspnea scale
PNA: Pneumonia

[1] mMRC (modified Medical Research Council) is a dyspnea scale based on the British Medical Research Council. See mrc.ukri.org for more details.

[2] CAT (COPD Assessment Test) is a questionnaire that evaluates the effect of COPD currently on daily life. See catestonline.org for details.

COPD Foundation Management of COPD[1]
Adapted from COPD Foundation (copdfoundation.org)

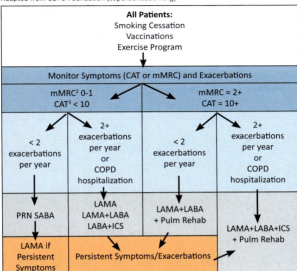

CAT: COPD Assessment Test
ICS: Inhaled Corticosteroid
LABA: Long-Acting Beta Agonist
LAMA: Long-Acting Muscarinic Antagonist
mMRC: modified Medical Research Council dyspnea scale
SABA: Short-Acting Beta Agonist

[1] The COPD foundation also differentiates Asthma-COPD Overlap (ACO) when a patient has COPD with a history of asthma or allergies and shows reversibility in FEV$_1$. Either LABA + ICS or LAMA + ICS should be considered. If persistent symptoms, consider LAMA + LABA + ICS. More information can be found at copdfoundation.org.
[2] mMRC (modified Medical Research Council) is a dyspnea scale based on the British Medical Research Council. See mrc.ukri.org for more details.
[3] CAT (COPD Assessment Test) is a questionnaire that evaluates the effect of COPD currently on daily life. See catestonline.org for details.

COPD Exacerbations

An exacerbation is a worsening of symptoms that results in at least 1 additional therapy to manage. Adapted in part from GOLD 2020 guidelines (goldcopd.org)

Criteria	No Respiratory Failure	Acute Respiratory Failure	
		Non-Life-Threatening	Life-Threatening
Respiratory Rate	20-30	> 30	> 30
Accessory Muscles	No	Yes	Yes
Mental Status	No Change	No Change	Worsening
Hypoxemia	Improved with Venti 24-35%	Improved with Venti 24-35%	Not Improved or needs O₂ > 40%
	Do not withhold oxygen from a patient with COPD who is hypoxemic (maintain minimum acceptable O₂)		
Hypercarbia ($PaCO_2$)	Baseline	Increased (50-60 mm Hg if normal baseline)*	Increased (> 60 mm Hg if normal baseline)* or pH 7.25 or below
Management	Add-on therapies (pharmacologic or other) as indicated by presentation	• Assess severity • Give oxygen • SABA + SAMA • ICS • Oral antibiotics • Consider NIV or High-Flow • Watch fluids • Consider heparin • Treat comorbidities	Consider indications for noninvasive vs invasive management, especially if hemodynamic instability or respiratory arrest is imminent

* $PaCO_2$ should be evaluated by looking at comparison to that patient's baseline, if known. The pH will be an important indicator of status of failure.

Indications for NIV vs Invasive Ventilation

1. Consider NIV or high-flow therapy* as a first-line treatment whenever possible	Respiratory acidosis: • pH 7.35 or below • PaCO$_2$ > 45 mm Hg Severe dyspnea/fatigue/↑ WOB Persistent hypoxemia (despite ↑ therapy)
2. Consider invasive mechanical ventilation when necessary *Trial NIV unless any of these conditions are evident* *Do not delay intubation once it becomes necessary*	• Unable to tolerate NIV • Failed NIV after a trial • Evidence of cardiac arrest • Evidence of respiratory arrest • Decreased mental status • Massive aspiration • Persistent vomiting • Inability to manage secretions • Severe hemodynamic instability (unresponsive to therapy) • Severe arrhythmias
3. If very severe COPD, consider the following	• Likelihood of reversibility of cause of respiratory failure • Patient's desires • Availability of ICU facilities

* High-flow oxygen (HFO, HFNC) up to 60 L/min, may be an alternative to standard oxygen therapy or NPPV. GOLD 2020 (goldcopd.org)

Cystic Fibrosis

A progressive, genetic disease caused by a mutation in the CFTR gene. This affects mucus and sweat glands, most notably causing thick, tenacious mucus in the lungs, but also affects the pancreas, liver, intestines, sinuses, and sex organs.

Pathophysiology

Dysfunction of the cystic fibrosis transmembrane conductance regular (CFTR) protein. This results in transport issues of chloride, sodium, and other ions, structurally altering secretions in the intestines, liver, lungs, pancreas, and reproductive tracts, as well as altering sweat gland secretions.

Etiology

Recessive genetic disorder

Diagnosis*

Clinical presentation of the disease (at least one):

- Positive newborn screening test (test completed since 2010)
  May be asymptomatic
- Chronic pulmonary disease
- Chronic sinusitis
- Gastrointestinal/nutritional abnormalities
- Salt loss syndromes
- Obstructive azoospermia
- History of CF in a sibling

Evidence of CFTR gene dysfunction (at least one):

- Elevated sweat chloride
  - 60+ mmol/L: positive test result (consistent with CF diagnosis)
  - 30-59 mmol/L: inconclusive (more testing needed)
  - < 30 mmol/L: negative test result (less likely CF)
- Two CFTR gene mutations known to cause CF on separate alleles
- Abnormalities in *Nasal Potential Difference* testing

---

* Based in part on: Farrell, P. M., White, T. B., Ren, C. L., Hempstead, S. E., Accurso, F., Derichs, N., . . . Sosnay, P. R. (2017). Diagnosis of Cystic Fibrosis: Consensus Guidelines from the Cystic Fibrosis Foundation. The Journal of Pediatrics, 181. doi:10.1016/j.jpeds.2016.09.064

Clinical Manifestations

Note: This section has a primary focus on respiratory symptoms despite the disease often affecting multiple body systems.

Physical Exam	Persistent, productive cough. Difficulty managing thick, tenacious secretions Barrel chest (air-trapping) Digital clubbing (severe disease) Pursed lip breathing (from air-trapping) Sinus disease (congestion, headache) Exacerbations: Worsening of normal symptoms, but may include: cough, tachypnea, dyspnea, increased sputum production. These may lead to respiratory arrest, so careful monitoring is needed.
Auscultation	Coarse crackles (secretions) are common Decreased breath sounds Wheezes/Bronchial breath sounds are not uncommon
Pulmonary Function Testing	Obstructive pattern ↓ $FEF_{25-75\%}$ (small airway involvement)
Chest Imaging	Air-trapping is common cor pulmonale Bronchiectasis*
ABGs	May be normal with less severe forms Progresses to Compensated Respiratory Acidosis with Hypoxemia
Labs	Chronic colonization of sputum (most common: *S. aureus*, *H. influenzae*, *P. aeruginosa*)

*After repeated infections, patients may develop Bronchiectasis secondary to their Cystic Fibrosis.

Management

Respiratory Components of Chronic Management
A vigorous combination of regular airway clearance techniques (mechanical assistance with clearing secretions) and pharmacological therapies are required several times a day.

Airway Clearance
Multiple options should be introduced/provided to ensure compliance with therapies outside of the hospital environment
- Assistive devices (most common as they can be integrated into a normal routine most easily):
  - Airway/chest wall oscillation (percussive vests/wraps)
  - PEP therapies
- Chest physiotherapy (postural drainage, percussion, vibration)
- Autogenic drainage
- Active Cycle of Breathing
- Huff coughing

Pharmacology
- CFTR Modulators - certain genotypes
- dornase alfa (DNase)
- SABA
- Inhaled antibiotics for chronic colonization
- Hypertonic solution (hydration of secretions)
- All vaccinations should be kept up to date
- The use of steroids is discouraged for chronic management

Exacerbation
An exacerbation is an acute episode of worsening pulmonary status (which is individualized, depending on the patient's baseline)

- Supplemental oxygen to maintain PaO_2 60-70 mm Hg (SpO_2 88-92%)
- May consider use of systemic steroids (data varies)
- Consider use of systemic antibiotic therapy
- SABA when evidence of bronchospasm
- Maintain aggressive, scheduled chest physiotherapy.
- NPPV, high-flow oxygen, invasive ventilation may become necessary- monitor clinical conditions, intubate when necessary
- Multiple exacerbations may lead to chronic lung changes (including bronchiectasis)

Cystic Fibrosis Drugs: Order of Delivery and Mixing

Not all drugs are listed, only those with clinical relevance or for which sufficient data is available.

Therapies in Suggested Order of Administration[2]	albuterol	ipratropium	hypertonic sol	dornase alfa	tobramycin	aztreonam
1. Bronchodilators (open the airways)						
albuterol	gray	green	red	red	red	red
ipratropium bromide[3]	green	gray	red	red	green	red
2. Mucolytics/Mucokinetics (mobilize, thin secretions)						
mannitol	DPI - do not mix					
hypertonic solution	red	red	gray	red	red	red
dornase alfa	red	red	red	gray	red	red
3. Airway Clearance[4] - CPT, IPV, Flutter valve, etc.						
4. Antibiotics (better deposition in infected areas)						
tobramycin	green	green	red	green	gray	red
aztreonam	red	red	red	red	red	gray
azactam	red	red	red	red	red	red
5. Steroids (if indicated)[5]						

[1] Green boxes have evidence to support the mixing of the drugs in the same nebulizer set-up. Red boxes indicate contraindication or lack of sufficient evidence

[2] Suggested order of administration as supported by Cystic Fibrosis Foundation, and supported by other major Cystic Fibrosis clinics

[3] Evidence is insufficient to recommend for or against long-term use

[4] Airway clearance is recommended in this order when chest physiotherapy (percussion with postural drainage) is being done. When a vest-based system is being used, it is recommended that drug delivery occur while the vest-based system is running (according to Cystic Fibrosis Foundation)

[5] Little data exists to support the use of inhaled steroids in patients with CF

Diabetic Ketoacidosis (DKA)

A potentially life-threatening complication of diabetes that results in an often severe metabolic acidosis (with respiratory implications), characterized by ketoacidosis and hyperglycemia.

Etiology
Infection (pneumonia, urinary tract infection, etc.)
Inadequate insulin intake
Undiagnosed disease (new onset)
Drugs (dobutamine, terbutaline, etc.)

Diagnosis

Based on 2009 American Diabetes Association criteria

	Mild	Moderate	Severe
Serum Glucose (mg/dL)	> 250 (typically 350-500)		
Arterial pH	7.25 - 7.30	7.00-7.24	< 7.00
Serum HCO$_3^-$ (mEq/L)	15-18	10-14	< 10
Ketones	+	+	+
Anion Gap (mEq/L)	> 10	> 12	> 12
Mental Status	Alert	Drowsy	Stupor/Coma

Clinical Manifestations
Presents rapidly (over 24-hrs). If slower, consider hyperosmolar hyperglycemic state (HHS) instead.
- Respiratory pattern: Kussmaul's (hyperventilation as a respiratory compensation to a metabolic acidosis)
- Decreased mental status
- Decreased skin turgor
- Fruity breath/odor (due to high ketones)

Treatment
- Correct acidosis (consider sodium bicarb if pH < 6.90)
- Support respiratory status (may tire abruptly)
- Correct electrolyte and fluid abnormalities
- Insulin administration (low-dose, unless potassium 3.3 or higher)

Drowning

A process that results in respiratory impairment from submersion or immersion in a liquid. Several other terms (near-drowning, nonfatal drowning, submersion injury) have been used previously but their use is discouraged by the AHA due to lack of consistency in usage.

Clinical Manifestations

Major symptoms may appear immediately or may be delayed (by as many as 6 hours).

Physical Exam	<ul><li>Hypoxemia</li><li>Shortness of breath</li><li>Change in levels of consciousness (cerebral edema, ischemia)</li><li>Cardiac arrhythmias</li></ul>
Auscultation	Coarse crackles (if pulmonary edema) Wheezing (bronchospasm)
Chest Imaging	Varies from normal-appearing to extensive atelectasis, pulmonary edema, interstitial infiltrates
ABGs	Metabolic or respiratory acidosis is common

Treatment

- Support respiratory status. Consider use of supplemental oxygen (SpO_2 > 94%), high-flow oxygen, NPPV, or invasive ventilation depending on clinical status (intubate if unable to maintain SpO_2 > 90% on other therapies)
- Treat pulmonary edema with positive pressure (high-flow oxygen, NPPV, invasive ventilation with PEEP)
- Treat bronchospasm with SABA
- If patient is hypothermic consider prolonged resuscitation (neurological outcomes are more promising)
- If danger of cerebral herniation, consider a short period of hyperventilation to reduce intracranial pressure (do not use for a prolonged period)

Drug Overdose

Intentional or unintentional (including nosocomial) overdosage of a drug which may result in harmful clinical manifestations, including death.

Etiology
Most Common Overdoses: Ethanol (alcohol), benzodiazepines, opioids
Unintentional: Nosocomial (med error), accidental overdose by pt
Intentional: Attempt at self-harm

Clinical Manifestations
Varies by drug class and other factors (amount of drug, combination, etc.)
See pg 11-56 for Drugs that cause Respiratory Depression

Physical Exam	<ul><li>Change in mental status, behavior</li><li>Respiratory depression</li><li>Hemodynamic instability</li></ul>
Auscultation	Coarse crackles (if pulmonary edema) Wheezing (bronchospasm)
Chest Imaging	Indications of aspiration (especially if loss of consciousness)
ABGs	Metabolic or respiratory acidosis is common

Treatment
- Goals: identify drug(s) (using typical patterns of clinical manifestations), stabilize clinical status, and prevent further deterioration
- Consider reversal agents (such as naloxone for opioids) when available
- Support respiratory status. Intubation if indicated to protect airway, support respiratory depression, etc.
- Support hemodynamic status. ACLS to treat clinically significant arrhythmias, hypotension
- Consider prolonged resuscitation (neurological outcomes are more promising)

Fungal Disorders

An infectious process affecting pulmonary status, which may have elements of being short-term (acute) such as with fungal pneumonia, or more chronic.

Etiology
- Regional risk factors exist but should not be used definitively to rule out a particular fungal disorder
- Patients who are immunocompromised or immunosuppressed are at greater risk of all infection, including fungal infection

Diagnosis
Generally diagnosed by microbiology (sputum sample)

Clinical Manifestations
Fungal infections range from asymptomatic to life-threatening infection. The specific clinical manifestations associated with a fungus varies and often may be similar to other infections/disorders. For this reason, consider ruling out fungal causes if suspected before treating other disorders.

See next page for specific clinical manifestations found with common fungi

Treatment
- Treat underlying fungus, often with antifungals
- Consider fungal infections in critically ill patients with influenza who are immunocompromised or who have received corticosteroids (CDC)
- Support respiratory status. Fungal disorders range in severity.
  - Support oxygen for hypoxemia
  - Support ventilation for respiratory failure
  - Consider airway clearance when clinically indicated

Clinical Practice Guidelines for various fungal infections can be found at the Infectious Diseases Society of America (idsociety.org)

Common Fungal Infections

Fungus	Fungus and Association	Regions Fungi Common[1]	Clinical Manifestations[2]
Aspergillosis	*Aspergillus fumigatus* Can be found in soil, decomposing matter, household dust, food, water, etc.	Considered common in most environments	Cough with minimal mucoid sputum, hemoptysis, fever, recurrent infections
Blastomycosis	*Blastomyces dermatitidis* Spores found in soil and decaying organic matter Transmission: Inhalation	US: midwestern, south-central, and southeastern states, esp. Ohio, Mississippi River valleys Other: Africa, India, Canada	Similar to pneumonia: cough, purulent sputum, chest pain, fever, joint/muscle aches, may progress to ARDS
Coccidioidomycosis	*Coccidioides immitis* Spores common after disturbance of soil (excavation, earthquakes, dust storms)	US: southwestern states, especially southern Arizona and San Joaquin Valley (California) Other: Mexico, South America	Similar to common cold: fever, chest pain, cough, headaches, malaise
Cryptococcosis	*Cryptococcus neoformans* Spores found in soil, decaying matter, bird droppings	Considered common in most environments	Cough with mucoid sputum, dyspnea, hemoptysis, pleuritic chest pain, fever
Histoplasmosis *(most common)*	*Histoplasma capsulatum* Bird excretions Route: Inhalation	US: central, eastern states, esp Ohio, Mississippi River valleys Other: Central, South America, Africa, Asia, Australia	Similar to tuberculosis: Cough, fatigue, fever, night sweats, hemoptysis

[1] Regional information from CDC.gov [2] Common manifestations presented but there is much variability and often multiple types of each disorder

Flail Chest

Three or more adjacent ribs with fractures in at least two places each, resulting in a floating segment. This section moves in the opposite direction (paradoxical) of the rest of the chest wall during respirations.

Etiology
Blunt chest trauma

Diagnosis
Usually visible on chest images, or may be able to visualize paradoxical segment with some patients

Flail sternum: fracture of the sternum in two places) may have similar effect

Clinical Manifestations

Physical Exam	• Paradoxical movement at flail segment (may be difficult to visualize) • Dyspnea • Hypoxemia • Increased work of breathing • Pain/splinting at flail segment
Auscultation	Coarse crackles (if pulmonary edema) Wheezing (bronchospasm)
Chest Imaging	Rib fractures evident: 3+ adjacent ribs should be fractured in at least 2 locations each. Underlying pulmonary contusion may be apparent.

Treatment
- Watch closely for respiratory failure - may trial NPPV to stabilize chest wall. Watch closely for respiratory failure; intubate if necessary.
- Adequate pain management to encourage deep breathing
- Monitor for indications for airway clearance, lung expansion

Heart Failure (by type)

Failure of the heart to function effectively, which can be divided into right-sided heart failure, left-sided heart failure, or biventricular heart failure (see diagram below for definitions, arrows indicate wrong-direction movement/pooling of blood)

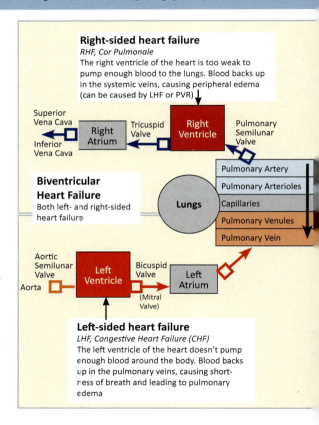

Left-sided Heart Failure (LHF, Congestive Heart Failure)

Diagnosis
Evaluation of signs and symptoms within the context of a history and physical

Clinical Manifestations

Physical Exam	<ul><li>Tachycardia (may be irregular)</li><li>Orthopnea</li><li>Dyspnea on exertion</li><li>Hypoxemia</li><li>Cough (pink, frothy secretions possible)</li><li>Pulsus alternans</li><li>Edema in legs, ankles, feet</li><li>If ↓CO, poor peripheral perfusion may be evident (hypotension, mental status, narrowed pulse pressure)</li></ul>
Auscultation	Persistent wheezing in some Coarse crackles if pulmonary edema
Chest Imaging	Cardiomegaly Increased pulmonary vasculature Kerley B lines May show signs of pulmonary edema

Treatment
- Supplemental oxygen to treat hypoxemia
- Respiratory interventions
- Consider CPAP for hypoxemia (esp. if increased work of breathing)
- Consider NPPV for hypoxemia with hypercapnia
- Optimize hemodynamics: ↓afterload, adequate preload, ↑ myocardial contractility, prevent dysrhythmias. May include inotropes, beta blockers, vasodilators
- Keep HOB > 10-45 degrees
- Correct any anemia or electrolyte imbalances

Right-sided Heart Failure (RHF, Cor Pulmonale)

Diagnosis
CVP > 10 with evidence of right-sided heart dysfunction

Etiology
- Left-sided heart failure: The most common cause of right-sided heart failure (pressure and volume overload, either acute or chronic)
- Cardiac (right heart disease/disorder): cardiomyopathy, ischemia, infarction, congenital or valvular disease
- Pulmonary (cor pulmonale, which is often as a result of pulmonary hypertension):
  - Acute: pulmonary embolism, ARDS
  - Chronic: hypoxemia, acidosis, obstructive or restrictive lung disease, obstructive sleep apnea

Clinical Manifestations

Physical Exam	- Dyspnea - Tachypnea - Fatigue, including dyspnea on exertion - Cough - Jugular venous distention (JVD) - Angina (usually unresponsive to nitrates) - Peripheral edema - Hypoxemia, possibly cyanosis
Auscultation	Abnormal if underlying pulmonary disease
Chest Imaging	Right ventricular hypertrophy

Treatment
- Treat causes of pulmonary hypertension when possible (pulmonary vasodilators, etc.)
- Reduce right ventricular afterload (diuretics), augment right ventricular function
- Treat underlying lung processes (PE, ARDS, COPD, etc.)
- Consider ECMO, ventricular-assist devices, transplantation

Immunocompromised

Patients who have an impaired immune system either due to disease (AIDS, autoimmune disorders, etc.), therapy (radiation, some drugs, etc.), or other process (burn, malnutrition, corticosteroids, transplantation, etc.) which increases risk of infection.

Clinical Manifestations
- Respiratory infections, primarily pneumonia, are common
- Pathogens may be typical or unusual. Be aware of opportunistic viral, bacterial, or fungal infections, as well as cytotoxic drug reactions.
  - Begin with broad-spectrum antimicrobial therapy
- Clinical signs may be decreased if neutropenic (fever may be the only sign of an infection)

Treatment
- Strict use of "reverse isolation" appropriate to the situation (all caretakers perform vigorous hand hygiene, wear gown, gloves, mask; avoid patient care if any sign of caretaker illness)
- At any sign of respiratory deterioration (acute respiratory failure), consider causes, treat early and aggressively due to high mortality in these patients
- Use noninvasive diagnostics when possible (there is a correlation between bronchoscopy/BAL and respiratory deterioration*)
- Use noninvasive therapies when possible (NIV) to prevent risk of ventilator-associated pneumonia

---

* Azoulay, E., Mokart, D., Kouatchet, A., Demoule, A., Lemiale, V. (2019). Acute respiratory failure in immunocompromised adults. The Lancet Respiratory Medicine, 7(2), 173-186. doi:10.1016/s2213-2600(18)30345-x

Interstitial Lung Disease (ILD)

A large variety of 200+ diffuse infiltrative disorders characterized by injury to the alveolar wall, leading to interstitial and alveolar exudates, the formation of hyaline membranes, and usually extensive scarring which causes pulmonary fibrosis

Types
- Idiopathic interstitial pneumonia
- Occupational lung disease
- Autoimmune Disease (lupus, rheumatoid arthritis)
- Sarcoidosis

Clinical Manifestations
Vary depending on severity, from asymptomatic to life-threatening, and by specific cause (when known), but there are several common manifestations:
- Progressive breathlessness with exertion
- Persistent nonproductive cough
- Auscultation: usually abnormal but nonspecific
- Chest imaging: reticular pattern is most common
- PFT that is restrictive in nature (at least in part); DLCO may be decreased

Treatment
- Treatment strategies vary some (specific drugs recommended, etc.) but most center on supporting symptoms versus treating the cause
- Smoking cessation education is critical to preserve lung function
- Avoiding causes/triggers may help prevent further damage (esp. if occupational)
- Long-term oxygen therapy (LTOT) may be necessary in more severe cases
- Pulmonary rehab and lung transplantation are general considerations for severe cases of ILD

Common Interstitial Lung Diseases

Disease	Etiology	Clinical Manifestations	Management
Idiopathic Pulmonary Fibrosis	*Cause unknown, but risk factors include: age, genetics, lung exposures, infections, etc.*	Typically 60+ yrs-old Chronic dyspnea on exertion, chronic cough (unproductive), fatigue, "velcro-like" crackles on auscultation	Long-term oxygen therapy Pulmonary rehab Drug therapy
Hypersensitivity Pneumonitis	*Hypersensitivity to environmental/occupational antigens*	Cough, dyspnea, fatigue, chest tightness, hypoxemia, crackles/wheezing	Corticosteroids (acute) Antigen avoidance If fibrosis: immunosuppression
Pneumoconiosis	*Inhalation of dust or particles (coal dust, silica, asbestos, cotton, etc.), largely occupational*	Cough (may be productive), shortness of breath, fatigue, dyspnea on exertion	Long-term oxygen therapy Avoid all causative agents Supportive care (treat symptoms)
Sarcoidosis	*Cause unknown*	Dyspnea on exertion, cough, chest pain, fever, anorexia	NSAIDs (non-steroidal anti-inflammatory drugs) Corticosteroids

Lung Abscess

A necrosis of the pulmonary tissue with the formation of cavities that contain necrotic debris or fluid caused by a microbial infection. Multiple abscesses may be referred to as a "necrotizing pneumonia."

Etiology
- Acute: less than 4-6 weeks old
- Chronic: older than 4-6 weeks old
- Primary abscess: caused by an aspiration (mouth anaerobes that enter lungs during an aspiration event) or pneumonia
- Secondary abscess: caused by another condition (bronchiectasis, immunocompromised patient, lung cancer, etc.)

Clinical Manifestations

Physical Exam	May have a periodic cough with expectoration of large amounts of purulent, fetid, bloody sputum Pleurisy Fever Night sweats Anorexia/weight loss Digital clubbing
Auscultation	Decreased breath sounds over infected area(s) Bronchial breath sounds Coarse crackles Dullness to percussion
Chest Imaging	Irregularly shaped cavity Aspiration: • posterior segment of upper lobes • superior segments of lower lobes

Treatment
- Treat underlying infection (antibiotics)
- Patient positioning (keep good lung up to avoid draining infectious secretions into good lung)
- Drainage of abscess/empyema is sometimes needed
- Complications include empyema (rupture into pleural space), bronchopulmonary fistula, respiratory failure, etc.

Neuromuscular Disorders

A number of disorders that affect the nerves that control voluntary muscles. These disorders have the potential to affect respiratory muscles, resulting in respiratory insufficiency (and possibly respiratory failure)

Etiology
Common neuromuscular disorders include::
- Amyotrophic Lateral Sclerosis (ALS)
- Duchenne Muscular Dystrophy (DMD)
- Guillain-Barré Syndrome (GBS) - see pg 10-51
- Multiple Sclerosis (MS)
- Myasthenia Gravis (MG) - see pg 10-51

Clinical Manifestations

Physical Exam	May be primarily nocturnal or generalized: Dyspnea Orthopnea Decreased tidal volume (↑ RR in an attempt to maintain adequate minute ventilation) Accessory muscle use Paradoxical breathing (see-saw breathing)
Auscultation	Decreased, especially in bases Secretions: coarse crackles Atelectasis: fine inspiratory crackles
Chest Imaging	Low lung volumes, atelectasis Evidence of aspiration Evidence of secretions (possible)
ABGs	Respiratory acidosis (uncompensated if acute, compensated if chronic) if insufficiency with Hypoxemia
PFTs	Restrictive pattern ↓ residual volume FVC while supine is ↓ versus upright (20-30% may indicate diaphragm weakness) ↓ MVV ↓ MIP (inspiratory muscles, diaphragm) ↓ MEP (expiratory muscles)

Management

- Assessment is a major aspect of management:
  - Perform PFTs or bedside parameters (pg 6-15) for all at-risk patients
  - Assess for: respiratory sufficiency (FVC), respiratory muscle strength (MIP, MEP), ability to cough and protect airway (MEP, CPF*)
  - If acute deterioration, NPPV may be an option (evidence is inconsistent) but do not delay intubation to protect airway, especially if further deterioration is expected (intubate proactively, not emergently)
  - Polysomnography study if primarily nocturnal
- Airway Clearance
  - Use of mechanical insufflator/exsufflator (Cough Assist, etc.) or thoracoabdominal compression may assist with secretion clearance
  - Tracheostomy to facilitate chronic management
- Respiratory Insufficiency
  - NIV vs invasive ventilation
  - Nocturnal vs constant

*Cough Peak Flow: Patient is instructed to cough as forcefully as possible, ensuring a good seal either with a mouthpiece or by face mask. This is measured by spirometry or peak flow meter (peak flow meter may underestimate ability[1])
Unassisted: patient demonstrates independent ability to cough
Assisted: patient demonstrates ability to cough with an adjunct (mechanical insufflator-exsufflator or thoracoabdominal compression)

[1] Kikuchi, K., Satake, M., Kimoto, Y., Iwasawa, S., Suzuki, R., Kobayashi, M., . . . Shioya, T. (2018). Approaches to Cough Peak Flow Measurement With Duchenne Muscular Dystrophy. Respiratory Care, 63(12), 1514-1519. doi:10.4187/respcare.06124

	Guillain-Barré Syndrome (GBS)	Myasthenia Gravis (MG)
Definition	An immune response to a preceding infection resulting in ascending muscular paralysis and autonomic dysfunction	Chronic autoimmune neuromuscular disorder of the voluntary (skeletal) muscles (including respiratory muscles)
Etiology	Idiopathic Commonly 2-4 weeks following a respiratory or GI infection	Idiopathic Genetic predisposition Certain drugs may induce or exacerbate
Clinical Manifestations	Symmetrical, ascending muscular weakness, pain, and paralysis, including the diaphragm and supporting respiratory muscles Decreased or absent reflexes in affected arms or legs Difficulty swallowing, risk of aspiration (choking, coughing) Severe BP, HR and rhythm fluctuations Bronchorrhea	Descending weakness pattern Weakness, fatigue in muscles as they are used (recover with rest) Dysphagia with weak cough Respiratory insufficiency requiring intubation Tensilon Test: improvement in symptoms with administration (no longer used in U.S.) Ice Pack Test: place bag of ice on closed eyelids, improvement in symptoms if MG Myasthenic crisis: acute, transient worsening usually with respiratory compromise
Treatment	Monitor bedside parameters closely (see pg 6-15). Intubate if signs of respiratory failure. Airway clearance and lung expansion as needed Plasmapheresis or immune globulin therapy	Crisis: Monitor bedside parameters closely (pg 6-15) Intubate if signs of respiratory failure Chronic: Anticholinesterase drugs Immunosuppressants Plasmapheresis

Oxygen Toxicity

Damage to the lungs and other systems caused by being exposed to high concentrations of oxygen for a short period of time, or being exposed to any supplemental oxygen for a prolonged duration

Clinical Manifestations

Physical Exam	**Pulmonary** Cough (non-productive) Hemoptysis Hypopnea May progress to ARDS, pulmonary fibrosis **Central Nervous System** Headache/dizziness Hyperventilation Nausea/Vomiting Changes in vision (blurring, tunnel-vision) Changes in hearing (tinnitus, hearing disturbances)
Chest Imaging	Pulmonary edema/inflammation

Treatment
- Minimizing unnecessary oxygen exposure should be a clinical priority.
- Set upper alarm of SpO_2 under 100% to trigger reminders to wean oxygen
- Prioritize strategies to optimize oxygenation:
    - Patient positioning (see pg 5-11)
    - Use of high-flow oxygen, CPAP/NPPV, or PEEP when unresponsive to supplemental oxygen (refractory hypoxemia)
    - Optimize lung recruitment (deep breathing, IS, etc.)

Pleural Effusion

Accumulation of excess fluid in the pleural space. The amount and type of fluid determines the impact on pulmonary function.

Types/Etiology:
- Chylothorax: damage to thoracic duct (milky white)
- Empyema: pus in the pleural space (pneumonia, abscess)
- Hemothorax: bloody fluid (trauma)
- Iatrogenic: feeding tube or central line malpositioned

Transudative: Increased hydrostatic pressure and/or decreased plasma oncotic pressure.
  Common: heart failure, hypoalbuminemia, cirrhosis

Exudative: Increased capillary permeability, contains fluid, protein, cells, etc.
  Common: pneumonia, cancer, PE, tuberculosis

Clinical Manifestations

Physical Exam	Dyspnea Cough Chest pain Tachypnea ↓ Tactile fremitus Tracheal deviation if massive (> 300 mL)
Auscultation	Decreased Dull to percussion (affected side)
Chest Imaging	Blunting of costophrenic angles Mediastinal shift (if more severe)

Treatment
- Small/asymptomatic: observe
- Larger/symptomatic: thoracentesis, chest tube
- Chronic/malignant: pleurodesis, treat underlying cause, long-term chest tube (PleurX catheter)

*A pleurodesis is the process of inserting a chemical or drug into the pleural space to cause the two layers to adhere to one another

Pleuritis (Pleurisy)
Inflammation of the lung pleura

Etiology:
Autoimmune disease (lupus, rheumatoid arthritis)
Drugs (procainamide, hydralazine, isoniazid)
Bacterial or viral pneumonia
Pulmonary embolism

Clinical Manifestations

Physical Exam	Abrupt onset Sharp, stabbing pain worsened during inspiration or coughing, usually unilateral
Auscultation	Pleural friction rub
Chest Imaging	Pleural thickening may be visible

Treatment
- Correct underlying cause, as able
- Treat pain (pain may result in shallow breathing, leading to hypoventilation atelectasis - see pg 10-18)

Pneumonia (PNA)

Acute inflammation of the lungs caused by a bacteria, virus, or fungus which results in abnormal airways/alveoli, often fluid- or pus-filled

Causes:
- Aspiration (see pg 10-56)
- Bacterial: Gram +, Gram -, Atypical (see pg 10-57)
- Viral: RSV, SARS (including COVID) (see pg 10-75)
- Hypersensitivity (see pg 10-46)

Sources:
- Community-acquired pneumonia (CAP): acquired outside the hospital, typically bacterial
- Nosocomial pneumonia: acquired in the hospital
  - Hospital-acquired pneumonia (HAP) - 48+ hrs after admission
  - Ventilator-associated pneumonia (VAP) - 48+ hrs after intubation and mechanical ventilation

Clinical Manifestations

Physical Exam	Fever Chest pain Cough, (incessant, abnormal secretions) Shortness of breath GI symptoms (nausea/vomiting/diarrhea)
Auscultation Percussion	Coarse + fine crackles Wheezes Decreased Dullness to percussion
Chest Imaging	Infiltrates, usually localized to where infection is centered (although more severe pneumonia may become bilateral, more diffuse, transitioning into ARDS)
ABGs	Vary but respiratory acidosis may be expected for moderate-to-severe pneumonia with hypoxemia (may be refractory to oxygen)
Labs	↑ Serum lactate (mod-to-severe)

Aspiration Pneumonia

Etiology:
- **Aspiration pneumonia**: chronic aspiration of colonized oropharyngeal secretions
- **Aspiration pneumonitis**: acute aspiration of gastric contents
- **Ventilator-associated pneumonia (VAP)**: aspiration (and micro-aspiration) usually around the ET tube cuff (vocal cords are held open by the airway, allowing both GI and oropharyngeal secretions)
- Periodontal disease, putrid sputum, ETOH history all may increase risk of anaerobic infection

Contributing factors are many, including: impaired mental status, dysphagia, GERD, inadequate cough, seizures, CPR

Clinical Manifestations
See general manifestations page 10-55, plus:

Pneumonia	Signs and symptoms of infection with purulent sputum
Pneumonitis	Sudden tachypnea and dyspnea, cough, crackles, wheezing, cyanosis, hypoxemia, may progress to respiratory failure.
Chest Imaging	Segmental consolidation (dependent, varies based on position during aspiration)

Treatment
- Prevent aspiration when able (head of bed at 30°, NPO when high-risk, intubation, etc.)
- Airway clearance (suction)
- Support symptoms (oxygen, therapeutic bronchoscopy, antibiotics, hydration, etc.)

Bacterial Pneumonia

Etiology:
- Bacterial infection (many bacteria) broken down into
  - Gram + (*S. aureus, S. pneumoniae*) which are generally more responsive to treatment
  - Gram - (*P. aeruginosa, E. coli, K. pneumoniae, H. influenzae*) which may be more resistive to treatment (and more likely to be hospital-acquired)
  - Atypical: difficult to detect through standard microbiology (*C. pneumoniae, Legionella, Mycoplasma pneumonia*)

Clinical Manifestations
See general manifestations page 10-55, plus:

Physical Exam	Fever more likely
Labs	↑ WBC Banding may be present (immature neutrophils)

Treatment
- Antibiotics to treat bacterial pneumonia
- Antipyretics to treat fever
- Support symptoms (oxygen, airway clearance, therapeutic bronchoscopy, antibiotics, hydration, etc.)

Pneumothorax (Air Leak Syndromes)
Accumulation of air or gas in the pleural space which compresses against the lung, impacting pulmonary and hemodynamic function

General Clinical Manifestations
See next page for specific manifestations. Clinical manifestations range from asymptomatic (small pneumothorax) to life-threatening (massive or tension pneumothorax)

Physical Exam	Pleuritic chest pain (may be sudden or gradual) Tachypnea Tachycardia Hypoxemia Hypotension Decreased chest expansion (affected side) Decreased tactile fremitus (affected side)
Auscultation Percussion	Decreased (affected side) Hyperresonance to percussion
Chest Imaging	Absent bronchovascular markings (affected side) Lung border may be visible on edge of pneumothorax (when compressed) **Small spontaneous** = < 3 cm apex-to-cupola **Large spontaneous** = > 3 cm apex-to-cupola

Treatment
- See next page for specific strategies
- In general: if small/asymptomatic observe and allow to self-resolve. If larger/symptomatic evacuate air if able, consider chest tube
- Supplemental oxygen (> 3 L/min) may help resorb the air in the pleural space at a rate faster than normal
- Avoid use of high-flow oxygen, CPAP, NPPV, ventilator when possible (positive pressure may worsen pneumo)
- Use of a Heimlich valve (a one-way valve that allows air to travel away from the leak)
- Recurrent pneumothorax: thoracoscopy, pleurodesis, bullectomy as clinically appropriate

Types of Air Leak Syndromes

Type	Description/Etiology	Specific Clinical Manifestations	Management
Non-spontaneous Pneumothorax	*Trapped air in pleural space. May occur with no apparent lung disease (primary) or with apparent lung disease (secondary)*	See general considerations, previous page	If small: monitor/observe. If large/symptomatic: evacuate air, chest tube esp if trauma or lung disease
Spontaneous	*Likely the spontaneous rupture of a bleb or bulla. Tall, thin patients are at ↑ risk. Various correlations.*	No clinical signs prior to pneumo. Acute onset of chest pain. Dyspnea (usually mild)	Resolve without intervention the majority of the time (~24 hrs), unless larger (see general considerations, previous page)
Tension	*A one-way valve is formed, allowing air into the pleural space on inspiration, but having no way to escape on exhalation. Compresses lung, ↓ venous return to the heart. Causes: PPV, trauma, iatrogenic*	May quickly progress to life-threatening: Hypotension, Hypoxemia, Dyspnea/chest pain, Tracheal shift (away from pneumo)	Immediate needle decompression using a large-bore (14- or 16-gauge) needle placed into the 2nd intercostal space at the midclavicular line
Pneumo-pericardium	*Presence of air/gas in the pericardial sac*	Can lead to cardiac tamponade	Evacuate air
Pneumo-mediastinum	*Accumulation of air/gas in the mediastinal space*		Usually resolves without intervention

Pulmonary Edema
Accumulation of excessive fluid in the alveolar walls and space of the lungs

Types:
Interstitial – Fluid moves only into the interstitium
Alveolar – Fluid moves into the interstitium, plus the alveoli

High-pressure pulmonary edema (cardiogenic, hydrostatic)	Permeability pulmonary edema (non-cardiogenic, neurogenic)
Transudation: volume/ pressure overload of the pulmonary circulation *Causes*: acute MI, arrhythmias, CHF, infection, hypervolemia, LVF, renal failure, shock	*Exudation*: ↑permeability of the pulmonary capillary membrane. *Causes*: ARDS, CNS (hemorrhage, trauma, stroke, tumors, ↑ ICP), drowning, smoke inhalation, oxygen toxicity

Clinical Manifestations
Varies with severity of underlying cause

Physical Exam	Restlessness/anxiety Orthopnea Hypoxemia with cyanosis Tachypnea Tachycardia Cough (varies - may be pink, frothy or dry)
Auscultation	Coarse crackles Wheezing
Chest Imaging	**Interstitial:** Haziness of vasculature and hilum **Alveolar:** Irregular, "butterfly" or "bat wing" pattern

Treatment
- Varies by underlying cause: support respiratory, support CO, monitor fluid status:
- See ARDS, pg 10-5
- See left-sided heart failure, pg 10-43

Pulmonary Embolism

The blockage of an artery in the lungs usually due to a thrombus (clot), reducing blood flow (or stopping it), potentially leading to V/Q mismatch, and hemodynamic compromise

Etiology:
- Lack of blood movement: bed rest, CHF, obesity, pregnancy, birth control pills, post-operative
- Fat (bone marrow): fractures, esp. long bones (leg), soft tissue
- Vessel wall abnormalities: trauma, phlebitis, infection
- Iatrogenic: air from CVP placement, indwelling catheters
- Foreign body: drug abuse, tumors

Clinical Manifestations *Varies with degree of blockage*

Physical Exam	Dyspnea Pleuritic chest pain (sharp, sudden) Restlessness, anxiety (usually sudden) Cough (may include hemoptysis) Tachypnea, Tachycardia Hypotension* Hypoxemia - may lead to cor pulmonale Diaphoresis
Auscultation	Coarse Crackles Wheezing Pleural friction rub
Chest Imaging	May be normal Pulmonary artery may be ↑
Lab Tests	D-Dimer: See pg 4-10

If BPsys < 90 mm Hg for > 15 min, drop of BP > 40 mm Hg, need for vasopressors, or evidence of shock: patient is hemodynamically unstable

Treatment
- Compression stockings, ambulation are prophylactic in higher-risk patients
- Vena cava filter (prophylactic, high bleed risk, or recurring PEs)
- Thrombolytics if hypotension but no significant bleeding risk
- Anticoagulation (heparin, etc.)
- Embolectomy if massive (and unstable)

Diseases

Pulmonary Hypertension

Hypertension of the pulmonary arteries (high blood pressure in the lungs), forcing the right-side of the heart to work more strenuously to pump blood through

Etiology (5 Categories):
1. Idiopathic, genetic, drugs, congenital heart disease
2. Left-sided heart disease
3. Hypoxia, lung disease (obstructive and restrictive)
4. Pulmonary artery obstructions (thromboembolic disease, tumors)
5. Multi-factorial, blood or metabolic disorders

Clinical Manifestations

Physical Exam	Progressive exertional dyspnea and fatigue Atypical chest discomfort Signs of right ventricular failure (JVD, hepatomegaly, peripheral edema, ascites)
Chest Imaging	Enlargement of central pulmonary arteries, right-ventricular enlargement, pleural effusions

Management
- Treat predisposing factors
- Treat respiratory failure (intubate if necessary)
- Careful fluid balance (overload may worsen hypertension)
- Pharmacology (phosphodiesterase inhibitors, prostacyclins, nitric oxide)

Respiratory Failure

The inability of the respiratory system to maintain adequate gas exchange, either in oxygen delivery and/or carbon dioxide removal

	Type 1 (Hypoxemic)	Type 2 (Hypercapnic)
Definition	The failure of lungs and heart to provide adequate oxygen to meet metabolic needs	The failure of the lungs to eliminate a sufficient amount of carbon dioxide
Criteria	$PaO_2 < 60$ on 50% oxygen $PaO_2 < 40$ any O_2 level + hypoxemia symptoms	pH < 7.30 with ↑ in $PaCO_2$ $PaCO_2 > 50$ (normal baseline) + symptoms of hypercapnia
Basic Causes	Right-to-left shunt V/Q mismatch Alveolar hypoventilation Diffusion defect Inadequate FiO_2	Pump failure (drive, muscles, WOB) ↑ CO_2 production Right-to-left shunt ↑ Dead space
Clinical Manifestations	**Acute**	
	Cyanosis Change in mental status Tachypnea Tachycardia	Change in mental status (↑ confusion, somnolence) Dyspnea Headache
	Chronic	
	Digital clubbing Polycythemia	Dyspnea on exertion Fatigue, irritability ↑ HCO_3^- (compensation)

Treatment	Supplemental oxygen
	Optimize oxygenation
	  Patient positioning
	  CPAP/PEEP
	Optimize
	  hemodynamics
		Correction of underlying
		  (such as drug overdose)
		
		Support failing ventilation:
		NPPV
		Invasive ventilation
		resp stimulants (neonate)

Diseases

Restrictive Lung Disease

A disease or disorder characterized by decreased lung volumes and capacities

Etiology:
Parenchymal:
  Compression: fibrosis, pleural effusion, pneumothorax, tumor
  Infiltration: edema, infection, secretions, hyaline membranes
  Volume Loss: atelectasis, ARDS, lobectomy
Chest Wall: musculoskeletal (kyphoscoliosis, obesity, etc.), neuromuscular

Nervous system control: depression of respiratory drive, paralysis

Clinical Manifestations
Most vary by underlying cause, of which there are many

Physical Exam	Dyspnea Hypoxemia (leading to cor pulmonale) Cyanosis
Auscultation	Decreased
Chest Imaging	Decreased lung volumes
PFTs	Lung volumes (TLC) decreased ↓ vital capacity (more so than FRC, RV) Flows likely normal (FEV_1, FVC)

Treatment
- Manage or treat underlying condition

Shock

A life-threatening condition of circulatory failure, commonly manifested as hypotension, causing inadequate oxygen delivery to meet cellular metabolic needs, resulting in cellular and tissue hypoxia (which progresses to cellular/tissue death).

Clinical Manifestations
Varies according to cause

Physical Exam	Hypotension (may be life-threatening) perfusion to vital organs likely affected Tachycardia, Tachypnea Cool, clammy skin with cyanosis Oliguria Abnormal mental status
ABG	Metabolic acidosis

Types of Shock (Causes and Management)

Type	Causes	Management *(support failing systems +)*
Anaphylactic	Life-threatening allergic reaction (blood, drugs, foods, environmental, etc.)	Remove/stop the cause Give epinephrine (IM) Manage airway
Cardiogenic	Acute MI, severe hypoxemia, arrhythmias, tension pneumothorax	Support cardiac output Antiplatelets, heparin Invasive interventions
Hypovolemic	Burns, dehydration, hemorrhage, trauma	Correct problem Replace lost volume Give blood as needed Inotropes, vasopressors
Neurogenic	Anesthesia, brain trauma, insulin shock, severe pain	Correct problem Vasopressors if hypovolemia
Septic	Pancreatitis, trauma, infection, immunoincompetence	Antibiotics IV fluids, vasopressors Supportive care

Sleep-Disordered Breathing

Abnormal respirations that occur during the sleep cycle, by physical obstruction of the airway and/or a lack of signal from the brain to initiate a breath

Etiology:
There are 60+ sleep disorders with varying etiologies
Body mass index (BMI): ↑ BMI = ↑ risk of sleep-disordered breathing
Anatomic alterations
Secondary to disease: CHF, stroke, brain lesions, etc.

Clinical Manifestations
Daytime somnolence, headache (AM), memory loss, personality changes, depression, inability to concentrate, decreased mental acuity, potential arrhythmias, pulmonary hypertension

	Obstructive Sleep Apnea (OSA)	Central Sleep Apnea (CSA)
During Sleep:	Obstructive apneas, hypopneas, and respiratory effort-related arousal caused by repetitive collapse of the upper airway	Repetitive cessation/decrease of both airflow and ventilatory effort
Resp. Effort	Yes	No
Symptoms	Snoring Gasping/choking/snorting	Milder snoring Cheyne-Stokes pattern for some patients
Treatment	Treat as chronic disease CPAP/APAP: 5+ events/hr w/ symptoms or >15/hr even if no symptoms Surgery (less common)	Treat underlying cause CPAP* (unless EF < 45%) NPPV* Supplemental oxygen Phrenic nerve pacemaker?

EF: Ejection Fraction; APAP: Autotitrating Positive Airway Pressure
*CPAP is recommended for hyperventilation-related CSA, while NPPV is recommended for hypoventilation-related CSA

Smoke Inhalation/Thermal Burns

Inhalation of smoke, fumes, or other caustic agents into the tracheobronchial tree with potential tissue injury resulting (burns or toxins)

Clinical Manifestations
If headache, nausea, confusion, suspect CO poisoning (see pg 10-21)

Upper Airway (symptoms within minutes, maybe hours)
Thermal burns are primary concern
- Stridor (if edema)
- Redness
- Ulcerations

Lower Airway (symptoms often delayed unless severe injury)
Thermal burns are less likely (heat dissipates)
Chemicals in smoke cause injury
- Cough (persistent, productive, may contain soot)
- Wheezing (persistent, chemical-triggered bronchoconstriction)
- Increased secretions leading to atelectasis
- Impaired surfactant leading to atelectasis

Treatment
- Directly examine airways
  - Laryngoscopy to examine upper airway
  - Bronchoscopy to examine lower airway
- Intubate if any signs of soot in the upper airways (nares, posterior pharynx, etc.) as increasing edema is likely.
  - Burns to face/neck may distort and compress airway
- Give humidified oxygen if not intubating
- Airway clearance may be necessary
  - Chest physiotherapy
  - Percussive ventilation (IPV, etc.)

Tracheoarterial Fistula
(Tracheoinnominate artery fistula, TI-fistula)
A rare, life-threatening abnormal passageway between the trachea and most often the innominate artery (although others are possible) which is almost always a complication related to artificial airways

Etiology
Presence of tracheostomy tube (more common) or endotracheal tube (less common). May be caused by the cuff or the tube tip. Note: less common now due to changes in tracheostomy positioning.

Clinical Manifestations
Massive hemoptysis

Treatment
- This is a life-threatening emergency with poor survival
- DO NOT DELAY CARE. If suspected:
  - Immediately over-inflate the cuff
  - If that fails: place finger in the stoma, distally towards the lungs, then pull finger towards sternum with enough pressure to lift the torso slightly off bed. Maintain pressure until transport to surgery (while providing bag-valve-mask ventilation)

Tracheoesophageal Fistula (TEF, or TE-fistula)
Bronchoesophageal Fistula (BEF)
A fairly rare abnormal passageway between the trachea and the esophagus (termed a TEF) or the major bronchi and the esophagus (termed a BEF)

Etiology
Congenital (may rarely be discovered as an adult)
Malignant (esophageal or lung cancer)
Iatrogenic (prolonged intubation, surgery, granulomas)

Clinical Manifestations
Coughing (frequent, may follow nutritional intake)
Aspirations (recurrent), possibly with infections
Malnutrition

Treatment
- Unlikely to self-resolve
- Patient should be NPO - remove NG/OG tubes (may need TPN)
- Head of bed up (45° or higher if possible)
- Treat underlying infections (pneumonia from aspirations)
- Intubated Patients
  - Extubate if possible; otherwise advance ET tube or place longer trach tube.
  - Consider waiting until after wean/extubation/decannulation due to concern of post-op complications
- Surgical repair is usually indicated (stent, etc.)

Trauma

A physical injury that may result in harm (bleeding, fractures, disfigurements, burns, etc.) of a wide severity, and may impact on cardiopulmonary status.

Etiology
Many cases/categories, including: head/brain trauma, chest trauma (penetrating, blunt force)

General Management
Always evaluate fully (ABCDE) to ensure nothing is missed, prioritizing life-threatening injuries.

Airway	**Verify patency; establish airway if any doubt** Airway obstruction is common Elevate head as clinically able Check for injury to teeth/tongue, other blockages If airway already, reconfirm placement/position
Breathing	**Verify adequacy of oxygenation/ventilation** Inspect chest (paradoxical movement/flail) Auscultate Palpate (subcutaneous emphysema, etc.) Check for emergencies*, penetrating trauma
Circulation	**Verify sufficient hemodynamics** Check central pulses (carotid, femoral) If impaired, consider emergencies* Control life-threatening hemorrhage Hypotension may indicate bleeding
Disability/ Neuro	**Verify level of consciousness (GCS)** Check pupillary size/reaction, sensation, etc
Exposure	**Verify no (significant) injuries are missed** Trauma patients should be completely undressed (exposed), all areas checked thoroughly for injury

* Thoracic emergencies include: tension pneumothorax (see pg 10-58); hemothorax (see pg 10-53); cardiac tamponade (see pg 10-22)

Traumatic Brain Injury (TBI)

Types
- **Epidural Hematoma**: bleeding between the dura mater and the skull: skull fracture tears an underlying blood vessel
- **Subdural Hematoma**: bleeding between inner layer of the dura mater and the surface of the brain, quickly compressing the brain. This is usually a result of severe head injury
- **Intracerebral Hemorrhage**: bleeding from a blood vessel in a specific area of the brain (basal ganglia, cerebellum, pons, etc.)

Management
Intracranial Pressure (ICP): Monitor if GCS 8 or below
- Normal: < 15 mm Hg
- Therapeutic Goal: maintain < 23 mm Hg
- Increased ICP can trigger "Cushing's Triad":
  - Bradycardia
  - Respiratory depression
  - Hypertension
- Systolic BP: maintain at 100-110 or above
- PaO_2: maintain above 60 mm Hg (avoid hyperoxygenating)
- Consider intubation if GCS < 8 (under 8: intubate), inability to protect airway, SpO_2 < 90 despite supplemental O_2, clinical signs of cerebral herniation)
- Ventilator: maintain $PaCO_2$ 35-45 mm Hg, only hyperventilate as a very temporary measure to reduce ↑ ICP (do not prophylactically)

Chest Trauma

Types

Blunt Force Trauma (motor vehicle, industrial, etc.)
- Fractures (ribs, sternum, scapula) See below and Flail Chest (pg 10-41)
- Contusions (pulmonary, chest wall)

Penetrating Trauma (gunshot wound, stabbing, shrapnel, etc.)
- Pneumothorax (see pg 10-58)

General Chest Trauma (can be Blunt and/or Penetrating)
- Cardiac Tamponade (see pg 10-22)
- Hemothorax (see pg 10-53)

Management
- **Rib Fractures, Chest Wall Contusion** (contusion to outside of chest wall - bruising)
  - Pain management to allow for adequate respiratory effort
  - Lung expansion (IS, deep breathing)
  - Airway clearance (if unable to cough effectively)
  - Many patients can self-manage, but may need intubation/ventilation if pain management is an issue
- **Pulmonary Contusion (contusion to lung tissue)**
  - Initially may appear less severe than it is (chest imaging, oxygenation, etc.)
  - 12-24 hrs post-injury: hypoventilation/hypoxemia may progressively worsen resulting in a need to intubate
  - May further progress to ARDS
  - Monitor patient status closely
- **Bleeding/Hemothorax**
  - Chest tube placement for evacuation of blood
  - Surgical intervention if massive

Tuberculosis

Chronic, progressive droplet infection caused by Mycobacterium tuberculosis which often affects the lungs but may affect other body systems. An initial (primary) infection is often asymptomatic is followed by a dormant (latent) period, which may or may not be followed by periods of active infection.

Etiology
Caused by exposure to *Mycobacterium tuberculosis*

Diagnosis
Screening: Mantoux tuberculin skin test (PPD) screens for active or latent infection or Interferon gamma release assay (IGRA), a blood test for latent infection.

Lab Test: Acid-fast bacilli (AFB) smear and culture from a sputum sample.

Clinical Manifestations
Tuberculosis may progress through various stages, including:
Primary TB: Often asymptomatic or minimally symptomatic
Latent TB: Asymptomatic and non-contagious period
Active TB: Most likely to be symptomatic, including:

Physical Exam	Cough (mucoid or mucopurulent sputum) Hemoptysis Chest tightness with dull pain Dyspnea Night sweats Fatigue Fever (usually low-grade)
Auscultation	Coarse crackles Wheezes Bronchial breath sounds Dull to percussion
Chest Imaging	May be similar to pneumonia (primary TB) Nodules (around the clavicle can indicate active TB; more calcified may indicate old infection)

Treatment

- Infection control: negative pressure room, N-95 type masks. Continue isolation until 3 consecutive negative AFB smears
- Initial treatment with antibacterial drug therapy, usually 4 drugs given together (first-line approach) over 2 months initially (intensive phase)
  - isoniazid
  - rifampin
  - pyrazinamide
  - ethambutol
- Some patients with latent TB should receive a therapy approved specifically for latent TB.
- Some cases of TB result in dissemination (spreading, including to other body systems)

Viral Infections

An infection, often with pulmonary effects, caused by the introduction of a virus with a range in illness from asymptomatic to life-threatening.

Types:
- Upper respiratory infection: largely affects the upper airway with nasal congestion, cough, sore throat (rhinovirus, adenovirus, some coronaviruses)
- Lower respiratory infection: parainfluenza (croup), bronchiolitis (RSV)
- Lungs: (influenza, viral pneumonia [adenovirus, some coronaviruses, parainfluenza, bronchiolitis])

(Respiratory) Clinical Manifestations
Varies by virus, viral load, immune status, etc. (from asymptomatic to life-threatening)

Physical Exam	Minimal symptoms (often cough, sore throat, malaise, headache, muscle aches) More severe symptoms (shortness of breath, dyspnea, productive cough, chest pain, hypoxemia with respiratory failure) May progress to ARDS
Auscultation	Coarse crackles Wheezes
Chest Imaging	Scattered infiltrates, vary in severity

Treatment
- Infection control: often droplet, use appropriate PPE
- Support oxygenation: supplemental O_2, patient positioning (pg 5-11), high-flow oxygen, NIV, intubation/ventilator with recruitment strategies, ECMO
- Support ventilation: NPPV, intubation/ventilation
- Prevent lung injury: permissive hypercapnia, etc.
- Support hemodynamics: fluid management, inotropes, etc.
- Antiviral drugs: not all viruses respond to an antiviral, may shorten duration and severity of the infection.
- Monitor and treat comorbidities which often trigger a more severe illness

11 Pharmacology

Abbreviations Used in Drug Administration	11-4
JCAHO Do-Not-Use List	11-5
Drug Administration Procedures	11-6
Drug Calculations	
Solution and Dosage Problems	11-7
Conversion Within and Between Systems	11-8
Common Conversions	11-9
Receptors	
Alpha and Beta	11-10
Muscarinic	11-10

Drug Tables (by class and generic name)
How to Use	11-11
Abbreviations Used	11-11

Anti-Asthma
Mast Cell Stabilizers
cromolyn sodium	11-12

Antileukotrienes
montelukast	11-13
zarfirlukast	11-13
zileuton	11-13

Bronchodilators
Short-Acting Beta Agonists (SABAs)
albuterol	11-14
levalbuterol	11-15
terbutaline	11-16

Long-Acting Beta Agonists (LABAs)
arformoterol tartrate	11-17
formoterol fumarate	11-18
salmeterol	11-18

Ultra Long-Acting Beta Agonists (ULABAs)
indacaterol	11-19
olodaterol hydrochloride	11-19

Bronchodilators (continued)

Short-Acting Muscarinic Antagonists (SAMAs)
  ipratropium bromide 11-20
Long-Acting Muscarinic Anatgonists (LAMAs)
  aclidinium bromide 11-21
  glycopyrrolate bromide 11-21
  revafenacin 11-22
  tiotropium bromide 11-22
  umeclidinium bromide 11-22
Xanthines (Methylxanthines)
  aminophylline 11-23
  dyphylline 11-23
  oxtriphylline 11-23
  theophylline 11-23

Alpha-1 Antitrypsin Deficiency Disorder
  alpha 1 proteinase inhibitor 11-24

Anti-Infectives (Inhaled)
  aztreonam 11-25
  colistin 11-26
  pentamadine isethionate 11-27
  ribavirin 11-28
  tobramycin 11-29
  zanamivir 11-30

Mucoactives
  acetylcysteine 11-31
  dornase alfa-dnase 11-32
  mannitol 11-32
  saline (isotonic, hypotonic, hypertonic) 11-33

Inhaled Analgesics
  lidocaine 11-34
  morphine/opiates 11-34

Inhaled Epinephrine
  racemic epinephrine 11-35
  epinephrine 11-35

Phosphodiesterase Inhibitors

roflumilast 11-36

Pulmonary Vasodilators
epoprostenol 11-37
iloprost 11-38

Smoking Cessation
5 A's 11-39
varenicline 11-40
bupropion 11-40
Nicotine-Replacement Therapies (NRT) 11-41

Steroids (Inhaled Corticosteroids) (ICS)
beclomethasone 11-44
budesonide 11-45
ciclesonide HFA 11-46
fluticasone propionate 11-47

Combination Therapies
ICS + LABA
budesonide + formoterol 11-49
fluticasone + salmeterol 11-48
mometasone + formoterol 11-49
SABA + SAMA
albuterol + ipratropium bromide 11-52
LAMA + LABA
vilanterol + umeclidinium 11-53
glycopyrrolate + formoterol 11-53
olodaterol + tiotropium 11-53
glycopyrrolate + indacterol 11-53
ICS + LAMA + LABA
fluticasone + vilanterol + umeclidinium 11-54
budesonide + glycopyrrolate + formoterol 11-54

Drugs that Cause Respiratory Depression 11-56
Common Cardiac Drugs (by effect) 11-57

Select Abbreviations used in Drug Administration

Spell out abbreviations when possible to avoid confusion. If there is any doubt about an intended meaning of an abbreviation, seek clarification before administering the treatment.

$\bar{a}$	before	IM	intramuscular
Aa, $\bar{aa}$	of each	IN	intranasal
ac	before meals	instill.	instilled
ad	to, up to	IU	international unit
ad lib	as much as necessary	IV	intravenous
		L	liter or left
aq dist	distilled water	liq.	liquid
BID	twice daily	M	mix
$\bar{c}$	with	mEq	milliequivalent
cap	capsule	mL	milliliter
cc	cubic centimeter (equal to a mL)	mMol	millimole
conc	concentrate	n, noct.	in the night
dil.	dilute	NAS	intranasal
elix	elixir	nebul	spray
emuls	emulsion	NKA	no known allergies
et	and	NKDA	no known drug allergies
ex aq	in water		
ext	extract	non rep	do not repeat
fl, fld	fluid	NPO	nothing by mouth
ft	make	NS	normal saline
gel	gel or jelly	NTE	not to exceed
g	gram	OTC	over-the-counter
gr	grain	oz	ounce
gtt, gtts	drop, drops	$\bar{p}$	after
hs	hour of sleep	pc	after meals

per	by, through	q2h	every 2 hours
per neb	by nebulizer	q3h	every 3 hours
per os	by mouth	q4h	every 4 hours
po	by mouth	q6h	every 6 hours
prn	as needed	qt	quart
pr or rect	rectally	Rx	take
pulv	powder	s̄	without
q	every	sol	solution
QID	four times/day	solv	dissolve
QOD	every other day	sos	if needed (1x)
qd, q1d	every day	STAT	immediately
qh	every hour	tab	tablet
qhs	at each bedtime	TID	three times/day

JCAHO Drug Abbreviations to Not Use (Handwritten)

Due to high likelihood of errors (similar abbreviations), JCAHO (jointcommission.org) has established a "Do Not Use" list. This applies to handwritten orders, updated August 2020.

Excluded Abbreviations	Recommendation
U (unit)	Write "unit"
IU (International Unit)	Write "International Unit"
Q.D., QD, q.d., qd (daily)	Write: daily
Q.O.D., QOD, q.o.d., qod (every other day)	Write: Every Other Day
*A Trailing 0 (X.0 mg) A lack of leading 0 (.X mg)	Write: X mg (no 0 after decimal) Write: 0.X mg (use 0 before decimal)
MS, MSO$_4$, MgSO$_4$	Write "morphine sulfate" or Write "magnesium sulfate"

*Note that certain things are exempt from the use of a trailing zero, including lab results that show precision (pH 7.0), tube/catheter sizes (ET Tube 8.0), and imaging studies.

Pharmacology

Drug Administration Procedures

A systematic approach is the best way to avoid medication errors. Consider these steps in addition to using a barcode or similar safety system:

1. **Review the medical record**
   Verify all orders, assess clinical appropriateness of orders, verify allergies, medical history, etc.

2. **Verify right patient**
   Use multiple ways to confirm: name, medical record number, date of birth, ID bracelet, etc.

3. **Ensure you have the right drug**
   Confirm drug label for contents. If any doubt, contact pharmacy prior to administration.

4. **Ensure you have the right dosage and concentration**
   Double-check drug dosage in the form being given. Verify units and concentration.

5. **Ensure you have the right time**
   Be aware of a drug's peak time and the implications for giving drugs early or late

6. **Ensure you have the right route**
   Some drugs have multiple routes: nebulized, MDI, DPI, oral, instilled, IV, etc. Dosing can be route-dependent.

7. **Perform patient assessment**
   A general impression should be made (level of consciousness, attitude towards care, etc.) and then vital signs and auscultation noted before, during, and after treatment. If an adverse effect is noted, STOP treatment, assess, and consider appropriate modifications (different drug, reduced dosage, etc.) as clinically indicated.

8. **Perform patient education**
   Capitalize on opportunities to demo and coach a patient on home drugs (inhaler use, for example). Explain treatments being given in patient-appropriate terminology (aim for 5th grade explanations if unknown)

9. **Document administration in an objective and timely manner**

Calculating Solution and Dosage Problems

W/W% = $\dfrac{\text{grams solute}}{100 \text{ gm solution}}$

W/V% = $\dfrac{\text{grams solute}}{100 \text{ mL solution}}$

V/V% = $\dfrac{\text{mL solute}}{100 \text{ mL solution}}$

Concent 1:500 solution into mg/mL

1:500 = 1 gm/500 gm
= 1 gm/500 mL
= 1000 mg/500 mL
= 2 mg/mL

What % solution is 2 mg/mL

2 mg/mL = 200 mg/100 mL
= 0.2 gm/100 mL
= 0.2 gm/100 gm
= 0.2% solution

Find mg of drug if 0.25 mL (1:200) is diluted in 2.5 mL saline

1:200 = 1g/200 mL
= 1000mg/200 mL
= 5 mg/mL
0.25 mL × 5 mg/mL
= 1.25 mg of drug delivered in 2.75 mL solution

1 mL H2O = 1 gm H2O (spec gravity 1.0)   1 gm = 1,000 mg

Pharmacology

Conversion within Same Measuring System

1. Set up a proportion	How many mg are in 5 g? $$\frac{g}{mg} = \frac{g}{mg}$$
2. Use what is known	1 g = 1000 mg
3. Solve the equation	$$\frac{1\ g}{1000\ mg} = \frac{5\ g}{X\ mg}$$ $$(1)(X) = (1000)(5)$$ $$X = 5{,}000\ mg$$

Conversion between Measuring Systems

1. Set up a proportion	How many grains are in 5 g? $$\frac{\text{System 1 Known}}{\text{System 2 Known}} = \frac{\text{System 1 X}}{\text{System 2 X}}$$ X is unknown (note that you will have to know 1 - see example below - to solve the equation)
2. Determine what is known	1 g = 15 grains
3. Solve the equation	$$\frac{1\ g}{15\ grains} = \frac{5\ g}{X\ grains}$$ $$(1)(X) = (15)(5)$$ $$X = 75\ grains$$ There are 75 grains in 5 g

Common Conversions

1 cup (C)	240 mL 8 fluid ounces	1 kilogram (kg)	2.2 lb
1 milliliter (mL)	1 cc 16 drops (gtts)	1 milligram (mg)	1000 micrograms (mcg)
1000 mL	~1 quart 1 L	1000 mg	1 gram (g)
1 teaspoon (t)	5 mL 60 drops		
1 tablespoon (T)	3 teaspoons 15 mL		
1 fluid ounce (US)	30 mL 2 tablespoons		

---

1. Convert all measurements to the same unit
2. $\dfrac{\text{Original Strength}}{\text{Amount Supplied}} = \dfrac{\text{Desired Strength (dosage)}}{\text{Unknown amount to be supplied}}$

Example 1:
How many mL of a drug must be given to deliver 75,000 units (50,000 units/mL)?

$$\dfrac{50,000}{\text{mL}} = \dfrac{75,000}{X \text{ mL}}$$

$$X = \dfrac{75,000}{50,000} = 1.5 \text{ mL}$$

Example 2:
How many mLs of a drug, at a concent. of 25 mg/mL of solution, would be needed to provide 100 mg?

$$\dfrac{25 \text{ mg}}{\text{mL}} = \dfrac{100 \text{ mg}}{X \text{ mL}}$$

$$X = \dfrac{100 \text{ mg}}{25 \text{ mg}} = 4 \text{ mL}$$

Pharmacology

Alpha and Beta Receptors

Receptor*		Location *General action when receptor stimulated*
alpha-1	α1	Located in peripheral blood vessels *vasoconstriction*
alpha-2	α2	Located in central nervous system *Action varies (vasoconstriction/dilation)*
beta-1	β1	Located in heart *Primarily vasoconstriction in heart (neg feedback)*
beta-2	β2	Located in smooth muscle + cardiac muscle *Relax bronchial smooth muscle* (if bronchoconstriction, this will open the airways. If no bronchoconstriction, unlikely to be helpful)

* Receptor action:
- Receptors with a 1 after (α1, β1) cause excitation.
  We remember this as: 1 is fun
- Receptors with a 2 after (α2, β2) cause inhibition.
  We remember this as: 2 is blue

Muscarinic (Acetylcholine or ACh) Receptors

*Muscarinic drugs work by **blocking** cholinergic response at specific receptors. Note that M1-M2-M3 are primary targets, although M4 and M5 exist. M3 most directly produces bronchoconstriction and secretions.*

Receptor		Respiratory-focused Effects
AChM1R	M1	Bronchoconstriction, ↑ ciliary beat freq, limit histamine release from mast cells
AChM2R	M2	Inhibit smooth muscle relaxation (indirectly cause bronchoconstriction), ↓ ciliary beat frequency
AChM3R	M3	Cause smooth muscle contraction (directly causes bronchoconstriction), mucus secretion, vasodilation, ↑ ciliary beat freq, ↑ immune response

Using the Drug Tables

- **Drug information is constantly changing with drugs being added or removed, indications changing, and adverse effects being updated. Please confirm information in this pocket guide with a reliable source.**
- Drugs are presented by major category, then alphabetically
- Onset/Peak/Duration: When clinically applicable and available
  - Onset: length of time until a therapeutic effect is likely
  - Peak: length of time until maximum effectiveness is reached
  - Duration: length of time until drug loses therapeutic effect
- Adverse Effects: most drugs have long lists of potential adverse effects. We usually present the most common (those that are reported to occur 9-10% of the time, or higher) effects.
  - It is important to remember that many drug forms contain both the active drug(s) + excipients which are used for suspension, propulsion, and stability. These excipients may also cause adverse effects in sensitive patients.
  - For combination drugs, see each individual drug for adverse effects.

Abbreviations Used

ICS: Inhaled Corticosteroids
SABA: Short-Acting Beta Agonist (Relievers*)
SAMA: Short-Acting Muscarinic Antagonist (Anticholinergics)
LABA: Long-Acting Beta Agonist
LAMA: Long-Acting Muscarinic Antagonist (Anticholinergics)

DPI: Dry Powder Inhaler
MDI: Metered-Dose Inhaler
Neb: Nebulizer treatment
pMDI: Pressurized Metered-Dose Inhaler
SMI: Soft Mist Inhaler

*Global Initiative for Asthma (GINA) refers to these as SABAs or Relievers (2020)

Anti-Asthma: Mast Cell Stabilizers

Generic *Brand Names*	Dosage (by FORM and INDICATION as appropriate)	Indications *Mode of Action*	Adverse Effects *Notes*
cromoxyn sodium *Nalcrom* Rarely used, not available in some areas	**Nebulizer** 20 mg in 2 mL **2 yr – adult:** 20 mg 4x/day may ↓ to 2-3x/day when stable **Allergen or EIB*:** Administer single dose 10-15 min, but not > 60 min, before precipitating event.	- Prophylactic maintenance of mild-to-moderate asthma - **Not for acute exacerbations** - Not as effective as SABA for Exercise-Induced Bronchoconstriction (EIB) *Prevents release of inflammatory mediators from inflammatory cell types.*	**Adverse:** Bronchospasm, cough, local irritation, dry mouth, chest tightness, vertigo, unpleasant taste in mouth. Neb solution (may dilute) may be mixed with albuterol Must be used at regular intervals for 2-4 weeks to be effective Note that inhaled steroids are preferred for persistent asthma; cromolyn is an alternative option

*EIB: Exercise-Induced Bronchospasm

Anti-Asthma: Antileukotrienes

Generic *Brand Names*	Dosage (by FORM and INDICATION as appropriate)	Indications *Mode of Action*	Adverse Effects *Notes*
montelukast *Singulair*	**Asthma, seasonal or perennial allergic rhinitis (taken in PM):** 6 mos-5 yrs: 4 mg 1x/day 6-14 yrs: 5 mg 1x/day ≥ 15 yrs: 10 mg 1x/day **Bronchoconstriction, EIB (prevention):** Take 2 hours prior to exercise 6-14 yrs: 5 mg/dose (chewable tab) ≥ 15 yrs: 10 mg/dose (tablet)	Seasonal/perennial allergic rhinitis, prophylaxis and chronic treatment of asthma, prevention of exercise-induced bronchospasm *Leukotriene receptor antagonist blocks inflammatory mediators*	Headache, dizziness, dyspepsia, fatigue, fever Do not take an additional dose for exercise-induced bronchospasm
zafirlukast *Accolate*	Take 1 hr before or 2 hrs after eating 5-11 yr: 10 mg 2x/day ≥ 12 yr: 20 mg 2x/day **Tablet:** 10 mg, 20 mg	Leukotriene receptor antagonist blocks inflammatory mediators	Headache, dizziness, dyspepsia, fatigue, fever
zileuton *Zyflo*	≥ 12 yr: 600 mg 4x/day (tabs) 1200 mg 2x/day (ER tabs)	Leukotriene inhibitor: *Prevents formation of inflammatory mediators*	Headache, dizziness, dyspepsia, fatigue, elevated LFT's (≥ 3x upper limit norm)

Bronchodilators: Short-Acting Beta Agonists (SABAs)

Generic Brand Names	Dosage	Indications Mode of Action	Adverse Effects Notes
albuterol AccuNeb ProAir ProAir Digihaler ProAir HFA RespiClick Proventil HFA Ventolin HFA VoSpire ER[1]	See Below	**Bronchoconstriction, Acute and Maintenance** Stimulates β1 (minor), β2 (strong) | onset	5 min | | peak | 30-60 min | | duration | 3-8 hrs |	Slight CV and CNS, hyperglycemia, hypokalemia, tremors - Oral forms (tablet, oral) are generally discouraged (less effective bronchodilation, more systemic effects)[2] - Digihaler pairs with an app, but is not needed to dispense drug

Acute/Exacerbation

NEBULIZER: 5 mg/mL (0.5%); 2.5mg/3mL (0.083%), 1.25 mg/3mL (0.042%), 0.63 mg/3mL (0.021%).

<u>Child:</u> 0.15 mg/kg (minimum 2.5 mg), every 20 min x 3 doses, then 0.15-0.3 mg/kg (up to 10 mg), every 1-4 hrs as needed **or** 0.5 mg/kg/hr by continuous neb.

<u>Adult:</u> 2.5-5 mg every 20 min x 3 doses, then 2.5-10 mg, every 1-4 hrs PRN or 10-15 mg/hr by continuous neb.

MDI and DPI: 90 mcg/puff

<u>Child:</u> 4-8 puffs, every 20 min x 3 doses, then every 1-4 hrs PRN

<u>Adol:</u> 4-8 puffs, every 20 min (up to 4 hrs), then every 1-4 hrs PRN

Chronic/Stable

NEBULIZER:

<u>Child < 12 yrs:</u> 0.15-0.25 mg/kg (max 5mg), every 4-6 hrs prn

<u>> 12 yrs:</u> 2.5-5 mg, every 4-6 hrs PRN

MDI:

<u>Child < 12 yrs:</u> 1-2 puffs 4x/day

<u>Child > 12 yrs – Adult:</u> 2-4 puffs, every 4-6 hrs (max 12 puffs/day)

[1] VoSpire ER is a tablet taken orally with duration of up to 12 hr (technically it is a LABA) [2] GOLD Guidelines 2018; GINA Guidelines 2020

Generic Brand Names	Dosage (by FORM and INDICATION as appropriate)	Indications Mode of Action	Adverse Effects Notes
levalbuterol Xopenex Xopenex HFA	See Below	**Bronchoconstriction** R-isomer form of albuterol, stimulates Beta-2 (strong) | onset	15 min
---	---
peak	30-60 min
duration	5-8 hrs		Slight CV and CNS effects, hyperglycemia, hypokalemia
	ACUTE EXACERBATION (NAEPP 2020) **Nebulizer:** 0.31 mg/3 mL, 0.63 mg/3mL, 1.25 mg/3 mL, 1.25 mg/0.5 mL (concentrated dose) <u>Child</u>: 0.075 mg/kg (minimum 1.25 mg) every 20 min x 3 doses, then 0.075-0.15 mg/kg (up to 5 mg) every 1-4 hrs as needed <u>Adult</u>: 1.25-2.5 mg every 20 min x 3 doses, then 1.25-5 mg every 1-4 hours as needed **MDI:** (45 mcg/spray) <u>Child</u>: 4-8 inh every 20 mins x3, then every 1-4 hrs as needed <u>Adult</u>: 4-8 inh every 20 mins for up to 4 hours, then every 1-4 hrs as needed	**NON-ACUTE (MAINTENANCE)** **Nebulizer:** 4 and under: 0.31-1.25 mg every 4-6 hrs PRN 5-11 yrs: 0.31-0.63 mg, every 8 hrs PRN 12+ yrs: 0.63 mg, 3x/day (nebulizer) increase to 1.25 mg if ineffective **MDI:** 4+ yrs: 1-2 inh every 4-6 hrs as needed	

Generic *Brand Names*	Dosage (by FORM and INDICATION as appropriate)	Indications *Mode of Action*	Adverse Effects *Notes*
terbutaline *Brethaire* *Brethine* *Bricanyl*	**Not typically used clinically today** **Nebulizer** 1 mg/mL **Oral:** < 12 yrs: 0.05 mg/kg 3x/day (max 5 mg/day) 12-15 yrs: 2.5 mg 3x/day (max 7.5 mg/day) > 15 yrs: 5 mg 3x/day; reduce to 2.5 mg 3x/day **Continuous IV:** 2-10 mcg/kg loading dose, then (asthma) 0.08-0.4 mcg/kg/min titrate up to 5-10 mcg/kg/min **Continuous Neb (uncommon):** 0.2-0.6 mg/kg/hr	**Bronchoconstriction** **Pre-term labor (off-label)** *Stimulates β-1 (mild)* *β-2 (mod)* | onset | 30-45 min | | peak | 2-3 hrs | | duration | 6-8 hrs |	Nervousness, restlessness, hyperglycemia, hypokalemia, tremors

Bronchodilators: Long-Acting Beta Agonists (LABAs)

BLACK BOX WARNING

A Black Box Warning applies to single-ingredient LABAs. This warning (the strongest warning possible by the FDA) means there is some evidence to suggest that these drugs may increase the risk of serious asthma-related events, including hospitalization, intubation, or death. An update in 2018 removed this warning from combination LABAs with corticosteroids.

Generic *Brand Names*	Dosage (by FORM and INDICATION as appropriate)	Indications *Mode of Action*	Adverse Effects *Notes*
arformoterol tartrate *Brovana*	**Nebulizer** 15 mcg in 2 mL Adults: 15 mcg 2x/day (every 12 hrs) (do not exceed 30 mcg/day)	**Maintenance treatment of COPD** *Acts locally on beta-2 receptors in the lungs, resulting in relaxation of smooth muscle. Also helps inhibit inflammatory response (histamine, leukotrienes, etc.)*	**Black Box Warning** (see top of this page) Chest pain, back pain, diarrhea, sinusitis - *NOT indicated for acute bronchoconstriction or asthma treatment* - *Once opened must be refrigerated and protected from light*

Pharmacology

Generic *Brand Names*	Dosage (by FORM and INDICATION as appropriate)	Indications *Mode of Action*	Adverse Effects *Notes*
formoterol fumarate *Perforomist*	**Nebulizer** 20 mcg in 2 mL Adults: 20 mcg 2x/day (every 12 hrs) use with jet nebulizer *Foradil Aerolizer (to treat asthma, COPD) was discontinued in the U.S. on 10/2015*	**Maintenance treatment of COPD** *Acts on beta-2 receptors in the lungs, relaxing smooth muscle. Also inhibits inflammatory response.* | onset | 1-3 min | | peak | 30-60 min | | duration | 12 hrs |	**Black Box Warning** *(see pg 11-17)* **Diarrhea, nausea, nasopharyngitis, dry mouth, vomiting, dizziness, insomnia** *NOT indicated for acute bronchoconstriction*
salmeterol *Serevent Diskus*	**Dry Powder Inhaler** 50 mcg/dose > 4 yrs: 1 inh 2x/day, 12 hrs apart for: Asthma (>4 yrs; add-on, not monotherapy) COPD (adults) **PREVENTION OF EIB (> 4 yrs):** 1 inh (50 mcg) at least 30 minutes prior to exercise. Don't repeat within 12 hrs, and not to be used by patients on salmeterol 2x/day. Chronic use is discouraged (NAEPP)	**Long-Term management of Bronchoconstriction** *In addition to normal LABA action (see formoterol, above), may inhibit late-phase of allergen-induced bronchoconstriction* | onset | 10-20 min | | peak | 3-5 hrs | | duration | 12 hrs |	**Black Box Warning** *(see pg 11-17)* Nasopharyngitis, upper respiratory infection, bronchitis, cough, back pain - *NOT indicated for acute bronchoconstriction* - *Off-label use for treatment of HAPE[1]*

Bronchodilators: Ultra Long-Acting Beta Agonists*

Generic *Brand Names*	Dosage (by FORM and INDICATION as appropriate)	Indications *Mode of Action*	Adverse Effects *Notes*
indacaterol *Arcapta* *Neohaler*	**Dry Powder Inhaler (DPI)** 75 mcg per tablet Adults: inhale 75 mcg once daily	**Maintenance treatment of COPD** *See formoterol, above* onset: 5 min peak: 30 min duration: 24 hrs	**Black Box Warning** *(see pg 11-17)* Cough, oropharyngeal pain, nasopharyngitis, headache, nausea *NOT indicated for acute bronchoconstriction*
olodaterol hydrochloride *Striverdi* *Respimat*	**Metered-Dose Inhaler** 2.5 mcg per actuation Adults: 2 actuations once daily	**Maintenance treatment of COPD** *See formoterol, above* peak: 10-20 min duration: 24 hrs	**Black Box Warning** *(see pg 11-17)* Nasopharyngitis, upper respiratory infection, bronchitis, cough, back pain *NOT indicated for acute bronchoconstriction*

*An Ultra LABA is taken once daily instead of multiple times per day, a designation used by some to help differentiate usage.

Anticholinergics: Short-Acting Muscarinic Antagonists (SAMAs)

Generic *Brand Names*	Dosage (by Form, Age, Indication as approp.)	Indications *Mode of Action*	Adverse Effects *Clinical Notes*

ipratropium bromide
 	
Atrovent
Atrovent HFA
	Nebulizer
	(0.02%) (0.5 mg/2.5 mL)
	> 12 yr:
	  0.25–0.5 mg, 3–4x/day
	<12 yr: 0.25–0.5 mg, 3x/day
	
	MDI: (17 mcg/puff)
	<12 yr: 1–2 puffs, 3x/day
	  (max 6/day)
	>12 yr: 2–3 puffs, 4x/day
	  (max 12/day)
	
	Exercise-Induced
	Bronchospasm (MDI):
	9+ yrs: 2 puffs 15–30 min before exercise
		COPD (acute + maintenance): bronchospasm
		Asthma (acute): bronchospasm
		Off-label use for EIB for those who do not respond to SABAs (ATS)
		
		Non-selectively blocks muscarinic receptors. Results in decreased contractility of bronchial smooth muscle.
		
		| onset | 15–30 min |
		| peak | 1–2 hrs |
		| duration | 6 hrs |
			Avoid in patients with atropine hypersensitivity
			
			Dry mouth, bronchospasm, angioedema, laryngospasm
			
			May also be used to treat (nasal spray) rhinorrhea, rhinitis. Adverse effects include nasal dryness and epistaxis. Avoid contact with eyes.

Acute Exacerbation (Asthma, COPD) - typically as combination therapy with SABA			
Nebulizer > 12 yrs: 0.5 mg, every 20 min x 3, then every 2–4 hrs < 12 yrs: 0.25–0.5 mg, every 20 min x 3, then every 2–4 hrs. **MDI:** (all ages) (NIH Guidelines): 4–8 puffs, every 20 min as needed for up to 3 hrs			

Anticholinergics: Long-Acting Muscarinic Antagonists (LAMAs)

Generic *Brand Names*	Dosage (by Form, Age, Indication as approp.)	Indications *Mode of Action*	Adverse Effects *Clinical Notes*
aclidinium bromide *Tudorza Pressair*	**Dry Powder Inhaler** 400 mcg per inhalation Adults: 1 inh 2x/day	**Maintenance treatment of bronchospasm associated with COPD** *Nonselective action on M1-M5 receptors, resulting in bronchodilation (by preventing bronchoconstriction)* onset: 10 min peak: 0.5-2 hrs duration: 12 hrs	Headache, pharyngitis, cough, diarrhea, rhinitis **Contraindicated in patients with severe reactions to milk proteins** *Do not use to treat acute bronchospasm*
glycopyrrolate bromide *Lonhala Magnair VMN* *Seebri Neohaler DPI*	**Vibrating Mesh Nebulizer** 25 mcg in 1 mL 25 mcg 2x/day **Dry Powder Inhaler (DPI)** 15.6 mcg per inhalation 1 inhalation 2x/day	**Maintenance treatment for COPD** *See aclidinium, above* onset: 15-30 min peak: 1-2 hrs duration: 12 hrs	Dyspnea, urinary tract infection *Do not use to treat acute bronchospasm*

Generic *Brand Names*	Dosage (by Form, Age, Indication as approp.)	Indications *Mode of Action*	Adverse Effects *Clinical Notes*
revefenacin *Yupelri*	**Nebulizer** 175 mcg in 3 mL Adults: once daily	**Maintenance treatment of COPD** *See ipratropium bromide* onset: 45 min peak: 2-3 hrs duration: 24 hrs	Cough, nasopharyngitis, upper respiratory infection, headache, back pain *Do not use to treat acute bronchospasm*
tiotropium bromide *Spiriva (HandiHaler) (Respimat)*	**DPI (HANDIHALER):** 18 mcg COPD: 2 inh of 1 cap/day **SMI (RESPIMAT)** 1.25, 2.5 mcg COPD: 2 inh of 2.5 mcg daily Asthma: 2 inh of 1.25 mcg daily	**Maintenance treatment of COPD, Asthma** *See ipratropium bromide* onset: 30 min peak: 3 hrs duration: >24 hrs	Dry mouth, urinary retention, constipation, increased HR, blurred vision, glaucoma *Not to be used as a rescue inhaler*
umeclidinium bromide *Incruse Ellipta*	**DPI:** 62.5 mcg per actuation Adults: 1 inh once daily	**Maintenance treatment of COPD** *See ipratropium bromide* onset: 5-15 min peak: 1-3 hrs duration: 24 hrs	Nasopharyngitis, upper respiratory infection, cough *Do not use to treat acute bronchospasm*

Methylxanthines (Xanthines)

Generic *Brand Names*	Dosage (by Form, Age, Indication as approp.)	Indications *Mode of Action*	Adverse Effects *Clinical Notes*
aminophylline	**NEONATAL APNEA:** Load: 5 mg/kg over 30 inches Maintenance: 5 mg/kg/day, every 12 hrs **Bronchodilation:** Load: 6 mg/kg over 20-30 min (IV) **Maintenance:** **Neonate:** 0.2 mg/kg/hr **6 wk - 6 mo:** 0.5 mg/kg/hr **6mo – 12mo:** 0.6–0.7 mg/kg/hr	**Bronchoconstriction** **Neonatal apnea** *Stimulates rate and depth of respirations and causes pulmonary vasodilation* **1-9 yrs:** 1-1.2 mg/kg/hr **9-12 yrs:** 0.9 mg/kg/hr (+ young smokers) **> 12 yrs:** 0.7 mg/kg/hr (+ older nonsmokers)	↑CV and CNS effects, many systemic effects Toxicity > 20 mg/L (> 15 mg/L in neonates)
dyphylline oxtriphylline theophylline	Multiple forms exist (tablets, capsules, syrups, elixirs, etc.) Titrate to serum theophylline level: COPD: 5-10 mcg/mL Asthma: 5-15 mcg/mL	**Used primarily for management of bronchoconstriction** *Multiple theories on mode of action (adenosine antagonism, catecholamine release, phosphodiesterase inhibition)*	**Serum Level Effects:** Nausea (> 20), Cardiac dysrhythmias (> 30), Seizures (40-45) • *Different forms of the drug may vary in effect (there are different amts of theophylline present)* • *Metabolism of theophyllines varies by individual (narrow therapeutic window)*

Pharmacology

Alpha-1 Antitrypsin Deficiency

Generic *Brand Names*	Dosage (by Form, Age, Indication as approp.)	Indications *Mode of Action*	Adverse Effects *Clinical Notes*
Alpha 1 Proteinase Inhibitor	60 mg/kg once weekly For IV use only, infuse over 30 min. **Powder (reconstitute)** **Aralast NP:** 500 mg, 1000 mg vials **Prolastin:** 1000 mg vial **Zemaira:** 1000 mg vial **Glassia:** 1000 mg (50 mL) Injection solution	**Congenital alpha-1 antitrypsin deficiency** *Replaces enzymes lost in patients with this disorder*	↑ALT, AST, headache, musculoskeletal discomfort, pharyngitis, allergic reactions, fever, light-headedness

Anti-Infectives

Generic Brand Names	Dosage (by Form, Age, Indication as approp.)	Indications Mode of Action	Adverse Effects Clinical Notes
aztreonam Cayston	**Powder (reconstitute)** 75 mg in single-use vial 7+ yrs: 75 mg 3x/day x 28 days *Do not repeat for 28 days after completion*	**Management of P. aeruginosa infection in cystic fibrosis (improvement of pulmonary symptoms related to CF)** *Anti-infective*	**Bronchospasm, rash** • To reconstitute: open glass vial of drug (remove cap, metal ring, and rubber stopper); add the diluent ampule to the glass vial, then gently swirl (do not shake) until dissolved • Administer by Altera Nebulizer to ensure adequate dose is delivered • Do not mix with other drugs • Watch for bronchospasm

Generic Brand Names	Dosage (by Form, Age, Indication as approp.)	Indications Mode of Action	Adverse Effects Clinical Notes
colistin (colistimethate) *Coly-Mycin M*	**Nebulizer** 150 mg <13 yrs: 30 or 75 mg, 1-2 x/day Adult: 75 or 150 mg 1-2 x/day Pneumonia (ventilator-assoc.) 150 mg CBA by vent circuit every 8 hrs over 60 min x 14 days (or until weaned from ventilator)	Used primarily to treat multidrug resistant (MDR) gram-negative bacteria (especially P. aeruginosa, A. baumannii, K. pneumoniae) Bronchiectasis with evidence of colonization/infection in lungs in cystic fibrosis and non-cystic fibrosis patients (off-label) Hospital- or ventilator-acquired pneumonia (off-label) *Antibiotic for G-activity (pseudomonal activity)*	Bronchoconstriction (pre-treat with SABA), Nephrotoxicity, acute renal failure, neurotoxicity, apnea, respiratory distress - *Important dosage conversion (colistimethate sodium vs. colistin-base activity [CBA]). Consult pharmacist if any doubt.* - *Dilute dose in NS to 4 mL (1 mL drug + 3 mL NS)* - *Prepare immediately prior to administration (must be used within 24-hrs once mixed, conversion to bioactive colistin, may result in life-threatening dose of colistin)* - *Administer via Pari LC plus nebulizer & filter valve set*

Generic *Brand Names*	Dosage (by Form, Age, Indication as approp.)	Indications *Mode of Action*	Adverse Effects *Clinical Notes*
pentamidine isethionate *NebuPent*	Nebulizer (comes as a powder that needs to be reconstituted) **5+ yrs**: 300 mg every 3-4 wks **< 5 yrs**: 8 mg/kg/dose up to 300 mg 300 mg per 1 vial (reconstitute with 6 mL sterile water)	**Prevent and treat Pneumocystis pneumonia (PCP) primarily in patients with CD3 < 200 cells/mm³ as a secondary option for those who can't take co-trimoxazole** *The mode of action is not understood, although there are known antifungal characteristics*	Irritation, cough, fatigue, SOB, bronchospasm, metallic taste, systemic effects - *Delivered via Respirgard II nebulizer (5-7 L/min using a 40-50 PSI compressor. Do not use with compressors that deliver at less than 20 PSI)* - *Consider pre-treating w/ SABA* - *Minimize exposure of healthcare workers to the treatment: consider use of PPE, negative pressure*

Pharmacology

Generic *Brand Names*	Dosage (by Form, Age, Indication as approp.)	Indications *Mode of Action*	Adverse Effects *Clinical Notes*
ribavirin *Virazole*	**Note the use of various units of measurement below:** **Nebulizer:** **6 g in 1 vial** (reconstitute with 300 mL sterile water to 20 mg/mL) **Continuous:** 6 g over 12-18 hrs/day x 3-7 days **Intermittent:** 2,000 **mg** over 2-3 hrs/day for 3-7 days	Primary indication is for severe, life-threatening RSV in infants/children (AAP) in infants/children (not indicated for adults) Off-label for RSV with certain transplant recipients *Antiviral (inhibits replication of RNA and DNA viruses)*	**Sudden deterioration of respiratory function in infants (monitor, stop treatment if needed, consider co-treatment with SABA), cardiac, conjunctivitis** - *May interfere with ventilator function if intubated (due to crystalline deposits) - occlusion of circuit, trigger dyssynchrony. Avoid use or consider alternatives (VM[1], expiratory filters, one-way valves, etc)* - *Use with SPAG-2 nebulizer delivery system* - *Minimize exposure of healthcare workers, esp. if pregnant, to the treatment: consider use of PPE, negative pressure. Wear goggles if contact lenses.*

[1] Several studies (Hartman, et al; Walsh, et al) have suggested that a vibrating mesh (VM) nebulizer used within a closed ventilator circuit may deliver similar amounts of ribavirin as the SPAG-2, but with less ventilator concerns (expiratory filters still required), preferably with NS 0.9%

Generic Brand Names	Dosage (by Form, Age, Indication as approp.)	Indications Mode of Action	Adverse Effects Clinical Notes
tobramycin DPI: *Tobi Podhaler* Nebulizer: *Bethkis* *Kitabis Pak* *Tobi*	**Dry Powder Inhaler (DPI)** 28 mg per inhalation capsule 6+ yrs: Inhale the contents of 4 capsules (using Podhaler) 2x/day for 28 days on, 28 days off **Nebulizer** 300 mg in 4-5 mL 6+ yrs: 300 mg every 12 hrs, repeat in cycles: 28 days on, 28 days off	Management of *P. aeruginosa* and other gram negative organism infections especially in cystic fibrosis patients Off-label use for non-CF bronchiectasis (80 mg, 2-3x/day) in patients with 3 or more exacerbations/year requiring antibiotics *Antibiotic for G- activity (Pseudomonal activity)*	Bronchospasm, cough, dyspnea, oropharyngeal pain, hemoptysis, chest discomfort, nausea, headache • In general tobramycin should be administered after all other treatments/therapies (SABA, then CPT, then other nebs, then tobramycin) • Neb: Use PARI LC Plus, do not mix with other drugs • DPI: Use podhaler and blister pack. Each capsule is loaded separately, inhale twice for each capsule

Generic Brand Names	Dosage (by Form, Age, Indication as approp.)	Indications Mode of Action	Adverse Effects Clinical Notes
zanamivir Relenza Diskhaler	**Dry Powder Inhaler (DPI)** 5 mg per blister **Influenza Treatment:** ≥ 7 yrs: 2 inh (10 mg) 2x/day x 5 days. Doses on days 1+2 should be 2+ hrs apart. Days 3+4+5 should be 12 hrs apart **Prophylactic Treatment:** ≥ 5 yrs: 2 inh (10 mg) 1x/day x 10 days (start within 36 hrs of onset of symptoms) **Prophylactic for a Community Outbreak:** 2 inh (10 mg) 1x/day for 28 days (start within 5 days of outbreak)	**Prophylaxis or Treatment of influenza A or B infection**[1] *Antiviral (Neuraminidase Inhibitor) which may be used prophylactically and/or as treatment* [1]Note that recommendations (indications) for antiviral prophylaxis and treatment are complex - see the Advisory Committee on Immunization Practices (ACIP) for details	**Malaise, dizziness, fever, cough, sinusitis, change in appetite, etc. Anaphylactic reactions have been reported.** - *Use with diskhaler (breath-actuated inhaler). Each capsule is loaded separately, 2 capsules required for 10 mg* - *Not recommended for use in patients with underlying lung disease (COPD, asthma)* - *If giving SABA give before zanamivir*

Mucoactives

Generic *Brand Names*	Dosage (by Form, Age, Indication as approp.)	Indications *Actions*	Adverse Effects *Clinical Notes*
acetylcysteine *formerly:* *Mucomyst* *(brand name discontinued)*	**Nebulizer** 10% (100 mg/mL), 10 mL, 30 mL 20% (200 mg/mL), 10 mL, 30 mL **Nebulized Dosaging (3-4 x/day)** | Age	10%	20%
---	---	---
>12 yr:	1-10 mL	2-20 mL
Child:	6-10 mL	3-5 mL
Infant:	2-4 mL	1-2 mL | 10% is administered at full-strength 20% may be further diluted with NS or Sterile Water **Instilled (every 1-4 hrs):** 1-2 mL of 20% or 2-4 mL of 10%	**Tenacious mucus** *Mucolytic: breaks mucus disulfide bonds, decreases mucus viscosity* | peak	5-10 min
---	---
duration	> 1 hr		**Bronchospasm (administer bronchodilator before use), stomatitis, nausea, rhinitis, unpleasant odor/taste. Over-mobilization of secretions** - *Administer SABA 10-15 mins prior to administration of acetylcysteine* - *Administered in oral form for acetaminophen overdose. Dosing for this is beyond the scope of this text.* - *Not recommended for administration with cystic fibrosis*

Pharmacology

Generic Brand Names	Dosage (by Form, Age, Indication as approp.)	Indications Actions	Adverse Effects Clinical Notes
dornase alfa-dnase *Pulmozyme*	**Nebulizer** 1 mg/mL in 2.5 mL 3 mos↑: 2.5 mg, 1-2 x/day	**Tenacious mucus (decreases infection)** *Selectively cleaves DNA of purulent secretions*	Same as acetylcysteine *Do not mix or dilute with other drugs (may inactivate drug)*
mannitol *Bronchitol*	**Dry Powder Inhaler (DPI)** 40 mg per capsule 18+ yrs: 400 mg, 2x/day take 2nd dose at least 2-3 hrs before bedtime	**Add-on maintenance treatment for adults with Cystic Fibrosis** *Hyperosmotic with an unknown mechanism of action but is theorized to play in role in changing the viscosity/elasticity of tenacious mucous, increasing mucociliary activity.*	**Bronchospasm** • Pre-testing required: a Bronchitol Tolerance Test (BTT)* must be passed in order for drug to be prescribed • Administer SABA 5-15 min before administration even after passing the BTT **Hemoptysis** *Pediatric trials are being conducted at time of print - check with reliable sources for updates*

*This is a series of steps where a patient is administered Bronchitol in the presence of preferably an RT who monitors SpO₂ and FEV₁ during various phases.

Solution	Administration	Clinical Notes
Saline: Isotonic (0.9%)	Often used as a diluent for concentrated drugs as it is physiologically the same as the salinity of the airways	
Saline: Hypotonic (0.45%)	Sterile water is used as a diluent/reconstituent for some nebulized drugs. Be aware of its hypotonic property, potentially triggering bronchospasm, especially in patients susceptible to a reaction (asthma, for example)	Potential mucosal irritation, overhydration, bronchospasm
Water (hypotonic) sterile, distilled (0.0%)		
Saline: Hypertonic (3.5%–7%) HyperSal	May be indicated for thick, hard-to-cough secretions by both invoking a strong cough and hydrating thick, tenacious secretions. **Sputum Induction** **3.5%, 7%** *Administer 2–5 mL* Irritating to the airways (where normal saline level is 0.9%), resulting in a cough	**Bronchospasm, mucosal irritation, edema** • *Hypertonic saline is irritating to the airways and may induce a strong cough (intended effect) as well as bronchospasm (pre-treat with a SABA)* • *The effectiveness in reducing hospital days, etc., has been unproven*

Inhaled Analgesics

Generic *Brand Names*	Dosage (by Form, Age, Indication as approp.)	Indications *Mode of Action*	Adverse Effects *Clinical Notes*
lidocaine (off-label)	**Nebulizer** 2-4 mL of 1%-4% lidocaine Dosing varies greatly in literature	Pre-bronchoscopy. Pre-nasogastric tube insertion. Intractable cough. Has also been used to treat asthma. *Inhibits Na+ ion channels*	Airway irritation, reduced gag reflex leading to aspiration *Patient should be NPO until airway can be adequately protected (lidocaine dulls normal airway protection reflexes)*
morphine sulfate* (off-label)	**Nebulizer** 2-5 mg as needed, preferably by breath-actuated nebulizer (Higher doses and escalating frequency may be needed).	Dyspnea, pain and cough in palliative care patients (severe end-stage COPD, lung cancer, etc.) *Binds to opioid receptors, producing analgesia (opioid agonist).*	Bronchospasm, **respiratory depression**, constipation and nausea • *Consider pre-treating with a SABA* • *May more specifically treat dyspnea and cough without as many systemic adverse effects, but no strong evidence to support (consider a trial with assessment of dyspnea)*

Inhaled Epinephrine
(Ultra-Short-Acting Adrenergic)

Generic *Brand Names*	Dosage (by Form, Age, Indication as approp.)	Indications *Mode of Action*	Adverse Effects *Clinical Notes*
racemic epinephrine S2 *Asthmanefrin** *Primatene Mist HFA**	**Nebulizer** 22.5 mg per mL (0.5 mL) dose = 11.25 mg (2.25%) S2: 0.25-0.5 mL (2.25%) diluted in 3 mL NS Stridor (2.25%): < 5 kg: 0.25 mL/dose > 5 kg: 0.5 mL/dose	**Bronchoconstriction** **Tracheobronchial inflammation** (post extubation stridor, croup) Stimulates: alpha-1 (mild) beta-1 (medium) beta-2 (mild) | onset | 3-5 min | | peak | 5-20 min | | duration | 0.5-2 hrs |	Rebound airway edema, cardiac arrhythmias, chest pain, trembling, dizziness, headache (adverse effects are usually less severe than epinephrine) **Racemic epinephrine is available without a prescription. This is strongly discouraged by ATS, ACCS, ALS, AAAI, ATS, and AAAE as there are other SABAs that are more selective to B2 (less adverse effects) and longer-acting*
epinephrine	**Nebulizer** 1:100 Anaphylaxis IM 0.15 or 0.3 mg	May be used for acute asthma, but rare due to adverse effects Anaphylaxis	Tachycardia, increased BP, tremors

Pharmacology

Phosphodiesterase Inhibitors

Generic *Brand Names*	Dosage (by Form, Age, Indication as approp.)	Indications *Mode of Action*	Adverse Effects *Clinical Notes*
roflumilast *Daliresp*	**Tablets:** 500 mcg per tab **Adults:** 250 mcg 1x/day x 4 weeks then: 500 mcg 1x/day	COPD maintenance in patients who have persistent symptoms/exacerbations besides otherwise optimal COPD management *PDE-4 Inhibitor primarily has an anti-inflammatory action (decreasing action of pro-inflammatory cells), and may have a very slight bronchodilation effect*	Diarrhea, nausea, vomiting, sleep/mood disturbances, suicidal ideation - *There may be slight improvement in lung function and decreased risk of exacerbations* - *This is not meant as a solo therapy; use with LABA for maintenance + use SABA for rescue*

Pulmonary Vasodilators

Generic *Brand Names*	Dosage by Form, Age, and/or Indication	Indications *Mode of Action*	Adverse Effects *Clinical Notes*
epoprostenol *Flolan* *Veletri*	**Nebulizer** **Refractory Hypoxemia (ARDS) Off-Label** 20,000 ng/mL @ 8 mL/hr, titrate down to 10,000 (10-50 ng/kg/min if weight-based dosing) **Post-cardiothoracic surgery (w/ pulmonary hypertension, RV dysfunction, or refractory hypoxemia) Off Label** 20,000 ng/mL @ 8 mL/hr Then: drop dose by 50% every 0.5-4 hrs until @ 2500 ng/mL and stable. Nebulizer @ 8 mL/hr at all times	Rescue treatment when evidence of pulmonary vasoconstriction (ARDS, pulmonary hypertension, right-ventricular failure) *Affects prostaglandin I receptor, increasing intracellular cAMP which relaxes vascular smooth muscle.*	Flushing, tachycardia, hypotension, chest pain, headache, nausea/vomiting, flu-like symptoms (many others, less systemic with inhaled vs. other routes) Various interfaces: • Ventilator: inspiratory limb near ET tube (change expiratory filters every 2-4 hrs) • Face mask • High-flow nasal cannula • NPPV • *May have anti-thrombotic and anti-inflammatory effects* • *May be the preferred agent for high-risk patients with severe symptoms (WHO)*

Pharmacology

Generic / Brand Names	Dosage by Form, Age, and/or Indication	Indications / Mode of Action	Adverse Effects / Clinical Notes
iloprost *Ventavis*	**Nebulizer** 10 mcg/mL; 20 mcg/mL **Pulmonary Hypertension** Adult Initial: 2.5 mcg inhaled, then: 5 mcg, 6-9 x/day Max/day: 45 mcg May consider lower dose (1.25 mcg/dose) for infants/sm children **Post-op Pulmonary Hypertensive Crisis (Peds):** 0.5 mcg/kg over 10 min (increase to 1, then 2, if no response. Administer every 30 mins up to 5 doses)	Used as a treatment for pulmonary (arterial) hypertension Works by vasodilation of pulmonary vessels	Pulmonary edema (discontinue immediately), rebound pulmonary hypertension (avoid rapid wean/discontinuation, restart if noted), syncope (avoid use in pts with hypotension), bronchospasm, flushing, headache, nausea, cough - Must be used with specific nebulizer (I-neb AAD System) - May also be administered during acute vasodilator testing (with pulmonary hypertension) when considering calcium channel blockers (administer 5 mcg over 15 min)

5 A's of Smoking

ASK	Ask about any nicotine use or exposure (ever) - all forms, as well as past quitting attempts, basic history of use. Include secondhand smoke exposure
ADVISE	Directly advise patients to quit smoking/nicotine use in a non-judgmental way
ASSESS	Assess readiness to quit (if not ready, assess why, provide motivation, tie-in to lung health, etc.)
ASSIST	Develop a plan with the smoker to quit, set a date to quit, address any barriers, educate on nicotine withdrawal symptoms, discuss options to help (see next pages), recommend counseling, provide adequate materials: • Nicotine replacement therapy • Behavioral therapy • Psychiatric drug therapy • Alternative therapies (hypnosis, etc.)
ARRANGE	Know options for follow-up (local quit programs/hotlines, etc.) and arrange for proactive follow-up with patient

Smoking Cessation

These therapies are used to reduce underlying nicotine cravings and are nearly always prescribed with a nicotine-replacement therapy (NRT) - see next page

Generic *Brand Names*	Dosage by Form, Age, and/or Indication	Mode of Action	Adverse Effects *Clinical Notes*
varenicline *Chantix*	**Tablet:** 0.5 mg, 1 mg Initiate 1 week prior to quit date. 1mg 2x/day after a 1 week titration: Days 1-3: 0.5 mg daily Days 4-7: 0.5 mg 2x/day Day 8+: 1 mg 2x/day 12 wk course of treatment, repeat course if success	*Binds with neuronal nicotinic acetylcholine receptors. Produces agonist activity (blocks the reward/reinforcement a person may feel as a result of smoking).*	**Suicidal ideation, abnormal dreams, headache, insomnia, irritability, depression, nausea, vomiting, cardiovascular symptoms** *Usually administered with a nicotine-replacement therapy (NRT)*
bupropion *Alpenzin** *Forfivo** *Wellbutrin* *Zyban*	**Tablet:** 75-200 (varies by brand, also available as a 12-hr or 24-hr extended release in some brands) Start 2 wks before quitting 150 mg/day x 3 days then 150 mg 2x/day for 7-12 weeks	*Unknown, may have non-adrenergic or dopaminic effects (decreases some of the cravings for cigarettes, may decrease withdrawal symptoms)*	**Seizures (larger dosages), suicidal ideation, dry mouth, insomnia, weakness, abnormal dreams, change in appetite** • *Usually administered with a nicotine-replacement therapy (NRT)*

Nicotine-Replacement Therapies (NRT)

Nicotine replacement therapies decrease withdrawal symptoms by giving measured, smaller doses of nicotine and are available in multiple forms (patch, gum, lozenge, inhaler, nasal spray)

Generic Brand Names	Dosage by Form, Age, and/or Indication	Mode of Action	Adverse Effects Clinical Notes
Longer-Action: *considered to be the most consistent delivery of nicotine, but unable to titrate to effect during the day*			
Transdermal patch Nicotrol	15 mg/patch for 6 weeks >10 cigarettes/day: Apply 1 patch in the A.M.; remove before bed (don't wear overnight)	Patches are considered long-acting, slow-onset	Skin irritation, insomnia, headache, nausea, tachycardia • Usually replaced each morning, takes about 30 mins to onset (use another NRT until effect) • If insomnia, remove patch at night (or use 16-hr patch applied each morning) • Second NRT often needed (spray, etc.) to handle breakthrough cravings • Habitrol requires a prescription
Transdermal Patch NicoDerm CQ Habitrol (many generics)	Patch: 7, 14, 21 mg/ patch <10 cig/day: 14 mg for 16-24 hr x 6 wk then 7 mg for 16-24 hr x 2 wk >10 cig/day: 21 mg for 16-24 hr x 6 wk then 14 mg for 16-24 hr x 2 wk then 7 mg for 16-24 hr x 2 wk		

Pharmacology 11-41

Generic Brand Names	Dosage by Form, Age, and/or Indication	Mode of Action	Adverse Effects Clinical Notes
Shorter-action: nicotine replacement therapies may be fairly easily titrated to need.			
Nasal Spray *Nicotrol NS*	Nasal Spray: 0.5 mg nicotine per spray 1-2 doses per hour x 3 months Max:40 mg (80 sprays) per day	Short-term: Absorbed through the nasal mucosa Peak: 10 mins	**Nasal (94%) and throat irritation, rhinitis, tearing** Requires a prescription
Nicotine Gum *Various brands*	Gum: 2, 4 mg (max: ~24 pcs/day) 2-4 mg over 30 min q. 1-2 hr x 6wk, then q. 2-4 hr x 3 wk, then q. 4-8 hr x 3 wk Chew gum slowly to avoid adverse (GI) effects. Chew until taste of nicotine, then park gum between cheek/gum until taste is gone (~1 min), then repeat process for about 30 mins.	Short-term: Absorbed through the oral mucosa primarily Peak: 20 mins	• *Dizziness, bleeding gums, nausea, vomiting, ulcers, excess salivation* • *Various gums exist, not all intended for NRT - verify a reputable source* • *Avoid eating/drinking x15 min before/after. Avoid acidic beverages which may decrease intake absorption*

Generic / Brand Names	Dosage by Form, Age, and/or Indication	Mode of Action	Adverse Effects / Clinical Notes
Nicotine Lozenges / *Various brands*	Lozenges: 2, 4 mg < 30 mins to usual AM cig: 4 mg dose > 30 mins to usual AM cig: 2 mg dose 1-2 lozenges ever 1-2 hrs x 6 wks Then: reduce lozenges/day x 6 wks Max: 5 lozenges every 6 hrs, 20/day Allow lozenge to dissolve in mouth over 30 minutes	Short-term: Absorbed through the oral mucosa primarily Peak: 20 min	**Mouth irritation, ulcers, abdominal pain, nausea, headache** *Available in various flavors* *Option for patients with dentures or other oral issues that can't use gum*
Nicotine Inhaler / *Nicotrol*	10 mg cartridges, 4mg delivered 6-16 cartridges/day (1 cartridge is ~20 mins of inhalations) 10-20 min continuous inhalations Instruct in use of inhaler, ensuring shallow breaths (focus is on upper airway, not getting drug all the way to the lungs).	Short-term: deposits primarily on oropharynx, minimal absorption through lungs Peak: 15 min	**Bronchospasm, GI upset, cough, mouth irritation/ burning** - *Due to risk of bronchospasm, consider with caution in patients with reactive airways (asthma, COPD, etc.)* - *Cartridge is good for 24-hrs once opened*

Pharmacology

Inhaled Corticosteroids (ICS)

General Considerations with Inhaled Steroids

- Shared adverse effects: oral candida *albicans* (swish and spit), immunosuppression, adrenal suppression, growth effects in pediatric patients, glaucoma/cataracts (use minimum effective dose to minimize all)
- Once symptoms are stabilized, the dosage should be titrated to the lowest effective dose
- Inhaled steroids are contraindicated for rescue efforts (systemic steroids are more appropriate)
- Dosaging guidelines below have been cross-referenced with National Institute for Health (NIH), Global Initiative for Asthma (GINA), Global Initiative for Chronic Obstructive Lung Disease (GOLD) and individual manufacturer recommendations. Please refer to the disease chapter for specific disease-centered recommendations.

Generic *Brand Names*	Dosage by Form, Age, and/or Indication	Adverse Effects *Clinical Notes*
beclomethasone *QVAR*	**HFA (40 mcg/puff, 80 mcg/puff):** 5-11 yrs: 40-80 mcg twice daily ≥ 12 yrs: 40-320 mcg twice daily **NIH Asthma Recommendations:**	• Not FDA approved for < 5 yr-old • Do not shake HFA cannister before use • Prime HFA cannister by spraying 2x • Use cautiously: there is evidence to suggest a reduction in growth for pediatric patients when taking QVAR

Dosage Level	5-11 yrs	≥ 12 yrs
Low Dose	80-160 mcg/day	80-240 mcg/day
Medium Dose	160-320 mcg/day	240-480 mcg/day
High Dose	> 320 mcg/day	> 480 mcg/day

Generic Brand Names	Dosage by Form, Age, and/or Indication	Clinical Notes
budesonide *Pulmicort Respules* *Pulmicort Flexhaler*	**Pulmicort Respules (nebulized)** 0.25 mg/2 mL, 0.5 mg/2 mL, 1 mg/2 mL Inf: 0.25 mg 2x/day or 0.5 1x/day Other ages: 0.25-0.5 mg 2x/day or 0.5-1 mg 1x/day **Pulmicort Flexhaler** (DPI) 90 mcg, 180 mcg 6-17 yrs: 180-360 mcg 2x/day 18+ yrs: 180-720 mcg 2x/day	*There are nuances in dosing with asthma - see* *manufacturer information for further information* **Respules:** Shake gently with circular motion Do not mix with other drugs **Flexhaler:** Prime before first use, but at no other time Do not shake; do not use a spacer Do not exhale through mouthpiece

NHLBI Asthma Recommendations:

Dosage Level	≤ 4 yrs		5-11 yrs		≥ 12 yrs	
	Respules	Respules	Flexhaler		Flexhaler	
Low Dose	0.25-1 mg/day	0.5 mg/day	180-400 mcg/day		180-600 mcg/day	
Medium Dose	0.5-1 mg/day	1 mg/day	400-800 mcg/day		>600-1200 mcg/day	
High Dose	> 1 mg/day	2 mg/day	> 800 mcg/day		> 1200 mcg/day	

Pharmacology

Generic Brand Names	Dosage by Form, Age, and/or Indication	Adverse Effects Clinical Notes
ciclesonide HFA *Alvesco*	**Metered-Dose Inhaler (HFA)** 80 mcg, 160 mcg **Asthma** 2-4 yrs: 40-160 mcg once daily 5-11 yrs: 40-160 mcg once daily 12+ yrs: 80-640 mcg MAX daily **GINA recommendations:** | Low Dose	80-160 mcg/day | | --- | --- | | Medium Dose | 160-320 mcg/day | | High Dose | > 320 mcg/day |	See Shared Adverse Effects (pg 11-44), plus: Headache, nasopharyngitis, upper respiratory infection, nasal congestion - *Prime inhaler 3x initially and with extended non-use (more than 10 days)* - *This inhaler does not require shaking*

Generic Brand Names	Dosage by Form, Age, and/or Indication	Adverse Effects *Clinical Notes*
fluticasone propionate *Flovent Diskus*	**Dry Powder Inhaler (DPI)** *Dose based on previous therapy + asthma severity* 50 mcg, 100 mcg, 250 mcg per blister **Asthma (No prior ICS):** 4-11 yrs: 50 mcg 2x/day (max 100 2x/day) 12+ yrs: 100 mcg 2x/daily (max 1,000 2x/day) **NHLBI/GINA recommendations (mcg/day):** 	Dosage	<12 yrs	≥12 yrs
Low	88-176	100-250
Medium	>176-352	>250-500
High	>352	>500		See Shared Adverse Effects (pg 11-44), plus: headache, throat irritation, upper respiratory infection • *May increase dose after 2 weeks of therapy in patients who are not adequately controlled* • *The Diskus should be held in a level, flat position*
fluticasone propionate *Flovent HFA*	**Metered-Dose Inhaler (MDI - HFA)** *Dose based on previous therapy + asthma severity* 44 mcg, 110 mcg, 220 mcg per inhalation **Asthma (No prior ICS):** 4-11 yrs: 88 mcg, 2x/daily 12+ yrs: 88 mcg, 2x/daily (max 880 2x/day) **NHLBI/GINA:** See Flovent Diskus, above	See Shared Adverse Effects (pg 11-44), plus: headache, throat irritation, upper respiratory infection

Generic *Brand Names*	Dosage by Form, Age, and/or Indication	Adverse Effects *Clinical Notes*
fluticasone furoate Arnuity Ellipta	**Dry Powder Inhaler (DPI)** 50, 100, 200 mcg per blister **Asthma** 5-11 yrs: 50 mcg, 1 inhalation daily 12+ yrs: 100 mcg, 1 inhalation daily (max 200 mcg)	See Shared Adverse Effects (pg 11-44), plus: upper respiratory infection, nasopharyngitis, headache, cough
fluticasone propionate ArmonAir Digihaler	**Dry Powder Inhaler (DPI)** 55, 113, 232 mcg per inhalation **Asthma** | Prev ICS Dose	Recommendation
---	---
None	55, 113, or 232 mcg (depends on asthma severity) 1 inh, 2x/day
Low	55 mcg
Medium	113 mcg
High	232 mcg		See Shared Adverse Effects (pg 11-44), plus: upper respiratory infection, nasopharyngitis, headache, cough - While an app is not needed to take this drug, a built-in electronic module records and stores information about inhaler events (quality of inhalation, etc.), updating an app by Bluetooth - Drug should be disposed of 30 days after opening foil pouch, regardless of doses remaining - This is a DPI (despite the name); do not prime or use a spacer

Combination: ICS and LABA

Generic *Brand Names*	Dosage by Form, Age, and/or Indication	Indications *Mode of Action*	Adverse Effects *Clinical Notes*
budesonide and formoterol *Symbicort*	**Metered-Dose Inhaler (pMDI)** 80/4.5, 160/4.5 mcg **Asthma** 6-11 yrs: 80/4.5 mcg 2 inh 2x/day 12+ yrs: based on previous ICS: 	Prev ICS Dose	Recommendation
---	---
None	80/4.5 or 160/4.5 (depends on asthma severity) 2 inh 2x/day
Low-to-Medium	80/4.5 2 inh 2x/day
Medium-to-High	160/4.5 2 inh 2x/day | **COPD** 160/4.5 2 inh 2d/day	Asthma: 12+ yrs uncontrolled on an inhaled corticosteroid COPD: maintenance treatment and to reduce potential exacerbations *Combines action of systemic corticosteroid and LABA*	See Individual Drugs + nasopharyngitis, rhinitis, influenza, back pain, headache, upper respiratory infection, oral candidas Instruct patient to shake inhaler for a full 5 seconds prior to using to mix medications. Prime twice when needed, shaking 5 seconds between primes. Rinse mouth after use

Generic *Brand Names*	Dosage by Form, Age, and/or Indication	Indications *Mode of Action*	Adverse Effects *Clinical Notes*
fluticasone and salmeterol *Advair Diskus*	Dry Powder Inhaler (DPI) 100/50, 250/50, 500/50 **Asthma** (100/50, 250/50) **COPD** (250/50) 1 inhalation 2x/day, max 2/day	Maintenance treatment of asthma in persons > 12 yrs Maintenance treatment (250/50) of airway obstruction (COPD)	See adverse effects for each drug
fluticasone and salmeterol *Advair HFA*	Metered-Dose Inhaler (MDI-HFA) 45/21, 115/21, 230/21 12+ yr: 2 inh. 2x/day, max 4/day Consider disease and severity in determining appropriate dosage	Maintenance treatment of asthma in persons > 12 yrs	See adverse effects for each drug - *If inadequate response after 2 weeks, consider increasing dosage if not at maximum* - *Shake well for 5 seconds. Prime 4x the first time, then 2x any other time priming needed (inhaler dropped, out of use > 4 wks)*

Generic *Brand Names*	Dosage by Form, Age, and/or Indication	Indications *Mode of Action*	Adverse Effects *Clinical Notes*
fluticasone and salmeterol *AirDuo Respiclick*	**Dry Powder Inhaler (DPI)** 55/14, 113/14, 232/14 mcg 12+ yr: 1 inhalation 2x/day	Maintenance treatment of asthma in persons > 12 yrs	See adverse effects for each drug • *This is a DPI- do not use with a spacer; do not prime* • *This device looks similar to an MDI, but is a DPI - be sure to hold upright when opening the yellow cap (opening the cap loads the dose)*
	Prev ICS Dose / **Recommendation**		
	None / Less Severe: 55/14 Severe: 113/14 or 232/14		
	Low / 55/14 mcg		
	Medium / 113/14 mcg		
	High / 232/14 mcg		
mometasone and formoterol *Dulera*	**Metered-Dose Inhaler (pMDI)** 50/5, 100/5, 200/5 mcg per actuation 12+ yrs: 2 inhalations, 2x/day Max 4 inhalations/day Consider disease and severity in determining appropriate dosage	Maintenance treatment of asthma in persons > 12 yrs	See adverse effects for each drug

Combination: SABA with SAMA

Generic Brand Names	Dosage by Form, Age, and/or Indication	Indications Mode of Action	Adverse Effects Clinical Notes
albuterol and ipratropium bromide *Duoneb*	**Nebulizer** 2.5/0.5 mg in 3 mL **COPD** 2.5/0.5 mg 4x/day (max: 6x/day) **Asthma (exacerbation)** (off-label) 2.5/0.5 mg every 20 min x3, then PRN **Bronchospasm (quick-relief)** (off-label) 2.5/0.5 mg every 4-6 hrs	**COPD with bronchospasm** **Off-Label use with bronchospasm/asthma** *SABA and anticholinergic combined effects, which are thought to have a greater effect than either drug independently*	No common adverse effects, although cardiac arrhythmia, tachycardia are reported at higher doses
albuterol and ipratropium bromide *Combivent Respimat*	**Metered-Dose Inhaler (pMDI)** 103/18 mcg per actuation **COPD:** 1 inh 4x/day (max 6x/day) **Asthma (exac)**(off-label): 8 inh every 20 min for up to 3 hrs **Bronchospasm (quick-relief)**(off-label): 2-3 inh every 6 hrs		

Combination: LAMA and LABA

Generic *Brand Names*	Dosage by Form, Age, and/or Indication	Indications *Mode of Action*	Adverse Effects *Clinical Notes*
umeclidinium and vilanterol *Anoro Ellipta*	62.5 mcg/25 mcg per puff 1 inhalations, once daily	**COPD long-term maintenance** *LABA and anticholinergic combined effects, which are thought to have a greater effect than either drug independently*	**See Black Box Warning on pg 11-17** • *Do not use for acute symptoms* • *Not indicated for Asthma*
glycopyrrolate and formoterol *Bevespi Aerosphere*	9 mcg/4.8 mcg per puff steady state = 2-3 days 2 inhalations, 2x/day		
tiotropium and olodaterol *Stiolto Respimat*	3.1 mcg/2.7 mcg per puff (equiv to 2.5/2.5 mcg) 2 inhalations, once daily		
glycopyrrolate and indacaterol *Utibron Neohaler*	27.5 mcg/15.6 mcg per cap Inhale 1 cap every 12 hrs via Neohaler		

Pharmacology

Combination (Triple Therapies): ICS + LAMA + LABA

Generic *Brand Names*	Dosage (by Form, Age, Indication as approp.)	Indications *Mode of Action*	Adverse Effects *Clinical Notes*
fluticasone, umeclidinium, and vilanterol *Trelegy Ellipta*	**Adult Use Only:** Dry Powder Inhaler 100/62.5/25 mcg 200/62.5/25 mcg **Asthma:** 1 actuation daily (either strength) **COPD:** 1 actuation daily of 100/62.5/25 mcg	Long-term maintenance treatment for Asthma (prevent and control symptoms) Long-term maintenance for COPD: improve daily symptoms and reduce exacerbations *This is a triple-combination drug consisting of a corticosteroid (fluticasone), an anticholinergic (umeclidinium), and a LABA (vilanterol)* *Note that vilanterol is not approved to be used independently*	See individual drugs for adverse effects - *Should not be used as a rescue device* - *Due to steroid, patients should be instructed to rinse mouth without swallowing to avoid thrush*

Generic / Brand Names	Dosage (by Form, Age, Indication as approp.)	Indications / Mode of Action	Adverse Effects / Clinical Notes
budesonide, glycopyrrolate, and formoterol *Breztri Aerosphere*	Adult Use Only: pMDI 160/9/4.8 mcg COPD: 2 inh twice daily	**Long-term maintenance treatment for COPD** *This is a triple-combination drug consisting of a corticosteroid (budesonide), an anticholinergic (glycopyrrolate), and a LABA (formoterol)*	See individual drugs for adverse effects - *Should not be used as a rescue device* - *Due to steroid, patients should be instructed to rinse mouth without swallowing to avoid thrush*

Common (Acute Care) Drugs That May Cause Respiratory Depression

Interventions are indicated when clinically significant (RR < 8/min, ↓ SpO₂, change in LOC, etc.). Note that for many drugs, the risk and level of depression is dose-dependent. Always provide supportive care as needed (airway management, oxygen delivery, etc.)

Drug Class	Generic Names	Strategies to Intervene
Anesthetics	dexmedetomidine* ketamine propofol	Decrease (preferred) or stop dose
Antipsychotics	haloperidol* olanzapine risperidone	benztropine (for risperidone)
Barbiturates	pentobarbital phenobarbital thiopental	No specific antidote
Benzodiazepines	diazepam lorazepam midazolam	flumazenil
Opioid Analgesics	codeine fentanyl hydrocodone methadone morphine oxycodone remifentanil tapentadol tramadol	naloxone
Paralytics	cisatracurium pancuronium rocuronium** succinylcholine vecuronium**	neostigmine **sugammadex succinylcholine has no reversal Do not administer without appropriate sedation and airway management

*Less likely than other sedatives to cause respiratory depression

Common Cardiovascular Drugs

There are many drugs used to manipulate or treat cardiovascular abnormalities. Some common classes and drugs are presented here.

Drug Class	Common Drugs (generic name)	
Antiarrhythmics Used to treat and reduce symptoms related to heart rhythm disorders	acebutalol adenosine amiodarone atenolol betaxolol bisoprolol carvedilol digoxin diltiazem* disopyramide dofetilide doletilide esmolol ibutilide	lidocaine magnesium metoprolol mexiletine nifedipine nimodipine nisoldipine phenytoin procainamide* propafenone propanolol* sotalol* tocainide verapamil*
Positive Inotropics* Increase cardiac contractility to support cardiac function	amrinone digoxin dobutamine dopamine	epinephrine isoproterenol milrinone
Vasodilators Relax smooth muscles in blood vessels, generally decreasing BP	captopril enalapril fenoldopam isoproterenol isosorbide hydralazine labetalol metoprolol	minoxidil nesiritide nicardipine nitroglycerin nitroprusside phentolamine tolazoline
Vasopressors Induce vasoconstriction, generally increasing BP	ephedrine epinephrine metaraminol bitartrate	norepinephrine phenylephrine vasopressin

* Negative Inotropics decrease cardiac contractility to decrease cardiac workload (in angina, for example). They are presented with antiarrhythmics and are marked with asterisks.

Pharmacology

12 Resuscitation

Basic Life Support (in-Hospital) Algorithm.................... 12-2
CPR Components (Summarized).................................... 12-4
Automatic External Defibrillator (AED)........................ 12-5
Opioid-Associated Life-Threatening Emergencies 12-6
Special Situations
    Asthma.. 12-7
    Cardiac Surgery... 12-7
    Benzodiazepine Overdose 12-7
    Electrolytes... 12-7
    Pregnancy 12-7
Post ROSC Care... 12-8

This chapter has been updated with 2020 American Heart Association (AHA) recommendations for In-Hospital CPR (BLS) and aspects of ALS. While information in this chapter is consistent with ACLS guidelines, it is not comprehensive by any means.

The AHA currently releases guidelines annually with major releases usually every 5 years. Please check cpr.heart.org for the latest information.

Pediatric and Advanced Life Support (PALS) and Neonatal Resuscitation Program (NRP) can be found summarized in Oakes' Neonatal/Pediatric Respiratory Care Pocket Guide (respiratorybooks.com)

Basic Life Support (In Hospital) Algorithm

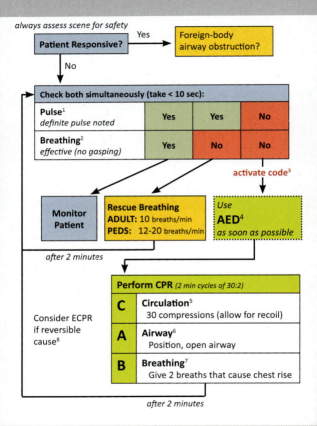

Notes from BLS Algorithm (previous page)

1- Check Pulse: If no definitive pulse within 10 sec, start CPR
　　　　　　　Adult/child: use carotid or femoral
　　　　　　　Infant < 1 yr: use brachial

2- Check Breathing: Simultaneously check breathing with pulse. Note that gasping/agonal breathing is NOT effective breathing.

3- Witnessed Collapse: Call code or send someone for help immediately
　　Unwitnessed Collapse in Peds: Give 2 mins CPR, then seek help/AED
　　　　　　　　　　　　　in Adults: Call code or send someone for help

4- AED: Focus is on use as early as possible but with minimal interruption to chest compressions. SEE PG 12-5 for in-depth AED info.

5- Chest Compressions: Equal compression/relaxation ratio. Avoid leaning on chest during relaxation phase (may restrict recoil)

   2 Rescuers:
   Unsecured airway - Pause compressions for ventilations. Begin compressions at peak inspiration of 2nd breath.
   Secured airway - Do not pause or synchronize for ventilations.
   Change roles every 2 mins to avoid tiring (↓ quality of compressions)

6- Open Airway
   Head tilt-chin lift: preferred when no evidence of head or neck trauma.
   Jaw thrust:
   　　　　　Primarily for C-Spine caution (do not tilt head)
   Open mouth and remove any visible foreign material, vomitus, or loose dentures. Blind finger sweeps are not indicated.

7- Provide Breathing; Avoid large, rapid or forceful breaths. Do not deliver more volume or force than is needed to produce visible chest rise. Use mouth to mouth/nose for infants.

8- ECPR: Extracorporeal CPR (initiation of extracorporeal circulation and oxygenation during resuscitation). This is not routinely recommended but could be used for potentially reversible causes that might benefit from this temporary cardiorespiratory support.

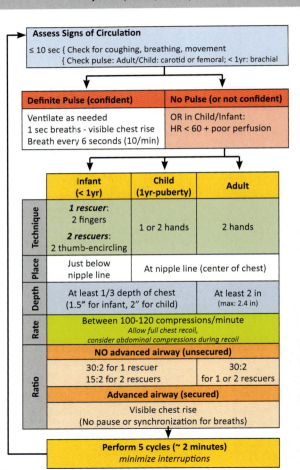

Automatic External Defibrillator (AED)

Witnessed Arrest	Unwitnessed Arrest
Use AED ASAP	Initiate CPR Use AED as soon as device is ready

Rhythms (child and adult only):
- Shockable Rhythm:
 Give 1 shock, immediately resume CPR (beginning with compressions), do not check pulse. Recheck rhythm in 2 minutes.
- Not Shockable Rhythm:
 Immediately resume CPR. Recheck rhythm in 2 minutes.

Placement: exposed chest, anterolateral or anteroposterior

Infants (< 1 yr)

1st Preference:	Manual Defibrillator
2nd Preference:	AED with pediatric dose attenuator
3rd Preference	AED without a dose attenuator may be used if above two are not available

Children

1st Attempt	2 Joules/kg
Subsequent Attempts	at least 4 Joules/kg, *not to exceed 10 Joules/kg or the adult maximum dose*

Ages 1- 8 yrs
use pediatric dose-attenuator system, if available.

Opioid-Associated Life-Threatening Emergencies*

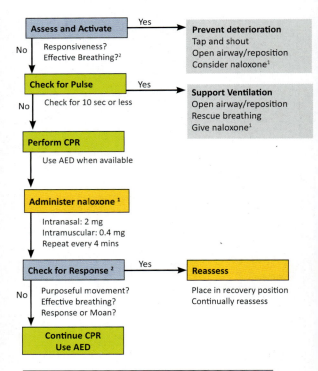

* Summarized from AHA 2020 Guidelines
[1] Cardiac arrest is usually secondary to respiratory arrest with opioids. Note that patients may awaken combative, so adequate supports need to be in place. The effects of naloxone may be shorter than the opioid (be aware of risk of decompensation 30-90 mins after administration)
[2] Do not delay CPR to await response to naloxone

Special Situations
Cardiac Arrest Due to Asthma
- Consider the possibility of a tension pneumothorax if a sudden increase in PIP or sudden difficulty in ventilation
- Utilize a low RR, low VT strategy due to concerns with auto-PEEP
- If auto-PEEP is noted (sudden decrease in BP, etc.), momentarily disconnect from bagging/ventilation to allow patient to exhale (relieving some of the auto-PEEP)

Cardiac Arrest after Cardiac Surgery
- The immediate goal is restoration of perfusion (using CPR)
- If witnessed, immediately defibrillate (VF/VT). Start CPR if defibrillation ineffective within 1 minute
- Resternotomy is indicated if available

Benzodiazepine Overdose
- Due to side effects of reversal, it is not recommended to administer flumazenil
- Provide support with bag-mask ventilation, then intubate

Electrolyte Abnormalities
- If hyperkalemia, IV calcium should be administered
- If hypomagnesemia, IV magnesium should be administered
- If hypermagnesemia, IV calcium should be administered
- If hypokalemia, do not routinely give IV calcium

Cardiac Arrest in Pregnancy
- Consider causes of arrest
    - A Anesthetic complications
    - B Bleeding
    - C Cardiovascular
    - D Drugs
    - E Embolic
    - F Fever
    - G General nonobstetric causes (normal Hs and Ts)
    - H Hypertension
- Provide continuous lateral uterine displacement (1-handed or 2-handed)
- Anticipate a difficult airway
- If no ROSC in 5 min, consider immediate perimortem cesarean delivery

Post-ROSC Care

Top priorities:
- Airway management,
- Management of respiratory parameters (SpO$_2$ 92-98%, PaCO$_2$ 35-45 mm Hg), and
- Management of hemodynamic parameters (BP$_{sys}$ > 90 mm Hg or
MAP > 65 mm Hg)
- Obtain a 12-lead ECG

If patient isn't following commands:
- Initiate Targeted Temperature Management (TTM): The goal is 32-36° C for 24-hrs using a cooling device while monitoring core temperature
- Brain CT Scan
- Monitor EEG
- Maintain normal oxygen, carbon dioxide, glucose level
- Use lung-protective strategies if ventilator

If patient is following commands:
- Continually monitor core temperature
- Maintain normal oxygen, carbon dioxide, glucose level
- Monitor EEG

Identify and treat ACS and other reversible causes

H's	T's
Hypovolemia	Tension pneumothorax
Hypoxia	Tamponade (cardiac)
Hydrogen ion (acidosis)	Toxins
Hypo/hyperkalemia	Thrombosis (pulmonary)
Hypothermia	Thrombosis (coronary)

13 Equations

Acid-Base	13-2
Oxygenation	13-4
Ventilation	13-12
Ventilator Calculations	13-15
Hemodynamics	13-20
Patient Calculations	13-26
Pulmonary Function	13-27
Miscellaneous	13-27

Drug Calculations.................SEE CHAPTER 11

This chapter is intended to be a quick reference for the most common equations used in patient care.

Many equations have multiple forms. We have chosen to present, in most cases, the form most helpful at the bedside as well as any reliable shortcuts.

Subscripts have been modified to make the equations as readable as possible.

Remember PEMDAS order of operations when solving equations:

Parentheses (Brackets)	simplify
Exponents	solve
Multiplication	from left to right
Division	from left to right
Addition	from left to right
Subtraction	from left to right

Equations 13-1

13-2 Equations

Equation	Explanation	Clinical Application
Acid-Base		
Anion Gap	AG: the difference between measured cations (+) and anions (−) (the unmeasured ions)	Indicates whether a metabolic acidosis is due to an increase of acid (rather than a decrease of base)
$AG = Na^+ - (Cl^- + HCO_3^-)$ (United States)	Normal: 12 (± 4) mEq/L	↑ AG = ↑ unmeasured anions (acid): ↑ **acid production:** lactate (hypoxia) ketones (diabetes) ↑**acid addition:** poisons (methanol, salicylates) ↓ **acid excretion:** renal failure
$AG = (Na^+ + K^+) - (Cl^- + HCO_3^-)$ (International adds K+)	Normal: 16 (± 4) mEq/L	↓ AG = ↓ unmeasured anions: albumin
Base Excess (BE)	To calculate base excess	May be used to help confirm validity of results
$BE = \dfrac{\Delta PaCO_2 + \Delta pH \times 100}{2}$	ΔPaCO₂: change from normal (40) ΔpH: change from normal (7.40)	Accurate only in ranges of: PaCO₂: 30-50, pH 7.30-7.50

Equation	Explanation	Clinical Application
Henderson-Hasselbach $$pH = 6.1 + \log\left[\frac{HCO_3^-}{0.03 \times PCO_2}\right]$$	6.1: a dissociation constant HCO_3^-: bicarb level from ABG 0.03: the CO_2 solubility constant PCO_2: the partial pressure of CO_2	Calculation of pH or $PaCO_2$
Rule of 8's (HCO_3^- Estimation) <table><tr><th>pH is:</th><th>multiply $PaCO_2$ by:</th></tr><tr><td>7.6</td><td>8/8</td></tr><tr><td>7.5</td><td>6/8</td></tr><tr><td>7.4</td><td>5/8</td></tr><tr><td>7.3</td><td>4/8</td></tr><tr><td>7.2</td><td>3/8</td></tr></table>	Example: pH: 7.4 $PaCO_2$: 40 mm Hg Multiply $PaCO_2$ by 5/8 Estimated HCO_3^-: 25 mEq/L	When given the pH and $PaCO_2$, this estimates HCO_3^-. Use especially for verifying if an ABG is valid (see *Oakes' ABG Pocket Guide*)
Winters' Formula ($PaCO_2$ Estimation) $PaCO_2$ predicted $= 1.54 \times HCO_3^- + 8.36\ (\pm 1)$	**Interpretation:** If actual $PaCO_2$ is greater than predicted, there is a mixed acidosis If actual $PaCO_2$ is less than predicted, there is a respiratory alkalosis	Measures respiratory compensation for metabolic acidosis

Equations

Oxygenation

Equation	Explanation	Clinical Application
A-a O2 Gradient $P(A-a)O_2$ $(A-a)DO_2$ $= P_AO_2 - P_aO_2$ **Estimate** Expected $P_aO_2 = 500 \times FiO_2$	Normal: 10 - 25 mm Hg (air) = 30 - 50 mm Hg (100% O_2) P_AO_2: Alveolar Air Equation (see below) P_aO_2: from ABG FiO_2: decimal form of O_2 Increases with age: Expected A-a gradient = (Age + 10) / 4	Assists in determining between a shunt and V/Q mismatch **Use when assessing hypoxia** (especially if unexplained or more severe than clinically expected) Increased Shunt, V/Q mismatch, alveolar hypoventilation, or ↓ diffusion
Alveolar Air Equation P_AO_2 $= ([P_b - P_{H_2O}] \times FiO_2) - P_aCO_2/RQ$	Normal on RA = 100 mm Hg on FiO_2 1.0 = 663 mm Hg P_b: barometric pressure (mm Hg) (sea level = 760) P_{H_2O}: water vapor pressure (normal = 47) FiO_2: decimal form of O_2 P_aCO_2: from ABG RQ: Respiratory Quotient (normal = 0.8)	The partial pressure of oxygen in the alveoli. This is an important value in determining how much oxygen is getting from the alveoli (P_AO_2) to arterial blood (P_aO_2). Assuming normal RQ, you can make this quicker by multiplying by an RQ of 1.25 instead of dividing by 0.8. Used in several equations: P(A-a)O_2 gradient, a/A ratio, and percentage shunt

Equation	Explanation	Clinical Application
Arterial/Alveolar O₂ Tension a/A Ratio $= PaO_2 / P_AO_2$	Normal: 0.8 - 0.9 at any FiO₂ (elderly may be lower, ~0.75) Index of gas exchange function or efficiency of the lungs	More stable than A-a gradient: A-a gradient changes with FiO₂, a/A remains relatively stable with FiO₂ changes. PaCO₂ or V/Q changes can alter <0.6 = shunt, V/Q mismatch, or diffusion defect; < 0.35 indicative of weaning failure <0.15 = refractory hypoxemia
Arterial-Venous O₂ Content Difference $C(a-\bar{v})O_2$ $= CaO_2 - C\bar{v}O_2$	Normal $C(a-\bar{v})O_2 = (20-15) = $ ~5 vol% Difference between arterial and mixed venous O₂ contents. CaO₂: Arterial O₂ Content 20 vol% CvO₂: Mixed Venous O₂ Content Normal = 15 vol%	Represents O₂ consumption by tissues, and an estimate of cardiac output **Increased** Decreased cardiac output Increased O₂ consumption (fever, etc.) **Decreased** Increased cardiac output Paralytics Peripheral shunting (sepsis, trauma)

Equations

Equation	Explanation	Clinical Application
FiO2 Estimation Desired FiO2 = $\dfrac{\text{Desired PaO}_2 \times \text{Known FiO}_2}{\text{Known PaO}_2}$	Desired FiO2: "new" FiO2 to set Desired PaO2: goal PaO2 Known FiO2: current FiO2 Known PaO2: current PaO2	Used to estimate the FiO2 needed to achieve a target PaO2. This is an estimate with some basic assumptions (for example, with a V/Q mismatch, increasing FiO2 may not adequately raise PaO2)
Oxygen Consumption (Demand) $\dot{V}_{O_2}$ $= CO \times C(a-\bar{v})O_2 \times 10$	CO: Cardiac Output $C(a-\bar{v})O_2$: $CaO_2 - C\bar{v}O_2$ Normal: 200-250 mL/min $\dot{V}_{O_2}I$ (**Oxygen Consumption Index**) can be calculated by replacing CO with CI (Cardiac Index). This takes into account body size. Normal = 110-165 mL/min/m²	Volume of oxygen consumed by the body tissues per minute. Indication of metabolic level and cardiac output **Increased** Increased metabolism Increased cardiac output **Decreased** Decreased metabolism Decreased cardiac output

Equation	Explanation	Clinical Application
Oxygen Content CaO_2 $C\overline{v}O_2$ CcO_2 (see each, below)	1.34: constant representing the amount of oxygen bound per gram of hemoglobin. Values from 1.34 - 1.39 are considered acceptable (references vary) Hgb: Hemoglobin 0.0031: constant representing the amount of oxygen dissolved in plasma	Oxygen Content represents the amount of oxygen bound to hemoglobin (the majority) + the amount of blood dissolved in plasma (minimal) Useful in determining how much oxygen is actually in blood. Unlike PaO_2 or SaO_2, incorporates hemoglobin.
(Arterial Oxygen Content) $CaO_2 =$ $(Hgb \times 1.34 \times SaO_2) + (PaO_2 \times 0.003)$	Normal: 15-24 mL/dL (vol%) SaO_2: calculated in ABG PaO_2: from ABG	Total amount of oxygen in arterial blood
(Mixed Venous Oxygen Content) $C\overline{v}O_2 =$ $(Hgb \times 1.34 \times S\overline{v}O_2) + (P\overline{v}O_2 \times 0.003)$	Normal: 12-15 mL/dL (vol%) $S\overline{v}O_2$: calculated in mixed venous blood gas $P\overline{v}O_2$: from mixed venous blood gas (PA catheter)	Total amount of oxygen in mixed venous blood
(Pulmonary Capillary Oxygen Content) $CcO_2 =$ $(Hgb \times 1.34 \times ScO_2) + (PAO_2 \times 0.003)$	ScO_2: is usually assumed to be 100% (so can be left out) PcO_2: PAO_2 for clinical purposes	Total amount of oxygen in capillary blood (before anatomical shunts)

Equations

Equation	Explanation	Clinical Application
Oxygen Delivery (Supply) $\dot{D}O_2$ $= CO \times CaO_2 \times 10$	Normal: 750–1000 mL/min CO: Cardiac Output CaO_2: O_2 Content (see equation) 10: conversion factor to mL/min $\dot{D}O_2I$ (**O_2 Delivery Index**) can be calculated by dividing $\dot{D}O_2$ by BSA (accounts for body size) Normal is 500–600 mL/min/m^2	The amount of oxygen is transported from the lungs to the circulation **Increased:** Hyperoxia, FiO_2, ECMO **Decreased:** Cardiac Output decreases (cardiac, hypovolemia, etc.), respiratory disorder (V/Q mismatch, diffusion issue, hypoventilation)
O_2 Extraction Ratio O_2ER $= \dfrac{O_2 \text{ demand } (\dot{V}O_2)}{O_2 \text{ supply } (\dot{D}O_2)}$ $= \dfrac{C(a-\bar{v})O_2}{CaO_2}$	Normal: ~25 % ($\dot{V}O_2$: ~250 mL/min, $\dot{D}O_2$: ~1 L/min) Ratio of the body's oxygen consumption ($\dot{V}O_2$) to systemic oxygen delivery ($\dot{D}O_2$) Actual O_2ER also varies by organ	Indicator of the adequacy of systemic oxygen delivery. Normal resting $\dot{D}O_2$ is usually more than adequate to meet $\dot{V}O_2$ (ensuring aerobic metabolism). As demand ($\dot{V}O_2$) increases or delivery ($\dot{D}O_2$) decreases, O_2ER increases to maintain aerobic metabolism until ~70% (max O_2ER), after this, anaerobic metabolism/tissue hypoxia is likely **Increased:** Decreased oxygen delivery or increased oxygen consumption **Decreased:** Increased oxygen delivery or decreased oxygen consumption

Equation	Explanation	Clinical Application
Oxygenation Index (Oxygen Index) OI $$= \frac{FiO_2 \times 100 \times \overline{Paw}}{PaO_2}$$	Normal = no defined normal, but lower is better (OI is close to 0 if all parameters are physiologic/normal) FiO_2: use decimal form Paw: Mean Airway Pressure* PaO_2: from ABG A noninvasive form of OI, Oxygen Saturation Index (OSI), substitutes SpO_2 for PaO_2.	Helpful in assessing severity of hypoxia. Unlike P/F ratio, takes mean airway pressure into account (PEEP, etc.) Used clinically to help guide therapies such as nitric oxide, surfactant and ECMO • Signs of refractory hypoxemia at around 10-15 • Higher OI (25 or higher) may indicate severe hypoxemic respiratory failure
Oxygen Reserve $= \dot{D}O_2 - \dot{V}O_2$	Normal: 750 mL/min $= CO \times C\overline{v}O_2 \times 10$	Venous O_2 supply: O_2 supply minus O_2 demand
Oxygen Saturation (mixed venous) $S\overline{v}O_2$ $= SaO_2 - \dot{V}O_2/\dot{D}O_2$	Normal: 75 % (60-80 %)	Percent of hemoglobin saturated with oxygen (in mixed venous blood)

*The abbreviation for mean airway pressure, $\overline{Paw}$ can also be written as MAP, but because that is also used to refer to mean arterial pressure, this book uses $\overline{Paw}$ to refer to mean airway pressure, MAP to mean mean arterial pressure

Equations

Equation	Explanation	Clinical Application
Oxygen Saturation SaO_2 $= HbO_2/\text{Total Hb} \times 100$	Normal: 95-100% HbO_2: Oxyhemoglobin Content	Percentage of hemoglobin that is occupied (usually by oxygen) May be falsely elevated by abnormal hemoglobins (carbon monoxide, etc.)
P/F Ratio (PaO_2/FiO_2 ratio, Horowitz Index) $= PaO_2 / FiO_2$	Normal: 400-500 mm Hg PaO_2: from ABG FiO_2: in decimal format	This is a basic estimate of the A-a gradient, used at bedside because it is a simple calculation. Used with other criteria for determining ARDS severity (Berlin definition): {P/F Ratio table below} Both mortality and ventilator days increase as the P/F ratio drops (especially below 200)

P/F Ratio	Severity
200-300	Mild
100-200	Moderate
< 100	Severe

Equation	Explanation	Clinical Application
Predicted PaO2 in Adults (based on age) Predicted PaO$_2$ = 109 − 0.4 (Age in Years)	<table><tr><th>Age</th><th>Expected PaO$_2$</th></tr><tr><td>30</td><td>97</td></tr><tr><td>40</td><td>93</td></tr><tr><td>50</td><td>89</td></tr><tr><td>60</td><td>85</td></tr><tr><td>70</td><td>81</td></tr><tr><td>80</td><td>77</td></tr></table>	Use this as a rough estimate (there are other equations that will produce slightly different numbers, but these are all estimates). PaO$_2$ decreases as people age due to changes in lung mechanics (such as a decreasing $\dot{V}/\dot{Q}$)
Respiratory Index RI = $P(A-a)O_2 / PaO_2$	Normal: < 1.0	Estimation of oxygenation 1.0 – 5.0 = V/Q mismatch > 5.0 = refractory hypoxemia due to physiological shunt
Respiratory Quotient (Exchange ratio) (RQ, RE) RQ = $\dfrac{\dot{V}CO_2}{\dot{V}O_2}$	Normal: 200 / 250 = 0.8 While VCO$_2$ and VO$_2$ are in mL/min, the actual quotient has no unit RQ = ratio of CO$_2$ produced to O$_2$ consumed (internal respiration) RE = the amount of O$_2$/CO$_2$ exchange in the lungs per minute (external respiration) RE = RQ in steady state condition	RQ is an indicator of the balance between O$_2$ being used and CO$_2$ being produced. Indirect calorimetry is used to collect the information needed

Equations

Equations

Equation	Explanation	Clinical Application
Ventilation		
Alveolar (Minute) Ventilation $\dot{V}_A$ $= \dot{V}_E - \dot{V}_D$	Normal: 4-6 L/min $\dot{V}_E$: Minute ventilation $\dot{V}_D$: Dead space ventilation As the equation shows, dead space ventilation is subtracted from minute ventilation, leaving alveolar ventilation	The volume of inspired air reaching the alveoli **per minute** By definition $\dot{V}_A < \dot{V}_E$ (due to dead space)
Alveolar Volume V_A $= \dot{V}_A / f$	$\dot{V}_A$: Alveolar ventilation f: Frequency (respiratory rate)	The volume of inspired air reaching the alveoli **per breath**
Dead Space Ventilation $\dot{V}_D$ $= \dot{V}_E - \dot{V}_A$	Normal: $1/3\ \dot{V}_E$ $\dot{V}_E$: Minute ventilation $\dot{V}_A$: Alveolar ventilation	The volume of wasted air (not participating in gas exchange) per minute

Equation	Explanation	Clinical Application
Dead Space Volume V_D $= V_T - V_A$ See nomogram, next page	Normal: 1/3 V_T Anatomical: 1 mL/lb IBW = 0.5 mL/lb with airway Mechanical: ~ 10 mL/inch of tubing	The volume of wasted air (not participating in gas exchange) per breath (V > Q) Increased: ↓ CO, pulmonary vasoconstriction, pulmonary embolus
Dead Space / Tidal Volume Ratio V_D / V_T **Physiological V_D/V_T Ratio (Bohr Equation)** $\dfrac{V_{Dphys}}{V_T} = \dfrac{P_aCO_2 - P_{\bar{E}}CO_2}{P_aCO_2}$ **Anatomical V_D/V_T Ratio:** $\dfrac{V_{Danat}}{V_T} = \dfrac{P_{et}CO_2 - P_{\bar{E}}CO_2}{P_{et}CO_2}$	Normal: 0.33 (150 V_D /450 V_T) $P_{\bar{E}}CO_2$: mixed expired Estimate: $V_{Dphys} / V_T =$ ($\dot{V}_E$ actual / $\dot{V}_E$ predicted) x (P_aCO_2 actual / 40) x 0.33 Pet: end tidal	$V_D/V_T > 0.5$ is indicative of respiratory failure *Technically, P_aCO_2 would best reflect deadspace but can't be measured reliably (and often varies from one alveolus to the next). Clinically, P_aCO_2 is used as a rough estimation of the impact of dead space. Many lung diseases (atelectasis, pneumonia, pulmonary edema, emboli, etc.) can exhibit changes in V_D (i.e, V_{DAlv}) without corresponding changes in P_aCO_2*

Nomogram to estimate minute ventilation required to maintain a given PaCO2 when VD/VT is known:

To obtain the required minute ventilation to achieve a given PaCO2, the minute ventilation is plotted against the PaCO2 (measured simultaneously) and the VD/VT ratio is read on the isopleth that corresponds to the intersection. The isopleth is then followed to the desired PaCO2 and the corresponding minute ventilation read off the vertical axis.

For example: A patient with a $\dot{V}_E$ of 5L and a PaCO2 of 60 mm Hg has an estimated VD/VT ratio of 0.40. To achieve a desired PaCO2 of 40 mm Hg, follow the 0.40 isopleth up to correspond to the PaCO2 of 40 on the horizontal axis. Then read the appropriate minute ventilation of about 8 L/min off the vertical axis.

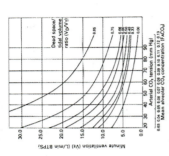

Equation	Explanation	Clinical Application
Minute Ventilation (Minute Volume) $$\dot{V}_E$$ $$= V_T \times f$$ see pg 13-12 for alveolar ventilation	Normal: 5 – 7 L/min V_T: Tidal Volume f: Frequency (Respiratory Rate)	Total amount of gas moved into (inhaled minute ventilation) or out of (exhaled minute ventilation) the lungs per minute

Equation	Explanation	Clinical Application
Ventilation/Perfusion Ratio $\dot{V}/\dot{Q}$ Ratio $$\dot{V}_A/\dot{Q}c = \frac{(C\bar{v}CO_2 - CaCO_2) \times 8.63}{PaCO_2}$$	Normal: $\frac{4 L/min}{5 L/min} = 0.8$ Ratio of minute alveolar ventilation to minute capillary blood flow Represents external respiration	Ratio changes represent the degree and type of respiratory imbalances ↓ Ratio (↓V/Q) = atelectasis, COPD, pneumonia, pneumothorax, N-M disorders, etc. ↑ Ratio (V/↓Q) = shock, pulmonary emboli, cor pulmonale, PPV
Ventilator Calculations *Additional equations can be found in Oakes' Ventilator Management Pocket Guide*		
Ventilator Rate Needed to achieve a desired $PaCO_2$ New RR = $\frac{(Current\ RR) \times (Current\ PaCO_2)}{(Desired\ PaCO_2)}$ Ventilator Minute Ventilation Needed to achieve a desired $PaCO_2$ New $\dot{V}_E$ = $\frac{(Current\ PaCO_2) \times (Current\ \dot{V}_E)}{(Desired\ PaCO_2)}$ New FiO_2 = See pg 13-6		This equation works best for patients on ventilator modes with consistent tidal volumes, rates (and assumes a steady state physiologically) For RR, be sure to calculate using the total rate (ventilator breaths + spontaneous breaths)

Equations

Equations

Equation	Explanation	Clinical Application
Airway Resistance R_{aw} $= PIP - Pplat / \dot{V}_I$ See also pg 5-5 and 6-14	Normal: 0.5 - 2.5 cm $H_2O/L/sec$ @ a flow of 0.5 L/sec (30 L/min) with ET tube (approp. size) = 4 - 8 cm $H_2O/L/sec$ PIP: Peak Inspiratory Pressure Pplat: Plateau Pressure $\dot{V}_I$: Inspiratory Flow in L/sec $\uparrow$PIP + $\uparrow$Pplat (P_{TA} constant) = $\downarrow$Cstat $\uparrow$PIP + same Pplat ($\uparrow P_{TA}$) = $\uparrow R_{aw}$ $\downarrow$PIP + $\downarrow$Pplat (P_{TA} constant) = $\uparrow$Cstat $\downarrow$PIP + same Pplat ($\downarrow P_{TA}$) = $\downarrow R_{aw}$	Represents frictional resistance of airflow (80%) and tissue motion (20%) **Increased airflow resistance:** trachea (normal resistance from turbulent airflow), airway collapse (tracheomalacia, etc.), edema, bronchospasm, secretions, artificial airway (esp. ET tube) **Increased tissue resistance:** pulmonary edema, fibrosis, pneumonia Small changes in radius will increase airway resistance dramatically Technically there exists both inspiratory resistance (R_I) and expiratory resistance (R_E). They approximate each other normally, but may vary with lung disease. This equation uses inspiratory flow) measures inspiratory airway resistance.

Equation	Explanation	Clinical Application
Compliance C $= \Delta V / \Delta P$ $C_T = C_L + C_{CW}$ $C_L = \Delta V / P_{alv} - P_{pl}$ $C_{CW} = \Delta V / P_{pl} - P_B$ See next pages for static/dynamic compliance See Also pg 5-5 and 6-14	Normal: 70 - 100 mL/cm H₂O Total compliance can be referred to as C_T: lung + thorax C_{rs}: (respiratory system) Compliances C_L: lung compliance C_{CW}: chest wall (thorax) compliance Pressures P_B = barometric pressure P_{pl} = pleural pressure P_{alv} = alveolar pressure	Represents the ease of distention of the lungs and thorax Includes elastic, functional, and tissue viscous resistance Ideal = 100 mL/cm H₂O Lungs and chest wall each = 200 mL/cm H₂O.

Equations 13-17

Equation	Explanation	Clinical Application
Static Compliance Cstat $= V_T / P_{plat} - PEEP$ See Also pg 5-5 and 6-14	Normal: 70 - 100 mL/cm H$_2$O Pplat: inspiratory hold on ventilator until pressure stabilizes (1-4 seconds) See Oakes' *Ventilator Management Pocket Guide* for more on Cstat, including details on tubing compliance (automatically compensated for with most current ventilators)	Represents the combination of lung elasticity and chest wall recoil **Increased** ↑ lung elasticity or ↑ chest wall recoil. **Decreased** ↓ lung elasticity or ↓ chest wall recoil. Trending Cstat has greater value than interpreting a single value
Dynamic Compliance Cdyn $= V_T / PIP - PEEP$ See Also pg 5-5 and 6-14	Normal: 40 - 70 mL/cm H$_2$O See Oakes' *Ventilator Management Pocket Guide* for more on Cdyn, including details on tubing compliance (automatically compensated for with most current ventilators)	Represents the combination of static lung compliance (Cstat) and airway resistance (Raw) Trending Cdyn has greater value than interpreting a single value

Remember Splat (S= Static, plat= reminder to put plateau pressure in equation); Dip (D=Dynamic, ip=PIP in equation)*

*Special appreciation to Misty Carlson, MS, RRT for this mnemonic

Equation	Explanation	Clinical Application
Driving Pressure ΔP $= Pplat - PEEP$	$\Delta P = V_T/C_{RS}$ (theoretical equation) Pplat: Plateau Pressure V$_T$: Tidal Volume C$_{RS}$: Respiratory System Compliance	May be a better measure of "functional" lung size (and is preferred by some in targeting safe V$_T$ - versus using PBW or IBW) > 15 may increase mortality
Mean Airway Pressure $\overline{P}aw$, mPAW, MAP Constant Flow Volume Ventilation: $= 0.5 \times (PIP-PEEP) \times (T_I/T_{tot}) + PEEP$	Average airway pressure (cmH$_2$O) during several breathing cycles For pressure ventilation, use same equation but do not multiply by 0.5	Usually measured during mechanical ventilation, often used to monitor and indirectly manipulate oxygenation. PEEP is a major determinant If inspiratory and expiratory airway resistance are different (such as with lung disease), mean alveolar pressure may vary from $\overline{P}aw$
Rapid Shallow Breathing Index RSBI $= f / V_T$	Measure f and V_T (in liters) while receiving no or minimal vent support (usually low PS/CPAP). Normal: <100 >105 = increased potential for weaning failure	Used as one determination of readiness to wean/extubate. If patient is breathing fast and shallow, score will be high (and likely to fail); if normal RR and normal V$_T$, score will be low, more likely to succeed.

Equations

Equation	Explanation	Clinical Application
Time Constant TC TC = Raw x Cstat Note: TC generally refers to inspiratory TC. Expiratory TC may be much longer than inspiratory TC in COPD.	1TC = 63% 2TC = 87% 3TC = 95% 4TC = 98% 5TC = 99% %: % of V_T entering lungs within each TC period Normal TC = 0.2 sec Normal T_I = 3 - 4 TC $\quad$ = 3 or 4 x 0.2 sec $\quad$ = 0.6 – 0.8 sec	TC_{inspir} indicates alveolar filling time. ↑ TC (> 0.2 sec) is usually indicative of ↑Raw (but may be ↑C_{LT}). ↓ TC (< 0.2 sec) is usually indicative of ↓C_{LT} (but may be ↓Raw) TC_{expir} indicates alveolar emptying time Less than 3 TC_{expir} will generally result in air-trapping TC_{expir} may be approximated with a flow-volume loop
Perfusion/Hemodynamic Monitoring		
Cardiac Output CO or $\dot{Q}_T$ = SV x HR	Normal: 4-8 L/min (at rest) See Fick equation below and *Oakes' Hemodynamic Monitoring Pocket Guide* for more information. Cardiac Index (CI) can be calculated by dividing CO by BSA (takes into account body size)	Amount of blood ejected from heart per minute. Indicator of pump efficiency and a determinant of tissue perfusion

Equation	Explanation	Clinical Application
Fick Equation $\dot{V}O_2$ $= CO \times Ca\text{-}\bar{v}O_2$	See Oakes' *Hemodynamic Monitoring: A Bedside Reference Manual* for more info.	Method of measuring cardiac output. Fick estimate: $CO = 125 \times BSA / Ca\text{-}\bar{v}O_2$
Left Ventricular Stroke Work LVSW $= (MAP - PCWP) \times SV \times 0.0136$	Normal: 60–80 gm/m/beat MAP: Mean Arterial Pressure PCWP: Pulmonary Capillary Wedge Pressure (aka PAOP) SV: Stroke Volume To calculate the Index (LVSWI) substitute SV with SVI (takes body size into account)	Measure of pumping function of left ventricle = left ventricular contractility
Mean Arterial (Blood) Pressure (MAP, $\overline{BP}$) $= \dfrac{Systolic + 2(Diastolic)}{3}$ See also page 1-11	Normal: 93 mm Hg (70–105) Systolic: top number in BP Diastolic: bottom number in BP	Average driving force of systemic circulation. A minimal MAP of about 60 is required to maintain sufficient perfusion to vital organs. Determined by cardiac output and total peripheral resistance.

Equation	Explanation	Clinical Application
Mean Pulmonary Artery Pressure PAP, PAMP $$= \frac{PASP + 2(PADP)}{3}$$	Normal: 10-15 mm Hg PASP: Pulmonary Artery Systolic Pressure PADP: Pulmonary Artery Diastolic Pressure	Average driving force of blood from the right heart to left heart (this is the pulmonary circulation)
Pulmonary Vascular Resistance PVR $$PVR = \frac{PAMP - PCWP}{CO} \times 80$$	Normal: 20-250 dynes•sec•cm^{-5} = 0.25-2.5 units (mm Hg/L/min) PAMP: Pulmonary Artery Pressure Mean PCWP: Pulmonary Capillary Wedge Pressure CO: Cardiac Output To calculate the Index (PVRI) substitute CO with CI (takes body size into account)	Resistance to right ventricular ejection of blood into pulmonary vasculature Indicator of RV afterload

Equation	Explanation	Clinical Application
Pulse Pressure PP = BPsys - BPdia	Normal: 40 mm Hg (20-80)	Difference between BP systolic and BP diastolic
Right Ventricular Stroke Work RVSW = (PAMP - CVP) × SV × 0.0136	Normal: 10-15 gm/m/beat PAMP: Pulmonary Artery Mean Pressure CVP: Central Venous Pressure SV: Stroke Volume To calculate the Index (RVSWI) divide RVSW by BSA (takes body size into account)	Measure of pumping function of right ventricle (RV contractility)

Equations

Equation	Explanation	Clinical Application
Shunt Equation $\dot{Q}s/\dot{Q}T$ **Clinical Equation (use if PaO2 > 150)** $= \dfrac{P(A-a)O_2 \times 0.003}{C(a-\bar{v})O_2 + P(A-a)O_2 \times 0.003}$ **Classical Equation (use if PaO2 < 150)** $= \dfrac{CcO_2 - CaO_2}{CcO_2 - C\bar{v}O_2}$ **Estimates** (ideal: FIO2 0.50 x 20 min before sampling/calculating) $= \dfrac{P(A-a)O_2}{20}$ $\dot{Q}s/\dot{Q}T = 5\%$ per every 100 mm Hg below expected	Normal: 2-5% (mostly from Thebesian veins) Ratio of shunted blood (Qs) to total cardiac output (QT) P(A-a)O2: A-a O2 Gradient (pg 13-4) C(a-v)O2: Arterial-Venous O2 Content (pg 13-5) CcO2: Pulmonary Capillary Oxygen Content CaO2: Arterial Oxygen Content CvO2: Mixed Venous Oxygen Content Estimate using PaO2/FIO2: > 300 = < 15% shunt 200 - 300 = 15 - 20% shunt < 200 = > 20% shunt $C(a-\bar{v})O_2$ can be assumed if a mixed venous sample cannot be obtained: 4.5 - 5% if good CO and perfusion 3.5% in critically ill patients	A measure of right-to-left shunted blood (passes from right side of heart to left side of heart without being oxygenated, either for anatomical or physiological reasons) Indicator or efficiency of pulmonary system: < 10% = normal lungs 10-20% = minimal effect 20-30% = significant pulmonary disease > 30% = life-threatening This is a complicated calculation that requires a PA catheter to be more than an estimate. While the equation is uncommonly used, the concept is critical to bedside care.

Equation	Explanation	Clinical Application
Stroke Volume SV = CO/HR × 1000	Normal: 60–120 mL/beat CO: Cardiac Output HR: Heart Rate To calculate the Index (SVI) divide SV by BSA (takes body size into account)	Amount of blood ejected by either ventricle per contraction
Systemic Vascular Resistance SVR = $\dfrac{\text{MAP} - \text{CVP}}{\text{CO}} \times 80$	Normal: 800–1600 dynes•sec•cm^{-5} MAP: Mean Arterial Pressure CVP: Central Venous Pressure CO: Cardiac Output To calculate the Index (SVRI) substitute CO with CI (takes body size into account)	Resistance to LV ejection of blood into systemic circulation. Indicator of LV afterload. mm Hg/L/min × 80 = dynes•sec•cm^{-5}

Equation	Explanation	Clinical Application
Patient Calculations		
Body Surface Area BSA $= (H^{0.725} \times W^{0.425}) \times 0.007184$	Average: 1.9 m² (males) 1.6 m² (females) H: Height in centimeters W: Weight in kilograms	When used with hemodynamic equations (usually then called an "index"), body size is at least partially accounted for (theoretically making the values more accurate)
Ideal Body Weight IBW (kg) F: 45.5 + [0.9(Height(cm) - 154)] M: 50 + [0.9(Height(cm) - 154)] **Estimate** (must convert to kg after) F: 100 + 5lb per inch over 5 ft M: 106 + 6lb per inch over 5 ft	Ideal body weight is a commonly used calculation (despite being based on a life insurance equation) 1 kg = 2.2 lb	For clinical purposes there is relatively little difference between IBW and PBW ARDSnet calculations are based upon PBW and some clinicians prefer using PBW for ventilator calculations There are other calculations: predicted normal weight, lean body weight, fat free mass, and adjusted body weight which are not presented here
Predicted Body Weight PBW (kg) F: 45.5 + [0.91(Height(cm) - 152.4)] M: 50 + [0.91(Height(cm) - 152.4)]	Predicted Body Weight (PBW) is the preferred equation for ARDS	

Equations

Equation	Explanation	Clinical Application
Pulmonary Function (Bedside)		
% Predicted $$\frac{Actual}{Predicted} \times 100$$	Calculation of actual vs predicted with pulmonary function	See PFT chapter for information on using Lower Limits of Normal (LLN) vs % Predicted
% Change $$\frac{post\ Measure - pre\ Measure}{pre\ Measure} \times 100$$	Calculation of percentage change comparing before and after	While this equation can be applied to multiple scenarios, it is particularly used for pre- and post- bronchodilator spirometry
Miscellaneous		
Fick's Law of Diffusion $$Diffusion = \frac{Area \times diffusion\ coefficient \times \Delta P}{Thickness}$$		Gas diffusion rate across the lung membrane

Equations

Equation	Explanation	Clinical Application
Combined Gas Law $$\frac{(P1)(V1)}{(T1)} = \frac{(P2)(V2)}{(T2)}$$	This is a **combination** of Boyle's, Charles', and Gay-Lussac's laws. 1 = Initial variable 2 = Final variable P1: Pressure 1 P2: Pressure 2 V1: Volume 1 V2: Volume 2 T1: Temperature 1 T2: Temperature 2	Solve for any 1. Anything (P1=P2, V1=V2, or T1=T2) held constant can be dropped from the equation.
Boyle's Law $$(P1)(V1) = (P2)(V2)$$	With temperature held constant, **pressure and volume** are inversely related (as one increases, the other decreases)	Ventilation (breathing!) Body plethysmography (PFTs) Blood gas measurements
Charles' Law $$\frac{(V1)}{(T1)} = \frac{(V2)}{(T2)}$$	With pressure held constant, **volume and temperature** are directly related (as one increases, the other increases)	ATPS to BTPS correction
Gay-Lussac's Law $$\frac{(P1)}{(T1)} = \frac{(P2)}{(T2)}$$	With volume held constant, **pressure and temperature** are directly related (as one increases, the other increases)	Cylinder pressures

Equation	Explanation	Clinical Application
Dalton's Law of Partial Pressures $P_{tot} = P_1 + P_2 + P_3 + ...$	The total pressure exerted by a mixture of gases is equal to the sum of the partial pressures of the gases	Used to determine partial pressure of specific gases (O_2) at different atmos. pressures: $P_B = P_{O_2} + P_{N_2} + P_{CO_2} + P_{(trace\ gases)}$
Helium/Oxygen (Heliox) Flow Conversion and Duration 80/20 actual flow = set flow × 1.8 70/30 actual flow = set flow × 1.6 60/40 actual flow = set flow × 1.4	80/20: 80% Helium, 20% Oxygen 70/30: 70% Helium, 30% Oxygen 60/40: 60% Helium, 40% Oxygen	When Heliox (a less dense gas) is run through an oxygen flowmeter, the flow is higher than the numbers indicate. Use the formula to calculate actual flow being delivered This equation is not necessary if using a properly calibrated Heliox flowmeter (that matches the mixture being used)
Law of LaPlace $P = 2T/r$	P: Pressure needed (dynes/cm²) T: Surface tension (dynes/cm) r: Radius (cm)	Particularly important in considering aerosol therapy (aerosol suspension)

Equations

Equation	Explanation	Clinical Application
Air-to-O2 Ratio (Air Entrainment) $\dfrac{Air}{O_2} = \dfrac{(100 - O_2\%)}{(O_2\% - 21)}$	Use to determine Air:Oxygen Ratio 1. Subtract 100-O2% = Air ratio part 2. Subtract 21-O2% = O2 ratio part (ignore any negative sign) 3. Put together Air:O2 4. Reduce by dividing both parts by the 2nd number Example: TF = 1.7 + 1 = 2.7 x 10 L/min = 27 L/min	Used in determining ratio of air to oxygen (such as with venturi masks)
Magic Box Shortcut for Air-to-O2 Ratio		Example: Calculate the Air:O2 ratio for 50% oxygen
Total Flow Calculation (L/min) = [(Air Ratio) + (O2 Ratio)] x O2 Flow	1. Take Air:O2 Ratio from above 2. Add ratio parts together 3. Multiply by O2 Flow	This calculates total flow of a high flow device (venturi masks, etc.)

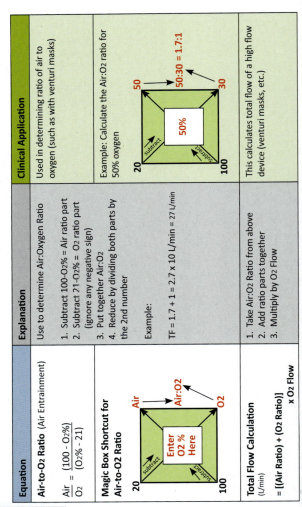

Equation	Explanation	Clinical Application
Gas Cylinder Duration Times Time (min) = $\dfrac{(\text{PSIG} - 500) \times \text{CF}}{\text{Flow (L/min)}}$	PSIG: Pressure from Cylinder 500: optional reserve (to ensure adequate supply, tank doesn't run dry) CF: conversion factor (L/psi)	**Oxygen Conversion Factors** D cyl: 0.16 (max PSIG: 2015) E cyl: 0.28 (max PSIG: 2015) H cyl: 3.14 (max PSIG: 2265) **Heliox Conversion Factors** E cyl: 0.23 (max PSIG: 2015) H cyl: 2.50 (max PSIG: 2265)
Duration of a Liquid System Amt of Gas (L) = $\dfrac{\text{Liquid Weight (lb)} \times 860}{2.5 \text{ lb/L}}$ Duration of Gas (min) = $\dfrac{\text{Amt of Gas (L)}}{\text{Flow (L/min)}}$	1 L liquid = 860 L gas Liquid Wt = Total Wt − Cylinder Wt	

Equations

Equation	Explanation	Clinical Application
Poiseuille's Law $$=\frac{\pi(P_1-P_2)r^4 t}{8\eta L}$$	P_1, P_2 = Pressure on either side of tube r = radius t = time η = coefficient of viscosity L = length of vessel	While not calculated often, this is the pressure required to produce a given flow (assuming laminar flow) Used for flow of air through airways
Reynold's Number $$Re = \frac{\text{(fluid velocity)} \times \text{(fluid density)} \times \text{(vessel diameter)}}{\text{viscosity of fluid}}$$		Indicator of turbulent vs. laminar flow Used for flow of blood through vessels. The higher the Reynold's number, the more likely flow is to be turbulent
Temperature Conversion $$F° = (C° \times 9/5) + 32°$$ $$C° = (F° - 32) \times 5/9$$	F°: degrees Fahrenheit C°: degrees Celsius	See Appendix (A-4) for temperature conversion charts
Tobacco Use Pack-Years $$= (PPD) \times (\text{\# Years Smoked})$$	PPD: Packs per day (there are 20 cigarettes in a pack) # Years Smoked: count total years smoked, taking into account any substantial periods of quitting	Generally this is used for tobacco (cigarettes) only. Other forms should be documented (vaping, cigars, marijuana, etc.), but should not be mixed into this equation.

A Appendix

Basic Units of Measure A-2
Gas Phase Symbols A-2
Blood Phase Symbols A-2
Conversions
   Metric A-3
   U.S./Metric Equivalents A-3
   Temperature (C ↔ F) A-4
   Weight (kg ↔ lb) A-4
   Height (ft ↔ in ↔ cm) A-4
Abbreviations A-5

Basic Units of Measure

cm H$_2$O	centimeters of water pressure
gm%	gram percent (number of grams per 100 grams of total weight)
kg	kilograms
kPa	kiloPascals (SI unit for pressure)
mg	milligrams
mL	milliliters
mm Hg	millimeters of mercury (pressure)
vol%	volume percent (number of mL in a substance per 100 mL of volume)
L/min	liters per minute
mEq/L	milliequivalents per liter
torr	unit of measure roughly equivalent to mm Hg

Gas Phase Symbols

D	Diffusion
F	Fractional concentration of a gas
P	Partial pressure of a gas
$\bar{P}$	Mean pressure of a gas
R	Respiratory exchange ratio
V	Volume of a gas
$\dot{V}$	Flow of a gas (volume/time)

Blood Phase Symbols

Q	Volume of blood
$\dot{Q}$	Blood flow (cardiac output) in L/min
C	Concentration (content in the blood phase)
S	Saturation in the blood phase

Conversions

Metric Measures

Linear			Weight			Volume		
kilometer (km)	m × 10³		kilogram (kg)	g × 10³		kiloliter		1 × 10³
decameter	m × 10		decagram	g × 10		decaliter		1 × 10
meter (m)			gram (g)			liter (L)		
decimeter	m × 10⁻¹		decigram	g × 10⁻¹		deciliter (dL)		1 × 10⁻¹
centimeter (cm)	m × 10⁻²		centigram	g × 10⁻²		centiliter		1 × 10⁻²
millimeter (mm)	m × 10⁻³		milligram (mg)	g × 10⁻³		milliliter (mL)		1 × 10⁻³
micrometer (μ)	m × 10⁻⁶		microgram (μg)	g × 10⁻⁶		microliter (μL)		1 × 10⁻⁶

U.S. Customary and Metric Equivalents

1 inch	2.54 cm	1 ounce (oz)	28.35g	1 ounce (fl)	29.57 mL
1 foot	.0348 m	1 pound	454 g	1 quart	0.9463 L
1 mile	1.609 km	1 gram	0.0352 oz	1 gallon	3.785 L
1 micron	3.937 × 10⁻⁵ in	1 kilogram	2.2 lb	cubic inch (in³)	16.39 mL
1 centimeter	0.3937 in			cubic foot (ft³)	28.32 L
1 meter	39.37 in			1 liter	1.057 qt

Temperature

$°C = (°F-32) \times 5/9$
$°F = (°C \times 9/5) + 32$

°F	°C
32	0
90	32.2
91	32.8
92	33.3
93	33.4
94	34.4
95	35.0
96	35.6
97	36.1
98	36.7
98.6	37.0
99	37.2
100	37.8
101	38.3
102	38.9
103	39.4
104	40.0
105	40.6
106	41.1
107	41.7
108	42.2
109	42.8

While 37 C is generally seen as "perfect normal" a range of normals is more appropriate

Height

1 Ft = 12 in
1 in = 2.54 cm

Ft	in.	cm.
5' 0"	60	152.4
5' 1"	61	154.9
5' 2"	62	157.5
5' 3"	63	160.0
5' 4"	64	162.6
5' 5"	65	165.1
5' 6"	66	167.6
5' 7"	67	170.2
5' 8"	68	172.7
5' 9"	69	175.3
5' 10"	70	177.8
5' 11"	71	180.3
6' 0"	72	182.9
6' 1"	73	185.4
6' 2"	74	188.0
6' 3"	75	190.5
6' 4"	76	193.0
6' 5"	77	195.6
6' 6"	78	198.1
6' 7"	79	200.7
6' 8"	80	203.2
6' 9"	81	205.7

Weight

1 kg = 2.2 lb

kg	lb	kg	lb	kg	lb
1	2.2	10	22.0	90	198.4
2	4.4	20	44.0	100	220.5
3	6.6	30	66.0	110	242.5
4	8.8	40	88.0	120	264.6
5	11.0	50	110.0	130	286.6
6	13.2	60	132.0	140	308.6
7	15.4	70	154.0	150	330.7
8	17.6	80	176.0	160	352.7

Abbreviations

Abbr.	Definition	Abbr.	Definition	Abbr.	Definition
AAP	American Academy of Pediatrics	BP$_{dia}$	Diastolic blood pressure	CO	Cardiac output
AARC	American Association of Respiratory Care	BP$_{sys}$	Systolic blood pressure	CO	Carbon monoxide
ABG	Arterial blood gas	B-P	Bronchopleural	CO$_2$	Carbon dioxide
A/C	Assist-Control Ventilation	BSA	Body surface area	COPD	Chronic obstructive pulmonary disease
ACCP	American College of Chest Physicians	BVM	Bag-Valve-Mask	CPAP	Continuous positive airway pressure
ACLS	Advanced Cardiac Life Support	CABG	Coronary artery bypass graft	CPG	Clinical Practice Guideline
ADH	Anti-diuretic hormone	CaO$_2$	Arterial oxygen content	CPP	Cerebral or coronary perfusion pressure
A-fib	Atrial fibrillation	Ca-$\bar{v}$O$_2$	Arterial-mixed venous O$_2$ content difference	CPT	Chest physical therapy
AG	Anion gap			CSF	Cerebral spinal fluid
AHA	American Heart Association	CBT	Continuous Bronchodilator Therapy	Cstat	Static compliance
		CC	Closing capacity	Ctubing	Compliance of the tubing
A-P	Anterior-Posterior	Ccw	Chest wall compliance	CV	Cardiovascular
ARDS	Acute respiratory distress syndrome	CHD	Congenital heart disease	CVA	Cerebrovascular accident
		CHF	Congestive heart failure	CvO$_2$	Venous oxygen content
ARF	Acute respiratory failure	Cdyn	Dynamic compliance	CVP	Central venous pressure
ASD	Atrial septal defect	CF	Conversion factor	CXR	Chest x-ray (radiograph)
ATS	American Thoracic Society	CF	Cystic fibrosis	DKA	Diabetic ketoacidosis
AV	Atrio-ventricular	CFF	Cystic Fibrosis Foundation	DLCO	Diffusion capacity for CO
a-v	arterio-venous	CI	Cardiac index	DO$_2$	Oxygen delivery
BE/BD	Base excess/deficit	CL	Compliance of the lung	DOE	Dyspnea on exertion
BLS	Basic Life Support	CLT	Compliance of the lung and thorax	DPG,2,3	2,3 diphosphoglycerate
BP	Blood pressure	cm H$_2$O	Centimeters of water	DPI	Dry powder inhaler
		CNS	Central nervous system	ECG	Electrocardiogram

ECMO	Extracorporeal membrane oxygenation
EDV	End diastolic volume
EEP	End expiratory pressure
ECG	Electrocardiogram
EPAP	Expiratory positive airway pressure
ERV	Expiratory reserve volume
et	End-tidal
ET	Endotracheal
ETS	Endotracheal suction
EIB	Exercise induced bronchospasm
f	Frequency (ventilator rate)
FDO$_2$	Fraction of delivered O$_2$
FECO$_2$	Fractional concentration of expired CO$_2$
FEF	Forced expiratory flow
FET	Forced Expiration Technique
FEV	Forced expiratory volume
FICO	Fraction of inspired CO
FIF	Forced inspiratory flow
FIO$_2$	Fraction of inspired oxygen

Abbr	Definition	Abbr	Definition	Abbr	Definition
FIVC	Forced inspiratory vital capacity	ILD	Interstitial Lung Disease	LV	Left ventricle	MEP	Maximal Expiratory Pressure
Fr	French	iNO	Inhaled nitric oxide	LHF	Left heart failure	MI	Myocardial infarction
FRC	Functional residual capacity	IPAP	Inspiratory positive airway pressure	LLN	Lower limits of normal	MIF	Maximum inspiratory force
F-T	Flow-time	IMV	Intermittent mandatory ventilation	LVF	Left ventricular failure	MIP	Maximum inspiratory pressure
FVC	Forced vital capacity			LVH	Left ventricular hypertrophy	MMAD	Mean mass aerodynamic diameter
Gaw	Airway conductance	IO	Intraosseous	LVEDP	Left ventricular end diastolic pressure	mm Hg	millimeters of mercury
GI	Gastrointestinal	I+O	Intake & output	LVEDV	Left ventricular end diastolic volume	MRI	Magnetic Resonance Imaging
H+	Hydrogen ion	IPPV	Intermittent positive pressure ventilation	LVESP	Left ventricular end systolic pressure	MRN	Medical Record Number
HbO2	Oxyhemoglobin	IPV	Intrapulmonary Percussive Ventilation	LVESV	Left ventricular end systolic volume	MvO2	Myocardial oxygen consumption
HCH	Hygroscopic condenser humidifier	IRV	Inspiratory reserve volume or Inverse ratio ventilation	LVSW	Left ventricular stroke work	MV	Mechanical ventilation
HCO3	Bicarbonate	IS	Incentive spirometry	LVSWI	Left ventricular stroke work index	MVV	Maximum voluntary ventilation
Hct	Hematocrit	IV	Intravenous	MAP	Mean airway pressure	NC	Nasal cannula
HFA	Hydroflouroalkane	J	Joule	MAP	Mean arterial pressure	NG	Nasogastric
HFO	High flow oxygen	JVD	Jugular vein distention	MBC	Maximum breathing capacity	NIF	Negative inspiratory force
HFV	High frequency ventilation	kg	Kilogram	MDI	Metered dose inhaler	N-M	Neuromuscular
Hgb	Hemoglobin	LA	Left atrium	MDO2	Myocardial oxygen delivery	NO	Nitric oxide
HME	Heat moisture exchanger	LABA	Long-acting beta agonist (or adrenergic)	MEF	Maximal expiratory pressure	NPPV	Noninvasive positive pressure ventilation
HR	Heart rate or heated reservoir	LAMA	Long-acting muscarinic antiadrenergic	MEFV	Maximal expiratory flow volume	NRB	Nonrebreather
I	Inspiration	LAP	Left atrial pressure			NSS	Normal saline solution
IC	Inspiratory capacity	LDH	Lactic dehydrogenase			N-STEMI	Non ST-elevation MI
ICP	Intracranial pressure	LOC	Level of consciousness			NTS	Nasotracheal suction
ICS	Inhaled corticosteroid	L-R	Left to right				
ID	Internal diameter						
I-E	Inspiratory/expiratory ratio						

O_2	Oxygen		occlusion pressure		dioxide
O_2ER	Oxygen extraction ratio	PAP	Pulmonary artery pressure	PEEP	Positive end-expiratory pressure
O_2 Sat	Oxygen saturation		Positive airway pressure	PEF	Peak expiratory flow
P	Pressure	PASP	Pulmonary artery systolic pressure	PEP	Positive expiratory pressure
PA	Pulmonary artery or posterior-anterior	PAT	Premature atrial tachycardia	PFT	Pulmonary function test
P(A-a)O_2	Alveolar-arterial oxygen partial pressure difference	Paw	Airway pressure	pH	Negative log of hydrogen ion concentration
PaCO_2	Partial pressure of arterial carbon dioxide	$\overline{Paw}$	Mean airway pressure	pHa	pH of arterial blood
PACO_2	Partial pressure of alveolar carbon dioxide	Pawo	Pressure at airway opening	pHv	pH of venous blood
PAC	Premature atrial contraction	PAWP	Pulmonary artery wedge pressure	PIF	Peak inspiratory flow
P-ACV	Pressure-assist/control ventilation	PB	Barometric pressure	PImax	Maximal inspiratory pressure
PAPD	Pulmonary artery diastolic pressure	PBW	Predicted body weight	PIO_2	Partial pressure of inspired oxygen
PAEPD	Pulmonary artery end-diastolic pressure	PCI	Percutaneous Coronary Intervention	PIP	Peak inspiratory pressure
Palv	Alveolar pressure	PCWP	Pulmonary capillary wedge pressure	PIT	Intrathoracic pressure
PAMP	Pulmonary artery mean pressure	Pcyl	Pressure in a cylinder	PIV	Intravascular pressure
PaO_2	Partial pressure of arterial oxygen	PE	Pulmonary embolism	PMI	Point of maximal impulse
PAO_2	Partial pressure of alveolar oxygen	PEA	Pulseless electrical activity	PNC	Premature nodal contraction
PAOP	Pulmonary artery	PECO_2	Partial pressure of expired carbon dioxide	PND	Paroxysmal nocturnal dyspnea
		PetCO_2	Partial pressure of end-expired carbon	PP	Pulse pressure
				PPE	Personal Protective Equipment
				P_{pl}	Intrapleural pressure
				P_{peak}	Peak inspiratory pressure
				PPHN	Persistent pulmonary hypertension of the newborn
				P_{plat}	Inspiratory plateau pressure
				PPV	Positive pressure ventilation
				PSTV	Paroxysmal supra-ventricular tachycardia
				pt	Patient
				PT	Prothrombin time
				PtcO_2	Transcutaneous partial pressure of oxygen
				PTL	Pharyngotracheal lumen airway
				Ptm	Transmural pressure
				PTT	Partial prothrombin time
				PV	Pressure ventilation
				PVC	Premature ventricular contraction
				PVD	Peripheral vascular disease
				P$\overline{v}O_2$	Partial pressure of oxygen in mixed venous blood
				PVR	Pulmonary vascular resistance

PVRI	Pulmonary vascular resistance index
P50	Pressure at 50% saturation
Q	Perfusion
Qc pul	Pulmonary capillary blood volume
Qpul	Pulmonary perfusion
Qs	Shunt
Qs anat	Anatomical shunt
Qs cap	Capillary shunt
Qs/Qt	Physiological shunt
QT	Total perfusion
R(RR)	Respiratory exchange ratio
Raw	Airway resistance
RA	Right atrium
RHF	Right heart failure
RAP	Right atrial pressure
RBC	Red blood cell
RFF	Ratio flow factor
RH	Right heart
RHF	Right heart failure
R-L	Right to left
ROSC	Return of spontaneous circulation
R pul	Pulmonary resistance
RQ	Respiratory quotient
RR	Spontaneous respiratory
RV	Right ventricle
RVEDP	Right ventricular end-diastolic pressure
RVEDV	Right ventricular end diastolic volume
RVESP	Right ventricular end systolic pressure
RVESV	Right ventricular end systolic volume
RVF	Right ventricular failure
RVSW	Right ventricular stroke work
RVSWI	Right ventricular stroke work index
SA	Sino-atrial
SABA	Short-acting beta agonist (or adrenergic)
SAH	Subarachnoid hemorrhage
SAMA	Short-acting muscarinic antiadrenergic
SaO2	Saturation of arterial oxygen
SBN2	Single breath nitrogen washout
SBT	Spontaneous Breathing Trial (weaning)
SCCM	Society of Critical Care Medicine
SOB	Shortness of breath
SPAG	Small particle aerosol generator
SpO2	Saturation of arterial oxygen by pulse oximeter
SV	Stroke volume
SVC	Slow vital capacity
SVI	Stroke volume index
SVN	Small volume nebulizer
SvO2	Saturation of oxygen in mixed venous blood
SVR	Systemic vascular resistance
SVRI	Systemic vascular resistance index
SW	Stroke work
SWI	Stroke work index
sx	Suction
TCO2	Total CO2
TE	Expiratory time
T-E	Tracheoesophageal
temp	Temperature
TF	Total flow
TI	Inspiratory time
TLC	Total lung capacity
TPN	Total parenteral nutrition
Ttot	Total cycle time
UO	Urinary output
USN	Ultrasonic nebulizer
V	Volume or ventricular
V̇	Flow
v	Venous
VA	Alveolar volume
V̇A	Alveolar ventilation
VC	Vital capacity
VCO2	Volume of carbon dioxide production
VD	Dead space volume
V̇D	Dead space ventilation
VD anat	Anatomical dead space
VD/VT	Deadspace/tidal volume ratio
V̇E	Minute ventilation
Vfib	Ventricular fibrillation
V̇I	Inspiratory flow
V̇O2	Volume of oxygen consumption
VSD	Ventricular septal defect
VT	Tidal volume
Vtach	Ventricular tachycardia
VTG	Thoracic gas volume
Vtubing	Volume loss to tubing
V/Q	Ventilation/perfusion ratio
WBC	White blood cell
WOB	Work of breathing

Index

ΔP 13-19

A

(A-a)DO₂: 13-4
A-a O₂ Gradient 13-4
AARC Guidelines
  Bland Aerosol Administration 9-5
  Humidification 9-58
  Incentive Spirometry 9-61
  IPPB 9-64
  Nasotracheal Suctioning 9-32
  Nonpharmacologic Airway Clearance 9-46
  Oxygen Therapy (Acute Care) 9-82
  Pharmacologic Airway Clearance 9-47
  Tracheostomy Care (Adults) 9-21
Abbreviations A-5
  basic units of measure A-2
  blood phase symbols A-2
  drug 11-4
  drug classes 11-11
  drug devices 11-11
  gas phase symbols A-2
ABCD Approach (COPD) 10-28
ABCDE Trauma Assessment 10-70
ABG. *See* Acid-Base
Abominal Paradox 1-6
Acapella 9-51
Accessory Muscles 1-16
Accolade 11-13
ACCP
  Airway Clearance 9-55
  Directed Cough 9-33
AccuNeb 11-14
Acetylcholine 11-10
acetylcysteine 11-31
ACh Receptors 11-10
Acid-Base
  accuracy check 2-19–2-20
  disorders 2-9–2-18
  equations 13-2
  interpretation 2-5–2-8
  normal values 2-2
Acid-Fast Smear and Culture 4-13, 10-73
aclidinium bromide 11-21
ACS. *See* Acute Coronary Syndrome

Active Cycle of Breathing 9-34
Acute Coronary Syndrome 10-4
  troponins 4-12
Acute Respiratory Distress Syndrome.
  See ARDS
Adenovirus 10-75
Adhesive Atelectasis 10-19
Adrenergic 11-35
Adult-Onset Asthma 10-9
Advair 11-50
Adventitious Breath Sounds 1-22
AED 12-5
Aerosol Therapy 9-4
  delivery devices 9-6
  selection and overview 9-8
  steps for administration 9-8
AFB 10-73
  lab test 4-13
Agonal Breathing 1-7
AIDS 10-45
Air Bronchogram 3-5
AirDuo 11-51
Air Entrainment
  equation 13-30
  ratios (chart) 9-85

Air Entrainment Mask 9-85
Air Leak Syndromes 10-58, 10-59
Air-to-O₂ Ratio 13-30
Airway Adjuncts 9-15
Airway Clearance 9-27
  active cycle of breathing 9-34
  assistive mechanical devices 9-48
  considerations 9-45
  directed/therapeutic cough 9-33
  selecting 9-28
Airway Management 9-14
  assessment 9-16
Airway Obstruction
  adjuncts 9-15
Airway Oscillations 9-50
Airway Pressure 5-3–5-4
Airway Resistance 5-5, 6-14
  equation 13-16
  normal value 6-3
albuterol 11-14
  to reduce potassium 4-4
albuterol/ipratropium bromide 11-52
A-Line. See Arterial Line Catheter
Allen Test 2-4

Allergic Asthma 10-9
Alpenzin 11-40
Alpha-1 Antitrypsin Deficiency 10-12, 10-23
  drug therapy 11-24
  lab test 4-11
Alpha 1 Proteinase Inhibitor 11-24
Alpha Receptors 11-10
ALS 10-49
Altera Nebulizer 11-25
Alveolar
  dead space 5-3
  pressure 5-3
  ventilation 5-6, 6-2, 13-12
  volume 13-12
Alveolar Air Equation 13-4
Alveolar Hypoventilation 10-8
Alvesco 11-46
  aminophylline 11-23
Amyotrophic Lateral Sclerosis 10-49
Anaerobic Infection
  aspiration 10-56
Anaerobic Metabolism
  equation 13-8
  lab indicator 4-6

Analgesics, Inhaled 11-34
Anaphylaxis 10-65
  shock 10-65
Anatomical Dead Space 5-7
Anatomical Vd/Vt Ratio 13-13
Anemia
  and oxyhemoglobin curve 9-73
Anemic Hypoxia 9-79
Anesthetics 11-56
Angina 1-28, 10-4
Anion Gap 13-2
  serum 4-11
Anoro Ellipta 11-53
Anterior-Posterior Diameter 1-15
Antiarrhythmics 11-57
Anti-Asthma Drugs 11-12–11-13
Anticholinergics 11-20–11-22
Anti-Infectives 11-25–11-30
Anti-Inflammatory Lung Function 10-10
Antileukotrienes 11-13
Antipsychotics 11-56
Aortic Regurgitation 7-10
Aortic Stenosis 7-10
Apnea 1-7
Apneustic Breathing 1-7

aPTT. *See* Partial Thromboplastin Time
Aralast 11-24
Arcapta Neohaler 11-19
ARDS 10-5
 Berlin definition 10-6
 chest radiograph 3-7
 hemodynamics 7-9
 IBW equation 13-26
 oxygenation target 9-81
 PBW equation 13-26
arformoterol tartrate 11-17
ArmonAir Digihaler 11-48
Arnuity Ellipta 11-48
Arterial/Alveolar O₂ Tension 13-5
Arterial Blood Gases. *See* Acid-Base
Arterial Blood Pressure 7-2
Arterial Line Catheter 7-6
Arterial-Venous O₂ Content Difference 13-5
Aspergillosis 10-40
Aspergillus fumigatus 10-40
Aspiration Pneumonia. *See* Pneumonia
Assessment
 acid-base 2-6
 cardiovascular 1-28
 chest radiograph 3-2

dyspnea 1-26
fluid and electrolyte 1-32
health history 1-1
hemodynamics 7-2
levels of consciousness 1-26
neurologic 1-30
oxygenation 9-68
systematic 1-14
Assisted Cough 9-33
Assistive Mechanical Devices 9-48
Asthma 10-9
 assessing control 10-15
 assessing severity 10-15
 cardiac arrest due to 12-7
 chest radiograph 3-7
 clinical manifestations 10-11
 diagnosis 10-10
 exacerbations 10-16–10-17
 heliox use 9-90
 pulmonary function 6-19
 sputum 4-16
 step treatment (GINA) 10-13–10-14
 time constant 5-5
Asthma-COPD Overlap 10-29
Asthmanefrin 11-35

Asystole 8-13
Ataxic Breathing 1-7
Atelectasis 10-18
 types of 10-19
Atrial
 fibrillation 8-11
 flutter 8-11
Atrovent 11-20
ATS Shortness of Breath Scale 1-27
Auscultation 1-13, 1-22
Autogenic Drainage 9-35
Autoimmune Disorders 10-45
Automatic External Defibrillator 12-5
A-V Nodal Rhythm 8-11
Axillary, term 1-19
aztreonam 11-25

B

Bagging. *See* Bag-Valve-Mask
Bag-Valve-Mask 9-14
Bands 4-9
Barbiturates 11-56
Barrel chest 1-15

Base Excess 2-2, 13-2
Basic Chemistry Panel 4-6
Basic Life Support 12-2
Basophils 4-9
BE. *See* Base Excess
beclomethasone 11-44
Bedside Parameters 6-15
 for neuromuscular disorders 10-50
BEF 10-69
Benzodiazepines 11-56
 overdose 12-7
Berlin Definition, ARDS 10-6
Beta Agonists 11-14–11-18
Beta Receptors 11-10
Bethkis 11-29
Bevespi Aerosphere 11-53
Bicarbonate 4-6
 critical values 4-2
Bilirubin 4-2
Biot's Respiration 1-7
Biventricular Heart Failure 10-42
Black Box Warning (LABA) 11-17
Bland Aerosol 9-4
Blastomyces dermatitidis 10-40
Blastomycosis 10-40

Bleeding Time 4-10
Blood Flow - Heart 7-5
Blood Gas. *See* Acid-Base
Blood Phase Symbols A-2
Blood Pressure 7-2
 abnormal 7-7
 mean 13-21
 mean arterial pressure 1-11
 pulse pressure 1-11
 ranges 1-5
Blood Sugar. *See* Glucose
Blood Urea Nitrogen 4-6
BLS 12-2
Blunt Force Trauma 10-72
BNP 4-11
Body Box. *See* Body Plethysmography
Body Plethysmography 6-7, 6-12
Body Surface Area 7-3, 13-26
Bohr Equation 13-13
Borg scale, modified 1-27
Boyle's Law 13-28
Bradycardia 1-5
Bradypnea 1-5, 1-7
Breathing Patterns 1-7

Breath Sounds
 abnormal 1-23
 normal 1-22
Brethaire 11-16
Brethine 11-16
Breztri Aerosphere 11-55
Bricanyl 11-16
Bronchial Breath Sounds 1-22
Bronchial Challenge 10-10
Bronchiectasis 10-20
 and lung abscesses 10-48
 percussive therapies 9-53
 sputum 4-16
Bronchiolitis 10-75
Bronchitol 11-32
Bronchodilator Responsiveness Testing 6-7
Bronchodilator Reversibility 10-10
Bronchodilators 11-14–11-18
 continuous 9-11
Bronchoesophageal Fistula 10-69
Bronchophony 1-25
Bronchoprovocation Challenge 6-7
Bronchovesicular Breath Sounds 1-22
Brovana 11-17
BSA. *See* Body Surface Area

B-type natriuretic peptide 4-11
Bubble Diffuser 9-57
budesonide 11-45
budesonide and formoterol 11-49
budesonide, glycopyrrolate, and formoterol 11-55
BUN 4-6
Bundle Branch Block 8-12
bupropion 11-40
Butterfly Pattern 3-5

C

Ca^{++}. *See* Calcium
Calcium 4-5
CaO_2 6-4, 9-75
Capillary Refill 1-16
Capping Trials 9-26
Carbogen 9-89
Carbon Dioxide
 cascade 9-74
 measured 9-89
Carbon Monoxide
 administered (DLCO) 9-89
Carbon Monoxide (CO) Poisoning 10-21
Carboxyhemoglobin 10-21
Cardiac
 hypertrophy 8-14
 infarct 8-15
Cardiac Index 7-3
Cardiac Monitoring 8-1
Cardiac Output 6-4, 7-3
 equation 13-20
 Fick Equation 13-21
Cardiac Surgery
 cardiac arrest after 12-7
Cardiac Tamponade 10-22
 hemodynamics 7-9
Cardiogenic Shock 10-65
Cardiomegaly 3-5
Cardiomyopathy 7-9
Cardiopulmonary Resuscitation 12-4
Carotid pulse 1-14
Cascade Humidifier 9-57
Cascade, O_2 and CO_2 9-74
CAT 10-28
Catheter, Transtracheal 9-88
$C(a-v)O_2$ 13-5
Cayston 11-25

CBC 4-8
CBT. *See* Continuous Bronchodilator Therapy
Cdyn 13-18
Celsius to Fahrenheit, Conversion 13-32
Central Line Catheter 7-6
Central Sleep Apnea 10-66
Central Alveolar Hypoventilation 10-8
CFTR Gene Dysfunction 10-32
Chantix 11-40
Charles' Law 13-28
Chest
 paradoxical movement 10-41
 symmetry 1-15
 topography 1-17
Chest Pain 1-28
Chest Physiotherapy 9-38
 postural drainage 9-38
Chest Radiograph 3-2
 AP vs. PA 3-5
 bat wing pattern 10-60
 butterfly pattern 10-60
 lateral 3-2
 PA film 3-3
 segmental infiltrates 3-9

tube and line position 3-10
water bottle shape 10-22
Chest Topography 1-17–1-20
Chest Trauma 10-72
Chest Wall Deformity 10-8
Chest Wall Oscillations 9-50
Cheyne-Stokes Breathing 1-8
Chloride 4-5
Chronic Bronchitis 10-25, 10-26
   PFT 6-19
   sputum 4-16
Chronic Obstructive Pulmonary Disease.
   See COPD
Chylothorax 10-53
ciclesonide HFA 11-46
Circulatory Hypoxia 9-79
Cl-. *See* Chloride
CL. *See* Compliance
Clotting
   bleeding time 4-10
   D-Dimer 4-10
   INR 4-10
   platelets 4-9
   PT 4-10
   PTT 4-10

CO. *See* Cardiac Output
Coagulation Studies 4-10
Coccidioides immitis 10-40
Coccidioidomycosis 10-40
codeine (nebulized) 11-34
Cof-flator 9-48
COHb 10-21
colistin (colistimethate) 11-26
Collateral Circulation (ABG) 2-4
Coly-Mycin M 11-26
Combined Gas Law 13-28
Combivent 11-52
Community-Acquired Pneumonia 10-55
Complete Blood Count 4-8
Compliance 5-5
   dynamic 5-5
   equation 13-17
   static 5-5
Comprehensive Metabolic Panel 4-6
Compressive Atelectasis 10-19
Congestive Heart Failure 10-42.
   See Left Heart Failure
   chest radiograph 3-6
Continuous Bronchodilator Therapy 9-11
   equation 9-11

Controlled Cough 9-33
Contusions 10-72
Conversion Equations 11-8
Conversions A-3
Conversions, Common 11-9
Cool Mist Aerosol 9-57
COPD
   ABCD approach (GOLD) 10-28
   chest radiograph 3-7
   clinical manifestations 10-25
   determining severity 10-24
   diagnosis 10-23
   ECG 8-14
   exacerbations 10-30
   heliox use 9-90
   hemodynamics 7-9
   hypoxic drive (O_2) 9-81
   management (COPD Foundation) 10-29
   management (stable) 10-27
   oxygenation target 10-27
   pursed-lip breathing 9-37
   supplemental O_2 10-27
CO Poisoning 10-21
Coronavirus 10-75
Cor pulmonale. *See also* Right Heart Failure

chest radiograph 3-5
hemodynamics 7-8
Costophrenic blunting 3-5
Cough
  directed or therapeutic 9-33
  huff (FET) 9-33
Cough Assist 9-48
Cough Peak Flow 10-50
COVID 10-75
CPAP 9-86
C. pneumoniae 10-57
CPR 12-4
CPT. *See* Chest Physiotherapy
Creatinine 4-7
Crepitus 1-16
Critical Lab Values 4-2
cromolyn sodium 11-12
Croup 10-75
Cryptococcosis 10-40
Cryptococcus neoformans 10-40
CSA 10-66
Cstat. *See* Static Compliance
CT scan, chest 3-11
Cuff
  tracheostomy tube 9-22

Cuirass 9-50
Culture and Sensitivity 4-13
Cushing's Triad 10-71
C$\bar{v}$O$_2$ 6-4
CVP
  abnormal 7-7
  catheter 7-6
CXR. *See* Chest Radiograph
Cyanosis 1-14
Cylinders
  color standards 9-66
  duration 13-31
Cystic Fibrosis 10-32
  active cycle of breathing 9-34
  airway clearance 9-46
  and bronchiectasis 10-20
  autogenic drainage 9-35
  chest physiotherapy 9-38
  clinical manifestations 10-33
  diagnosis 10-32
  drugs, order given 10-35
  exacerbations 10-34
  percussive therapy 9-53
  sputum 4-16

D

Daliresp 11-36
Dalton's Law of Partial Pressures 13-29
D-Dimer 4-10
Dead Space
  alveolar 5-7
  anatomical 5-7
  hypoxic hypoxia 9-78
  mechanical 5-7
  physiological 5-7
  types of 5-7
Dead Space/Tidal Volume Ratio 6-2, 13-13
Dead Space Ventilation 5-6, 13-12
Dead Space Volume 6-2, 13-13
Decannulation 9-26
Defibrillator 12-5
Demand-Flow Oxygen 9-87
dexmedetomidine 11-56
Diabetic Ketoacidosis 10-36
Diaphoresis 1-14
Diaphragmatic Exercises 9-36
Diaphragmatic Strengthening 9-37
Diastolic

arterial blood pressure 7-2
   pulmonary artery 7-2
Difficult Airway 9-16
Diffusing Capacity
   for carbon monoxide 6-7, 6-13
Digital Clubbing 1-16
Directed Cough 9-33
Diskhaler 11-30
Distension, ease of 5-5
DKA. *See* Diabetic Ketoacidosis
DLCO. *See* Diffusing Capacity
DMD 10-49
DO2 13-8
dornase alfa-dnase 11-32
Dosage Calculations 11-7
Double Cough 9-33
DPI. *See* Dry Powder Inhaler
Driving Pressure 10-7, 13-19
Drowning 10-37
Drug Administration 11-6
Drug Calculations 11-6
Drug Overdose 10-38
Drugs 11-1
   cardiocascular 11-57
   respiratory depression causing 11-56
   See Also Pharmacology

Dry Powder Inhaler 9-6, 9-13
Duchenne Muscular Dystrophy 10-49
Dulera 11-51
Dull (Percussion) 1-15
Duoneb 11-52
Dynamic Compliance 5-5, 6-14, 13-18
   equation 13-18
   dyphylline 11-23
Dyspnea 1-26
   assessing 1-26
   causes 1-26
   positional 1-26

E

ECG. *See* Electrocardiogram
E. coli 10-57
ECPR 12-3
E-Cylinder (duration) 9-67
EDD. *See* Esophageal Detector Device
Egophony 1-25
EKG. *See* Electrocardiogram
Elastance 5-5
Electrocardiogram
   12-lead 8-2
   15-lead 8-2

axis deviation 8-2
interpretation 8-6
interpreting, by PR interval 8-8
interpreting, by P wave 8-8
Interpreting, by rate 8-8
measuring ventricular rate 8-7
standard paper 8-7
summary of arrhythmias 8-9
waveform, explained 8-4
Electrolytes 4-3
   abnormalities 12-7
   affecting ventilation muscles 1-32
Emphysema 10-25, 10-26
   DLCO 6-13
   PFT 6-19
   sputum 4-16
Empyema 10-53
Endotracheal Tube 9-16
   sizing 9-16
End-tidal CO_2 Detector 9-19
Eosinophils 4-9
Epidural Hematoma 10-71
Epinephrine 11-35
   Inhaled 11-35
epoprostenol 11-37
Equations

acid-base 13-2
drug and dosage 11-7
oxygenation 13-4
patient calculations 13-26
perfusion/hemodynamic 13-20
pulmonary function 13-27
ventilation 13-12
ventilator calculations 13-15
ERV. *See* Expiratory Reserve Volume
Erythrocytes 4-8
Esophageal Detector Device 9-17
 verification 9-19
ETCO₂ 9-19
Eupnea 1-7
Exchange Ratio 13-11
Exercise Challenge 10-10
Exhalation 5-2
Expiration 5-2
Expiratory Reserve Volume 6-2
 description 6-6
External Respiration 9-75
Exudative 10-53

F

Fahrenheit to Celsius, Conversion 13-32
FEF 25-75 6-9
FEF 25%-75% 6-3
FEF 200-1200 6-9
 normal 6-3
fentanyl (nebulized) 11-34
FET. *See* Huff Cough
Fetid Sputum 4-15
FEV 1%
 normal 6-3
FEV1 6-3, 6-8
FEV1/FVC 6-8
Fever. *See* Hyperthermia
Fibrosis 10-64
 time constant 5-5
Fick Equation 13-21
Fick's Law of Diffusion 13-27
FIF 25%-75% 6-3
FiO₂ Estimation 13-6
Fissures (Lung) 1-17
 horizontal 1-17–1-18
 oblique 1-17–1-19

FIVC. *See* Forced Inspiratory Vital Capacity
Flail Chest 10-41
Flail Sternum 10-41
Flat (Percussion) 1-15
Flolan 11-37
Flovent 11-47
Flow, Laminar vs. Turbulent 13-32
Flow-Volume Loop
 description 6-10
 illustration 6-11
 interpretation 6-11
Fluid and electrolyte assessment 1-32
Fluid balance 1-32
fluticasone 11-47–11-48
fluticasone and salmeterol 11-50–11-51
fluticasone, umeclidinium, and vilanterol 11-54
Flutter Device 9-51
Forced Expiratory Flow 6-3
Forced Expiratory Technique 9-33, 9-34
Forced Expiratory Volume over Time 6-3
Forced Expiratory Volume Ratio 6-3
Forced Inspiratory Vital Capacity 6-2
Forced Midexpiratory Flow 6-3
Forced Midinspiratory Flow 6-3

Forced Vital Capacity 6-2, 6-8, 6-15
Forfivo 11-40
Fractures 10-72
FRC. See Functional Residual Capacity
Fremitus 1-16
Frog Breathing 9-45
Functional Lung Size 13-19
Functional Residual Capacity 6-2
  description 6-6
Fungal Disorders 10-39
Fungal Infection
  chest radiograph 3-6
FVC. See Forced Vital Capacity

G

Gas Cylinder Duration 13-31
Gases (Medical) 9-66, 9-89
Gas Laws
  Boyle's 13-28
  Charles' 13-28
  combined 13-28
  Dalton's 13-29
  Gay-Lussac's 13-28

Gas Phase Symbols A-2
Gay-Lussac's Law 13-28
GBS. See Guillain-Barré Syndrome
Glasgow Coma Score (GCS) 1-30
Glassia 11-24
Glossopharyngeal Breathing 9-45
Glottis (cough) 9-33
Glucose 4-/
  critical values 4-2
glycopyrrolate and formoterol 11-53
glycopyrrolate and indacaterol 11-53
glycopyrrolate bromide 11-21
GOLD (COPD) 10-24
Gram stain 4-13
Granulation Tissue 9-23, 10-69
Guarding (pain) 1-14
Guillain-Barré Syndrome 10-51

H

Habitrol 11-41
HAP. See Pneumonia
Hayek Oscillator 9-50

HCO_3^- 2-2
  estimation 13-3
Hct. See Hematocrit
H-Cylinder (duration) 9-67
Head Tilt-Chin Lift 12-3
Health History 1-1
Heart
  blood flow through 7-5
  compression of 10-22
  murmurs 1-29
Heart Block 8-12
Heart Failure 10-42
HEART Nebulizer 9-11
Heart Rate
  abnormal rhythms 1-9
  ranges 1-5
  strength 1-9
Heart Sounds 1-29
Heat & Moisture Exchanger 9-57
Height
  conversion table A-4
Heliox 9-89, 9-90
  equation 13-29
Helium Dilution 6-7, 6-12
Helium-Oxygen. See Heliox

Hematocrit 4-8
 critical values 4-2
Hemodynamic Monitoring 7-2
 abnormal 7-7
 catheters 7-6
 equations 13-20
Hemoglobic Hypoxia 9-79
Hemoglobin 4-8
 critical values 4-2
Hemoglobin Affinity 9-73
Hemothorax 10-53
Henderson-Hasselbach 13-3
Herniation, Brain 10-71
Hexaxial Reference System 8-2
HFCWO 9-50
Hgb. See Hemoglobin
High Altitude Pulmonary Edema (HAPE) 11-18
High Flow Oxygen (HFO) 9-86
High Frequency Chest Wall Oscillation 9-50
H. influenzae
Histoplasma capsulatum 10-40
Histoplasmosis 10-40
History of Present Illness 1-1
Histotoxic Hypoxia 9-79

HME. *See* Heat & Moisture Exchangers
Holding Chamber 9-6
Honeycombing (CXR) 3-5
HOPE Nebulizer 9-11
Horowitz Index 13-10
H's and T's (ACLS) 12-8
Huff Cough 9-33
Humidifiers
 bubble diffuser 9-57
 cascade 9-57
 HME 9-57
 passover 9-57
 wick 9-57
Humidity Therapy 9-56
 devices 9-57
hydromorphone (nebulized) 11-34
Hyperbaric Oxygen Therapy (HBOT)
 for CO poisoning 10-21
Hypercalcemia 4-5
 ECG 8-14
Hypercapnia
 neuro signs 1-31
 permissive 10-7
Hypercapnic Respiratory Failure 10-63
Hypercarbia. *See* Hypercapnia

Hyperchloremia 4-5
Hyperkalemia 4-4
 ECG 8-14
Hypermagnesemia 4-5
Hypernatremia 4-3
Hyperoxemia 9-72
Hyperphosphatemia 4-5
Hyperpnea 1-8
Hyperresonance 1-15
HyperSal 11-33
Hypertension 1-11
 pulmonary 10-62
Hyperthermia 1-12
Hypertonic solution 11-33
 sputum induction 4-14
Hypervolemia 1-32
Hypocalcemia 4-5
 ECG 8-14
Hypochloremia 4-5
Hypokalemia 4-4
 ECG 8-14
Hypomagnesemia 4-5
Hyponatremia 4-3
Hypophosphatemia 4-5
Hypopnea 1-8

Hypotensive 1-11
  shock 10-65
Hypothermia 1-12
Hypotonic solution 11-33
Hypoventilation Atelectasis 10-19
Hypovolemia 1-32
Hypovolemic Shock 10-65
Hypoxemia 9-76
  and cor pulmonale 10-44
  clinical manifestations 8-11
  diagnostic algorithm 9-77
  levels of 1-10, 9-76
  lung adequacy 9-72
  types, by abnormal value 9-80
  vs hypoxia 9-76
Hypoxemic Respiratory Failure 10-63
Hypoxia
  assessing (equation) 1-31
  neuro signs 13-4
  types of 9-78
  vs hypoxemia 9-76
Hypoxia (Chronic)
  oxygen conserving devices 9-87
Hypoxic Drive 9-81
Hypoxic Hypoxia 9-78

I

IBW 13-26
IC. *See* Inspiratory Capacity
Ice Pack Test 10-51
ICP 10-71
ICS 11-44–11-48
Ideal Body Weight 13-26
Idiojunctional rhythm 8-11
Idiopathic Pulmonary Fibrosis 10-47
I:E Ratio 1-15
IGRA 10-73
ILD. *See* Interstitial Lung Disease
iloprost 11-38
Immunocompromised 10-45
IMP2 9-50
Incentive Spirometry 9-60
  AARC Guidelines 9-61
InCourage 9-50
Incruse Ellipta 11-22
indacaterol 11-19
Indirect Calorimetry 13-11
In-Exsufflator 9-48

Influenza 10-75
  prophylaxis drug 11-30
Inhalation 5-2
Inhaled Corticosteroids (ICS) 11-44–11-48
iNO. *See* Nitric Oxide
Inotropics 11-57
INR. *See* International Normalized Ratio
Inspection 1-13
Inspiration 5-2
Inspiratory Capacity 6-2
  description 6-6
Inspiratory Reserve Volume 6-2
  description 6-6
Intake & Output 1-32
Intercostal 1-16
Interferon Gamma Release Assay 10-73
Intermittent Positive Pressure Breathing 9-63
  AARC Guideline 9-64
Internal Respiration 9-75
International Normalized Ratio 4-10
Interstitial Lung Disease 10-46
Intracerebral Hemorrhage 10-71
Intracranial Pressure 10-71
Intrapulmonary Percussive Ventilation 9-52

Intubation 9-17
  confirmation 9-18
  equipment 9-17
  procedure 9-17
IPPB. *See* Intermittent Positive Pressure Breathing
  ipratropium bromide 11-20
IPV. *See* Intrapulmonary Percussive Ventilation
IRV. *See* Inspiratory Reserve Volume
IS. *See* Incentive Spirometry
Isotonic Solution 11-33

J

Jaw Thrust 12-3
Jugular Venous Distension (JVD) 1-14

K

K⁺. *See* Potassium
Kerley B lines 3-6
ketamine 11-56
Kitabis Pak 11-29

K. pneumoniae 10-57
Kussmaul's Breathing 1-8, 10-36

L

LABAs 11-17
Lab Tests
  chemistry panels 4-6
  coagulation studies 4-10
  complete blood count (CBC) 4-8
  critical values 4-2
  electrolytes 4-3
  microbiology 4-13
  sputum 4-13
Lactate 4-6
LAMAs 11-21–11-22
Laminar Flow 13-32
LAP 7-3
LaPlace, law of 13-29
Laryngoscope 9-17
Law of LaPlace 13-29
Left Atrial Pressure 7-3
Left Heart Failure 10-42–10-43
  hemodynamics 7-8

Left Ventricular End Diastolic Pressure 7-3
Left Ventricular End Systolic Pressure 7-3
Left Ventricular Stroke Work 7-3
  equation 13-21
Legionella 10-57
Leukocytes 4-9
Leukocytosis 4-9
Leukopenia 4-9
levalbuterol 11-15
Levels of consciousness 1-31
Lidocaine 11-34
Liquid Cylinder Duration 13-31
Long-Acting Beta Agonists 11-17–11-19
Long-Acting Muscarinic Antagonists 11-21–11-22
Longhala Magnair VMN 11-21
Lower Limits of Normal 6-18
Lung Abscess 10-48
  sputum 4-16
Lung Adequacy 9-72
Lung Cancer
  sputum 4-16
Lung Distension
  compliance equation 13-17
Lung Expansion Therapy 9-59

selecting 9-59
Lung Flute 9-50
Lungs
external anatomy 9-39
fissures 1-17–1-20
lobes 1-17–1-21
Lung Segments
anterior 1-17
left lateral 1-19
posterior 1-18
right lateral 1-20
Lupus 10-46
LVESP 7-3
LVSW 7-3, 13-21
LVSWI 7-3
Lymphocytes 4-9

M

Magic Box (O_2) 13-30
Magnesium 4-5
Mallampati Score 9-16
mannitol 11-32
Mantoux Tuberculin Skin Test 10-73

Manually-Assisted Cough 9-33
Manual Ventilation. *See* Bag-Valve-Mask
MAP. *See* Mean Airway Pressure; *See* Mean Arterial Pressure
Mast Cell Stabilizers 11-12
Maximal Expiratory Pressure 6-3, 6-16
Maximal Inspiratory Pressure (MIP) 6-3
Maximum Voluntary Ventilation 6-3, 6-9
Mean Airway Pressure
equation 13-19
Mean Arterial Pressure 1-11, 7-2, 13-21
Mean Pulmonary Artery Pressure 7-2, 13-22
Mechanical Dead Space 5-7
Medication Administration 11-6
Medications. *See* Drugs
MEP. *See* Maximal Expiratory Pressure
Metabolic
acidosis 2-15
alkalosis 2-17
MetaNeb 9-50
Metered Dose Inhalers 9-6, 9-12
administration 9-12
Methemoglobinemia 4-8

Methylxanthines 11-23
Metric Conversions A-3
Mg^{++}. *See* Magnesium
Midclavicular, term 1-17
Mid-Sternal, term 1-17
Miliary Pattern 3-6
Minute Ventilation 5-6, 6-2, 13-14
MIP. *See* Maximal Inspiratory Pressure
Mitral Regurgitation 7-10
Mitral Stenosis 7-10
MMAD 9-5, 9-9
mMRC 10-28
Modified Allen Test 2-4
mometasone and formoterol 11-51
Monocytes 4-9
montelukast 11-13
morphine sulfate 11-34
mPAW. *See* Mean Airway Pressure
MRI Scan, Chest 3-12
MS 10-49
Mucoactives 11-31–11-33
Mucoid sputum 4-15
Mucomyst 11-31
Mucopurulent Sputum 4-15
Multiple Sclerosis (MS) 10-49

Muscles, Accessory 1-16
MVV. *See* Maximum Ventilatory Ventilation
Myasthenia Gravis 10-51
Myasthenic Crisis 10-51
Mycobacterium tuberculosis 10-73
Mycoplasma pneumonia 10-57
Myocardial Infarction (MI) 10-4
   hemodynamics 7-9

N

Na⁺. *See* Sodium
Nalcrom 11-12
naloxone 12-6
Nasal Cannula 9-83
Nasal Catheter 9-83
Nasal Flaring 1-14
Nasal Trumpet. *See* Nasopharyngeal Airway
Nasopharyngeal Airway 9-15
Nasotracheal Suctioning 9-31
   AARC Guideline 9-32
Near-drowning. *See* Drowning
Nebulizers 9-10

Nebuflent 11-27
Necrotizing Pneumonia 10-48
Needle Decompression 10-59
Negative Inspiratory Force. 6-3, 6-15
Neoplasm, sputum 10-65
Neurogenic Shock 10-65
Neurological Assessment 1-30
Neuromuscular Disorders 10-49
Neutrophils 4-9
NicoDerm 11-41
Nicotine
   gum 11-42
   inhaler 11-43
   lozenges 11-43
   stains 1-16
Nicotine-Replacement Therapies (NRT) 11-41–11-43
Nicotrol 11-41, 11-42
NIF. *See* Maximal Inspiratory Pressure
Nitric Oxide 9-89
   oxygen index 13-9
Nitrogen Washout 6-7, 6-12
Nitrous Oxide 9-89
Nodular Pattern 3-6
Non-allergic asthma 10-9

Noncardiogenic pulmonary edema
   ARDS 10-6
Nonfatal Drowning. *See* Drowning
Noninvasive Positive Pressure Breathing (NPPV) 9-86
Non-Obstructive Atelectasis 10-19
Non-Rebreathing Mask 9-84
Non-ST-Elevation MI (NSTEMI) 10-4
Normal Sinus Rhythm 8-9
Nosocomial Pneumonia 10-55
NPA. *See* Nasopharyngeal Airway
NPPV 9-86
NRB. *See* Non-Rebreathing Mask
NSTEMI 10-4

O

O₂ER 13-8
O₂ Extraction Ratio 13-8
Obesity 1-15
Obesity Hypoventilation Syndrome 10-8
Obstruction (upper airway)
   use of heliox with 9-90
Obstructive Atelectasis 10-19

Obstructive Sleep Apnea 10-66
OI 13-9
olodaterol hydrochloride 11-19
OPA. See Oropharyngeal Airway
Opioid Analgesics 11-56
Opioid-Associated Life-Threatening Emergencies 12-6
Opioids (nebulized) 11-34
Order of Operations 13-1
Oropharyngeal Airway 9-15
Orthopnea 1-26
OSA 10-66
Oscillatory PEP Therapy 9-50
Overdose, Drug 10-38
Oximetry, Pulse. See Pulse Oximetry
Oximetry, testing 6-7
oxtriphylline 11-23
Oxygen
  amount (equation) 13-7
  conserving devices 9-87
  content 2-2
  cylinder duration 9-67
  delivery devices 9-83
  low flow devices 9-83
  toxicity 10-52

Oxygenation 9-68
  assessment of 9-75
  cascade 9-74
  dissocation curve 9-73
  measures of 9-68
  partial pressure of 9-68
Oxygenation Index 13-9
Oxygen Consumption 13-6
  tissues 13-5, 13-6
Oxygen Content 13-7
  anemic hypoxia 9-79
  arterial 13-7
  mixed venous 13-7
  pulmonary capillary 13-7
Oxygen Delivery 7-4, 13-8
Oxygen Dissociation Curve 9-73
Oxygen Index 13-9
Oxygen Reserve 13-9
Oxygen Saturation 13-9, 13-10
Oxygen Therapy 9-81
  AARC Guidelines 9-82
  conserving devices 9-87
  delivery devices 9-83
  target, by disease 9-81
  toxicity 10-52

Oxygen Toxicity 10-52
Oxyhemoglobin Dissociation Curve 9-73

P

$P(A-a)O_2$ 13-4
PAC. See Premature Atrial Contractions
PA Catheter. See Pulmonary Artery Catheter
Pack-Years 13-32
$PaCO_2$
  critical values 4-2
  estimation 13-3
$PACO_2$ 6-4
P. aeruginosa 10-57
Palpation 1-13
Palpitations 1-28
PaO_2 9-68, 9-75
  critical values 4-2
  predicted 13-11
PAO_2 6-4, 13-4
PaO_2/FIO_2 Ratio 13-10
PaO_2/SpO_2 Relationship 9-72
Paradoxical Respirations 1-6
Parainfluenza 10-75

Paralysis 10-64
Paralytics 11-56
Paroxysmal Junctional Tachycardia 8-11
Paroxysmal Nocturnal Dyspnea 1-26
Partial Rebreathing Mask 9-84
Partial Thromboplastin Time 4-10
Passive Atelectasis 10-19
Passover Humidifier 9-57
Patient Assessment. See Assessment
PBW 13-26
PCO_2. 2-2
PDE-4 Inhibitor 11-36
Peak Expiratory Flow 6-3, 6-9
Peak flow 10-10
Peak Inspiratory Flow 6-9
Pectus
  carinatum 1-15
  excavatum 1-15
Pedal edema 1-16
PEF. See Peak Expiratory Flow
PEMDAS 13-1
Penetrating Trauma 10-72
pentamadine isethionate 11-27
Percent Change 13-27
Percent Predicted 13-27

Percussion 1-13, 1-15
Percussionator 9-50
PercussiveNeb 9-50
Percussive Vests/Wraps 9-53
Perforomist 11-18
Perfusion 5-9
  capillary 5-9
  shunt 5-9
  total 5-9
Perfusion Zones 5-10
Pericarditis 8-15, 10-22
Permissive Hypercapnia 10-7
$PETCO_2$. See End-tidal CO_2
P/F Ratio 13-10
pH 2-2
  critical values 4-2
Phosphate 4-5
Phosphodiesterase Inhibitors 11-36
Physiological Dead Space 5-7
Physiological Dead Space Ratio 6-3
Physiological shunt 5-9
Physiological VD/VT Ratio 13-13
Pitting Edema. See Pedal edema
Plasmapheresis 10-51
Platelet Count 4-9

Platypnea 1-26
Pleural Effusion 10-53
  thoracic ultrasound 3-14
Pleural Pressure 5-3–5-4
Pleural Rub
  breath sounds 1-24
Pleurisy 10-54
Pleuritic Chest Pain 1-28
Pleuritis 10-54
Pleurodesis 10-53
pMDI. See Metered Dose Inhalers
PMI 1-28
PNA. See Pneumonia
Pneumoconiosis 10-47
Pneumocystis Pneumonia
  pentamadine 11-27
Pneumomediastinum 10-59
Pneumonia 10-55
  and pleuritis 10-54
  aspiration 10-56
  bacterial 10-57
  chest radiograph 3-5
  community-acquired 10-55
  hospital-acquired (HAP) 10-55
  interstitial 10-46
  necrotizing 10-48

nosocomial 10-55
pneumocystis 11-27
sputum 4-16
ventilator-associated (VAP) 10-55
viral 10-75
Pneumonitis
 aspiration 10-56
 hypersensitivity 10-47
Pneumopericardium 10-59
Pneumothorax 10-58
 chest radiograph 3-6
 spontaneous 10-59
 tension 10-59
 thoracic ultrasound 3-14
PO_2 2-2
$PO_4^=$. See Phosphate
Point of Maximal Impulse 1-28
Poiseuille's Law 13-32
Polycythemia
 and oxyhemoglobin curve 9-73
Positioning, Head-Down 9-45
Positive Expiratory Pressure Therapy 9-49
Post-ROSC Care 12-8
Postural Drainage 9-38
modified positions (CFF) 9-41

Posture 1-15
Potassium 4-4
 critical values 4-2
PP. See Pulse Pressure
PPD. See Mantoux Tuberculin Skin Test
Predicted Body Weight 13-26
Predicted PaO_2 in Adults 13-11
Pregnancy
 cardiac arrest in 12-7
Premature Atrial Contractions 8-10
Premature Atrial Tachycardia 8-10
Premature Nodal Contractions 8-11
Premature Ventricular Contractions 8-12
Pressure, Dalton's Law 13-29
Pressure, Driving 13-19
Pressure Gradients 5-3–5-4
Primatene Mist 11-35
PR Interval 8-5
ProAir 11-14
Prolastin 11-24
propofol 11-56
Prothrombin Time 4-10
Proventil 11-14
PT. See Prothrombin Time
PtcCO₂. See Transcutaneous Monitoring

Ptt 5-4-5-5
PTT. See Partial Thromboplastin Time
Pulmicort 11-45
Pulmonary Artery Catheter 7-6
Pulmonary Artery Hypertension 10-62
Pulmonary Artery Pressure
 mean 13-22
Pulmonary Capillary Wedge Pressure (PCWP) 7-2
 abnormal 7-7
Pulmonary Contusions 10-72
Pulmonary Edema 10-60
 chest radiograph 3-5
 hemodynamics 7-9
 high-pressure 10-60
 permeability 10-60
 sputum 4-16
Pulmonary Embolism 10-61
 chest radiograph 3-6
 D-dimer 4-10
 ECG 8-14
 hemodynamics 7-9
Pulmonary Fibrosis 10-47
Pulmonary Function Testing
 abnormal 6-19
 average values 6-2

equations 13-27
  interpretation 6-17
  volumes and capacities 6-6
Pulmonary Hypertension 10-62
  chest radiograph 3-5
  oxygenation target 9-81
Pulmonary Vascular Resistance 7-3, 13-22
Pulmonary Vascular Resistance Index 7-3
Pulmonary Vasodilators 11-37–11-38
Pulmozyme 11-32
Pulse-Dose Oxygen 9-87
Pulse Oximetry 1-9, 9-68
  troubleshooting 9-69–9-70
  troubleshooting (quick) 1-10
Pulse Pressure 1-11, 13-23
Pulse Rate. *See* Heart Rate
Pulsus
  alternans 1-9
  paradoxus 1-9
  paradoxus, reverse 1-9
Pump Coughing 9-33
Pump Failure 10-63
Pupil Response 1-14
Pursed-Lip Breathing 9-37
Purulent Sputum 4-15
PVC. *See* Premature Ventricular Contrac-

tions
PVR 13-22. *See* Pulmonary Vascular Resistance
P wave 8-5

Q

QRS complex 8-5
Qs. *See* Shunt
QSphys. *See* Physiological shunt
QT 13-20
Quake 9-50
QVAR 11-44

R

racemic epinephrine 11-35
Radiating Pain 1-28
RAP. *See* Right Atrial Pressure
Rapid Shallow Breathing Index 13-19
RBCs. *See* Red Blood Cells
RE 13-11
Red Blood Cells
  labs 4-8
Referred Pain 1-28

Refractory Hypoxemia 9-76
  oxygen index 13-9
Relenza 11-30
Rescue Breathing 12-2
Reservoir Cannula 9-87
Residual Volume 6-2
  description 6-6
Residual Volume/TLC 6-2
Residual Volume/VC 6-2
Resistance, Airway
  airway 5-5
Resonance 1-15
Resorptive Atelectasis 10-19
RespiClick 11-14
Respiratory
  acidosis 2-11
  alkalosis 2-13
  pattern 1-6–1-8
  rate 1-5
Respiratory alternans 1-16
Respiratory Drive
  depression of 10-64
Respiratory Failure 10-63
  Type 1 (Hypoxemic) 10-63
  Type 2 (Hypercapnic) 10-63
Respiratory Index 13-11

Respiratory Muscle Strength 6-16
Respiratory Quotient 13-11
Respiratory Rate 6-2
Respirgard II nebulizer 11-27
Responsive Hypoxemia 9-76
Restrictive Disorders 6-19
Restrictive Lung Disease 10-64
Resuscitation 12-1
Reticular Pattern 3-7
Reticulocytes 4-9
Reticulogranular Pattern 3-7
Retrosternal 1-28
Return of Spontaneous Circulation (ROSC) 12-8
revefenacin 11-22
Reverse Isolation 10-45
Reversibility Testing. *See* Bronchodilator Reversibility
Reynold's Number 13-32
Rheumatoid Arthritis 10-20
Rhinovirus 10-75
RI 13-11
Rib
   angles 1-15
   ribavirin 11-28
   SPAG nebulizer 9-7

Rib Fractures 10-72
Right Atrial Pressure 7-2
Right Heart Failure 10-42–10-43
   hemodynamics 7-8
Right Ventricular End Diastolic Pressure 7-2
Right Ventricular End Systolic Pressure 7-2
Right Ventricular Stroke Work 7-3, 13-23
Right Ventricular Stroke Work Index 7-3
roflumilast 11-36
ROSC care, post 12-8
RQ. *See* Respiratory Quotient
RR. *See* Respiratory Rate
RSBI 13-19
RSV 10-75
Rule of 8's 13-3
Rule of 300 8-7
RV. *See* Residual Volume
RVEDP. *See* Right Ventricular End Diastolic Pressure
RVESP. *See* Right Ventricular End Systolic Pressure
RVSW 7-3, 13-23
RVSWI 7-3
RV/TLC 6-6

S

S2 11-35
SABAs 11-14
Saline, Nebulized 11-33
salmeterol 11-18
SAMAs 11-20
SaO_2 9-68, 13-10
Sarcoidosis 10-46, 10-47
   chest radiograph 3-7
S. aureus 10-57
Scapular, term 1-18
Seebri Neohaler DPI 11-21
Sepsis
   hemodynamics 7-10
Septic Shock 10-65
Serevent Diskus 11-18
Serum Bicarbonate 4-6
Shock 10-65
   hemodynamics 7-10
   types of 10-65
Short-Acting Beta Agonists 11-14–11-17
Short-Acting Muscarinic Antagonists 11-20
Shunt 5-9
   equation 13-24

hypoxic hypoxia 9-78
pulmonary 5-9
types of 5-9
Shunt Equation 13-24
Signet Ring Sign 3-6
Silhouette sign 3-6
Simple Mask 9-84
Single-Breath N₂ Test 6-3
Singulair 11-13
Sinoatrial Exit Block 8-10
Sinus
    arrhythmia 8-9
    bradycardia 8-9
    normal 8-9
    tachycardia 8-9
Sjögren Syndrome 10-20
Skin
    turgor 1-16
Skin Assessment 1-14
Sleep Apnea 10-66
Sleep-Disordered Breathing 10-66
Sleep Disorders 10-66
Slow Vital Capacity 6-2, 6-10
Small Particle Aerosol Generator (SPAG) 9-7

Small Volume Nebulizer 9-7
    jet 9-10
    mesh 9-10
    ultrasonic 9-10
SmartVest 9-50
SMI. *See* Soft Mist Inhaler
Smoke Inhalation 10-67
Smoking Cessation
    5 As (Counseling) 11-39
    drugs 11-40
    equation (pack-years) 13-32
Sodium 4-3
    critical values 4-2
Soft Mist Inhaler 9-6
Soot, presence of 10-67
Spacer 9-6
SPAG
    ribavirin 11-28
Speaking Valves 9-21
Spine Abnormalities 1-15
Spiriva 11-22
Spirometry 6-7, 6-8
S. pneumoniae 10-57
SpO₂. *See* Pulse Oximetry
SpO₂/PaO₂ Relationship 9-72
Sputum

    by disease 4-16
    characteristics 4-15
    collection 4-14
    induction 4-14
Stagnant Hypoxia 9-79
Static Compliance 5-5, 6-14
    of lungs 6-3
    of lungs and thoracic cage 6-3
ST depression 8-15
Steam Vaporizer 9-57
ST-Elevation 8-15, 10-4
STEMI 10-4
Sternocleidomastoid 1-14
Sternum Abnormalities 1-15
Stertor 1-24
Stiolto Respimat 11-53
Stoma Care 9-26
Stridor 1-24
    heliox 9-90
    thermal burns 10-67
Striverdi 11-19
Stroke Volume 7-3, 13-25
Stroke Volume Index 7-3
ST segment 8-5
Subcutaneous Emphysema 1-16
Subdural Hematoma 10-71

Subglottic Tubes 9-16
Submersion Injury. *See* Drowning
Substernal 1-16
Suctioning 9-29
   catheter size formula 9-30
   indications 9-29
   nasotracheal 9-31
   pressures 9-30
Suprasternal 1-16
SV 13-25. *See* Stroke Volume
SVC. *See* Slow Vital Capacity
SVI. *See* Stroke Volume Index
SVN. *See* Small Volume Nebulizer
SvO_2 13-9
SVR 13-25. *See* Systemic Vascular Resistance
SVRI. *See* Systemic Vascular Resistance Index
Swan Ganz. *See* Pulmonary Artery Catheter
Symbicort 11-49
Systemic Vascular Resistance 7-3, 13-25
Systemic Vascular Resistance Index 7-3
Systolic
   arterial blood pressure 7-2
   pulmonary artery 7-2

T

Tachycardia 1-5
Tachypnea 1-5, 1-8
Tactile fremitus 1-16
Tank Duration Charts 9-67
Targeted Temperature Management 12-8
TBI 10-71
TB Test. *See* Mantoux Tuberculin Skin Test
TCO_2 2-2. *See* Total Carbon Dioxide
TCOM. *See* Transcutaneous Monitoring
TEF 10-69
TE-fistula 10-69
Temperature 1-12
   conversion table A-4
   ranges 1-12
Temperature Conversion 13-32
Tension Test 10-51
Tension Pneumothorax 10-59
terbutaline 11-16
Thebesian 5-9
theophylline 11-23
Therapeutic Cough 9-33
Therapeutic Hypothermia 12-8
Thermal Burns 10-67

Thoracic Gas Volume 6-6
Thoracic Ultrasound 3-13
Thrombocytopenia 4-9
Thrombocytosis 4-9
Tidal Volume 6-2
   description 6-6
TI-fistula 10-68
Time Constant 5-5, 13-20
tiotropium and olodaterol 11-53
tiotropium bromide 11-22
TLC. *See* Total Lung Capacity
TLCO. *See* Diffusing Capacity
Tobacco Use
   equation 13-32
Tobi 11-29
tobramycin 11-29
Torsades de Pointes 8-13
Total Carbon Dioxide 4-6
Total Flow Calculation 13-30
Total Lung Capacity 6-2
   description 6-6
Tracheal Breath Sounds 1-22
Tracheal Deviation 1-14
Tracheal Stenosis
   heliox use with 9-90
Tracheoarterial Fistula 10-68

Tracheoesophageal Fistula 10-69
Tracheoinnominate Artery Fistula 10-68
Tracheostomy Tube 9-20
  care and monitoring 9-21
  care (nondisposable) 9-25
  considerations 9-25
  inner cannula 9-24
  replacing 9-24
  troubleshooting 9-22
Transairway Pressure Gradient 5-3–5-4
Transcutaneous Monitoring 9-68, 9-71
Transdermal Patch 11-41
Transpulmonary Pressure Gradient 5-3–5-4
Transthoracic Pressure Gradient 5-3–5-4
Transtracheal Oxygen 9-88
Transudative 10-53
Trauma 10-70
Traumatic Brain Injury 10-71
Trelegy Ellipta 11-54
Tremors 1-16
Tripod Position 1-15
Troponin 4-12
TTM 12-8
TTO. *See* Transtracheal Oxygen
Tuberculosis 10-73
  chest radiograph 3-6
  sputum 4-16
Tudorza Pressair 11-21
Turbulent Flow 13-32
Turgor 1-16
T wave 8-5
T-waves, peaked 4-4
Tympany 1-15

U

Ultrasound, thoracic 3-13
umeclidinium and vilanterol 11-53
umeclidinium bromide 11-22
Urine output 1-32
Utibron Neohaler 11-53
U wave 8-5

V

$\dot{V}_A$ 13-12
VAP. *See* Pneumonia
varenicline 11-40
Vasodilators 11-57
Vasopressors 11-57
VC. *See* Vital Capacity
VD 13-12
V_{Dalv} 5-7
V_{Danat} 5-7
V_{Dmech} 5-7
V_{Dphys} 5-7
V_D/V_T 6-3, 13-13
VE. *See* Minute Ventilation
Veletri 11-37
Venous Blood Gas 2-2, 2-4
Ventavis 11-38
Ventilation
  alveolar 5-6
  deadspace 5-6
  distribution of 5-8
  mechanics 5-2
  minute 5-6
Ventilation/Perfusion 5-11, 13-15
  aligning 5-11
  mismatch 5-11
Ventilator Calculations 13-15
  rate equation 13-15
Venti Mask. *See* Air Entrainment Mask
Ventolin 11-14
Ventricular
  fibrillation 8-13
  flutter 8-13

standstill 8-13
tachycardia 8-13
Venturi Mask. *See* Air Entrainment Mask
Venturi, Ratios 13-30
Vesicular breath sounds 1-22
Vest Therapy 9-53
Vfib. *See* Ventricular: fibrillation
Viral Infections 10-75
   sputum 4-16
Virazole 11-28
Vital Capacity 6-2, 6-15
   description 6-6
Vital Signs
   ranges 1-5
Vmax 50 6-3
VO_2 13-6, 13-21
Vocal Resonance 1-25
Voice Sounds 1-24
Volumes and Capacities
   illustration 6-5
VoSpire 11-14
V̇/Q̇. *See* Ventilation/Perfusion
Vt. *See* Tidal Volume
V-Tach. *See* Ventricular: tachycardia

W

Wandering Atrial Pacemaker 8-10
WBC. *See* Leukocytes
Weaning, Readiness (RSBI) 13-19
Wedge Pressure. *See* Pulmonary Capillary Wedge Pressure (PCWP)
Weight
   conversion table A-4
Wellbutrin 11-40
Whispered pectoriloquy 1-25
White Blood Cells. *See* Leukocytes
Wick Humidifier 9-57
Winters' Formula 13-3
Wolff-Parkinson-White Syndrome 8-6

X

Xanthines 11-23
Xopenex 11-15
X-ray Interpretation, Chest 3-2

Y

Yupelri 11-22

Z

zafirlukast 11-13
zanamivir 11-30
Zemaira 11-24
zileuton 11-13
Zyban 11-40
Zyflo 11-13